CORONARY ARTERY DISEASES

Edited by **Illya Chaikovsky**
and **Nataliia N. Sydorova**

Coronary Artery Diseases
Edited by Illya Chaikovsky and Nataliia N. Sydorova

Published by InTech

Janeza Trdine 9, 51000 Rijeka, Croatia

Publishing Process Manager Vedran Greblo

Technical Editor Teodora Smiljanic

Cover Designer InTech Design Team

Additional hard copies can be obtained from orders@intechopen.com

Coronary Artery Diseases, Edited by Illya Chaikovsky and Nataliia N. Sydorova
p. cm.
ISBN 978-953-51-0238-0

For EU product safety concerns:
IN TECH d.o.o., Prolaz Marije Krucifikse Kozulić 3, 51000 Rijeka, Croatia,
info@intechopen.com or visit our website at intechopen.com.

Meet the editors

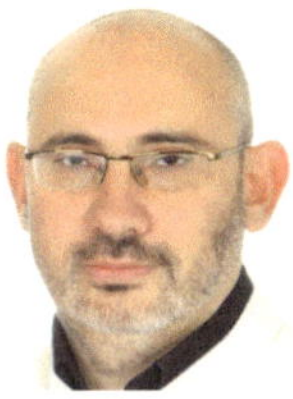

Dr Illya Chaikovsky was born in Kyiv, USSR in 1965. He graduated in general medicine in 1989, in internal medicine in 1991, in functional diagnostic in 1994, in medical cybernetics in 1997. He received his PhD in Medicine from University Duisburg-Essen (Germany) and PhD in medical and biological cybernetics and informatics from International Research and Training Center for Information Technologies and Systems of National Academy of Science (Kyiv, Ukraine). In 2000-2005 he was working as lead researcher in high-tech companies SQUID AG and MagScan GmbX (Germany). Currently, he is senior staff scientist in the field of medical cybernetics at International Research and Training Center for ITandS of NAS of Ukraine. He combines clinical work with research, focusing on advanced methods for analysis (including pattern recognition) of electrocardiogram , magnetocardiogram , heart rate variability and implementation of such approaches in clinical routine. His research in these areas has been presented at international congresses (ESC, AHA, ACC and many others) and has appeared in academic journals such as PACE, Clinical Cardiology, Annals of Noninvasive Electrocardiology, European Heart Journal, Biophysics etc. He is the author of the book (together with L. Fainzilberg) , devoted to analysis of ECG in phase space.

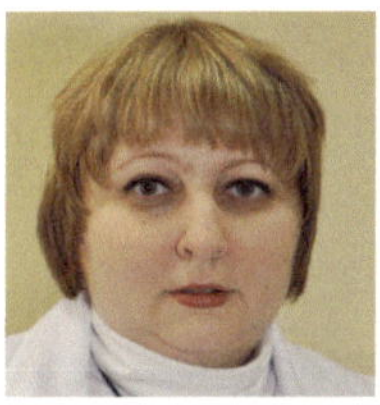

Dr Nataliia Sydorova was born in Kiev, Ukraine, in 1975. She got University Degree in General Medicine (1999) and earned her PhD in Cardiology (2003) at the Bogomolets National Medical University. She has been working as a cardiologist at Cardiological Clinic of Main Military Clinical Hospital of Ministry of Defence of Ukraine (Kiev) till 2001, and then – at Department of Military Common Practice and Family Medicine of the Ukrainian Military Medical Academy (Kiev). Her current position at this department is Associated Professor. In addition Dr. Sydorova was a Deputy Editor of the 'Journal of the American College of Cardiology. Ukrainian edition' from 2008 till 2010. At the present time she is a Deputy Editor of the 'Therapia. Ukrainian Medical Bulletin' journal (from 2010). She has got 12 patents for an invention and ca. 130 scientific publications.

Contents

Preface

This book has "wide geography" both literally and figuratively. First of all, this book brings together contributions from around the world, both from post-industrial countries and developing world.

This is natural, because coronary artery disease is becoming pandemic worldwide. CAD is the single most frequent cause of death in developed countries, causes about 1 in every 5 deaths.

Mortality from cardiovascular disease is predicted to reach 23.4 million in 2030. Moreover, in the developing world, cardiovascular disease tends to affect people at a younger age and thus could negatively affect the workforce and economic productivity. The morbidity, mortality, and socioeconomic importance of CAD make its diagnosis and management fundamental for all practicing physicians.

On another hand, the book widely represents "geography" of CAD itself, i.e. many various aspects of its pathophysiology, epidemiology, diagnosis, treatment are touched in this book.

Pathophysiologic mechanisms of CAD are well studied in general, but there are some details to be clarified. Oxidative stress is considered as one of important pathogenetic components of the atherosclerosis course, studies of its effect onto the atherosclerotic plaque formation and progression are still lasted. Section "Coronary artery disease: pathophysiology and epidemiology" includes the review "Coronary Artery Disease and Oxidative Stress"concerning this problem.

Another chapter in this Section is an epidemiological research demonstrating capabilities of the modern genetic risk factors in improvement of the ability to predict incident CAD beyond that afforded by traditional non genetic risk factors.

Section "Coronary artery disease: diagnostic features" begins with the chapter "Magnetocardiography in Unshielded Setting: Heart Electrical Image based on 2-D and 3-D Data in Comparison with Perfusion Image Based on PET Results", devoted to the promising technique of investigation of the cardiac electrical generator – magnetocardiography (MCG). Comparison is drawn of the cardiac imaging on the base of current density distribution maps, obtained by MCG and PET images. Two other articles of this Section are devoted to the different issues of the modern advanced resting electrocardiography, demonstrating that capabilities of this oldest technique of instrumental diagnosis in cardiology are far from completed. Exercise stress test is sometimes figuratively called "workhorse" in diagnosis of CAD. Authors of the chapter "Quantitative Functional Assessment of Ischemic Patients by Cardiopulmonary Exercise and Recovery Indices" emphasize important contribution of the cardiopulmonary indices for quantitative functional assessment of patients with CAD. Laboratory diagnostics is represented by the chapters "Oxidized low density lipoprotein, statin therapy and carotid stenosis", continuing the topic of oxidative stress impact onto the course of CAD and "Relationship Between the Serum 7-ketocholesterol Concentrations and Coronary Artery Disease" representing the measuring system for evaluation of the serum 7-ketocholesterol concentrations. Also clinical significance of 7KCHO is discussed.

Treatment of the coronary artery disease is continuously improved and developed. New evidences appear for effectiveness of modern therapeutic and surgical approaches. Section "Treatment for coronary artery disease" begins with the chapter "Evaluation of Anti-ischemic Therapy in Coronary Artery Disease" with detailed description of the modern treatment of patients with this disease. No doubt, that nowadays surgical revascularization – is one of the basic therapeutic interventions in CAD patients. In chapter "Coronary Arterial Drug-Eluting Stent: From Its Structure to Clinic" features and advantages of the drug-eluting stents available for clinical practice are discussed, demonstrating their future prospects. The subject with growing popularity of stem cells is covered in chapter "Pursuing Candidate Stem Cells for Candidate Regeneration in Patients Suffered from Acute Coronary Syndrome".

This book also contains the Section "Coronary artery disease and comorbidities" discussing such comorbidities as thyroid dysfunction ("Impact of Thyroid Dysfunction on Natural Course of Coronary Artery Disease", systemic vasculitis ("Coronary Artery Disease and Systemic Vasculitis: Case Report and Review"), professional stress ("Occupational Stress and Coronary Artery Disease"), migraine ("Endothelial Function in Migraine") and arterial hypertension ("Specific features of Target Organ Damage in Patients with Arterial Hypertension and Coronary Artery Disease") et al.

This book does not pretend on complete and integral description of the Coronary artery disease. Rather, it contains selected issues of this complex multifactorial disease. Nevertheless, we hope that readers will find *Coronary Artery Disease* useful for clinical practice and further research.

Illya Chaikovsky, MD PhD multiple, Senior research fellow, Assoc Prof,
International Research and Training Center for Informational Technologies and Systems of National Academy of Science, Kyiv, Ukraine

Nataliia Sydorova, MD PhD, Assoc Prof,
Ukrainian Military Medical Academy, Kyiv, Ukraine

Part 1

Coronary Artery Disease: Pathophysiology and Epidemiology

1

Coronary Artery Disease and Oxidative Stress

Mara S. Benfato, Tássia M. Medeiros and Tiago B. Salomon
LEO, Depto. de Biofísica, IBIO,
Programa de Pós-Graduação em Biologia Celular e Molecular,
Universidade Federal do Rio Grande do Sul,
Brazil

1. Introduction

O_2 arose on Earth in about 3.8 x 10^9 years ago due to the photosynthetic process in cyanobacteria hydrolyzed water. But it was only about 2.5 x 10^9 years ago that its levels rose to significant amounts. The increase in atmospheric concentrations of O_2 led to a great selective event, the first great mass extinction, due to stress on organisms that did not adapt to the new conditions. It also helped in the conquest of the land with the formation of O_3 (ozone) in the stratosphere, which filters the most harmful of the ultraviolet radiation (UV-C). In addition, using the O_2 as a substrate, the organisms generated much more energy (about 32 times more) but, in doing so, they started to generate reactive species in the process.

Reactive species (RS) are elements that react with biologically relevant organisms and although they act as cellular messengers, they also damage cellular components. In response to that, the organisms developed defences, which are now called antioxidants. The imbalance of the relation between RS and antioxidants is called oxidative stress. In this chapter we will study diseases related to oxidative stress but, in order to understand them, we first need to comprehend the radicals, their chemistry and the defences against such elements.

1.1 Reactive oxygen species (ROS) and reactive nitrogen species (RNS)

The RS are named according to the principal element in their composition, reactive oxygen species (ROS) and reactive nitrogen species (RNS), and are divided into radicals and non-radicals. Radicals have at least one unpaired electron in an open shell configuration and non-radicals are compounds that can generate radical species. Below we will see a list of the most important reactive species for human health (considered to date).

Note: Radicals are written with a dot attached to the upper right level representing the unpaired electron.

1.1.1 Reactive oxygen species

Hydroxyl radical ($HO^•$)

A hydroxyl radical is the most reactive radical known *in vivo* and the most harmful, to which the human body has no defence mechanism. But, because it is so reactive, it reacts immediately after formation (within 5 molecular diameters from its production site).

It can be formed mainly by the Fenton reaction, in which the hydrogen peroxide (see below) reacts with a transition metal (Fe^{2+} or Cu^+) forming two hydroxides, one of them a radical and the other just an ion (see equation below).

$$H_2O_2 + Fe^{2+} \rightarrow OH^- + OH^\bullet \quad (1)$$

The reaction is faster with Cu^+ (more than 60 times faster), but since it is not as bioavailable as Fe^{2+}, hydrogen peroxide reacts more with Fe^{2+} than with Cu^+ (Halliwell & Gutteridge, 2007). It can cause modification of DNA bases and strand breaks, inactivation of proteins and lipid peroxidation. As explained above, $HO^\bullet$ is too reactive to be enzymatically removed (it would attack the enzymes), hence the way to control its damages is to reduce its formation and repair the damage.

Superoxide ($O_2^{\bullet -}$)

Superoxide is both an anion and a radical formed when an electron is added to the O_2 molecule. It is produced mainly by the electron leakage in the mitochondrial electron transport chain, but there are also other sources (e.g. endoplasmatic reticulum). Superoxide is quite toxic and is used in the defence systems to control pathogens for being a pro-oxidant and precursor for other species, but this toxicity works both ways, damaging important cellular components, especially inactivate enzymes by oxidation or reduction of its Fe-S sites (Flint et al., 1993), such as in an aconitase enzyme (which converts citrate to isocitrate, in the Krebs cycle) with the superoxide which reduces its $(Fe_4S_4)^{2+}$ to $(Fe_4S_4)^+$.

Hydrogen Peroxide (H_2O_2)

Hydrogen peroxide is a covalent, pale-blue, viscous liquid. Mainly produced *in vivo* by superoxide dismutation (see 1.2), but other oxidases may produce it as well, it is also produced by the oxidation of long chain fatty acids in the peroxissome (Titorenko & Terlecky, 2011). It plays a part in the immune response via formation of hydroxyl radicals or via inactivation of the pathogens' enzymes. However, for reacting with transition metals, hydrogen peroxide (see Fenton reaction above) represents a major problem to living organisms.

1.1.2 Reactive nitrogen species

Nitric Oxide ($NO^\bullet$)

$NO^\bullet$ is a colourless monomeric gas stable in pure water. In physiological conditions the half-life of nitric oxide is only a few seconds. In mammals nitric oxide is produced by the oxidation of L-arginine catalyzed by nitric oxide synthase (NOS) (Mungrue et al., 2003). Nitric oxide has several physiological roles, especially in neural and vascular systems. In the neural system it works as a neurotransmitter, strengthens the most used synapses and has a role in long-term memory but in excess, may cause strokes and epilepsy. In the vascular system it controls the blood pressure (vasodilator), kills foreign organisms (e.g. Leishmania), in excess may cause chronic inflammation, septic shock and transplant rejection. It has a role in bladder control, penile erection and peristaltic movements.

Peroxynitrite

Peroxynitrite is formed by the reaction of the radicals superoxide and nitric oxide, the peroxynitrite is an unstable, short-lived, potent oxidant, non-radical.

$$O_2^{\bullet -} + NO^{\bullet} \rightarrow ONOO^- \quad (2)$$

Peroxynitrite causes damage to proteins (-sulfur groups), hydroxylation and nitration of aromatic compounds. It may damage DNA as well by strand breaks and damages 2-deoxyribose.

1.2 Antioxidant defences

As we observed in the last topic, reactive species play a great role in biological systems, but they tend to cause much damage as well. To defend against such damage organisms developed defences, generically called "antioxidants", and when such defences fail we also have a repair system. The antioxidants may be classified in two major groups, enzymatic and non-enzymatic or endogenous and diet-derived.

1.2.1 Enzymatic

Catalase

Catalase is a very reactive enzyme that dismutates hydrogen peroxide (H_2O_2) into water (H_2O) and O_2, as seen in eq. 3.

$$2H_2O_2 \rightarrow 2H_2O + O_2 \quad (3)$$

Located in intracellular organelles (mostly peroxissomes) that are known as high producers of hydrogen peroxide (H_2O_2), Catalase is a tetramer of four polypeptide chains, each over 500 amino acids long and containing one *Fe(III)-heme* group that allows the enzyme to react with the hydrogen peroxide. As hydrogen peroxide enters the active site, it interacts with the amino acids causing an oxygen transfer between the heme group and the peroxide. The free oxygen is bound to the heme group (eq. 4), later, it reacts with a second hydrogen peroxide molecule and produce water and oxygen (eq. 5).

$$H_2O_2 + \text{CAT-Fe(III)} \rightarrow H_2O + \text{Compound I} \quad (4)$$

$$H_2O_2 + \text{Compound I} \rightarrow 2H_2O_2 + \text{CAT-Fe(III)} + O_2 \quad (5)$$

Superoxide dismutase

Superoxide dismutases (SODs) are enzymes that dismutate superoxide in oxygen and hydrogen peroxide. In humans three forms of superoxide dismutase are present. SOD1 (CuZnSOD) is located in the cytoplasm, SOD2 (MnSOD) in the mitochondria and SOD3 (CuZnSOD) is extracellular. The CuZnSOD contains two protein subunits, each with a metal, a Cu in one and Zn in the other (hence the name CuZnSOD). The copper ions catalyze the dismutation of superoxide and the zinc only helps the stability of the enzyme. Although CuZnSOD, SOD1 and SOD3 are two different proteins encoded by different genes, SOD3 is synthesized containing a signal peptide that directs this enzyme exclusively to extracellular spaces (Halliwell & Gutteridge, 2007).

$$Cu^{2+}\text{-SOD} + O_2^{\bullet -} \rightarrow Cu^{+}\text{-SOD} + O_2 \quad (6)$$

$$Cu^{+}\text{-SOD} + O_2^{\bullet -} + 2H^+ \rightarrow Cu^{2+}\text{-SOD} + H_2O_2 \quad (7)$$

The MnSOD (SOD2) is quite different from CuZnSOD (not even having similar amino acid sequences), but performs the same reaction. It is more sensitive to denaturation (e.g. by heat) than the CuZnSOD. Each of its four protein subunits contains a manganese ion.

$$Mn^{3+}\text{-SOD} + O_2^{\bullet -} \rightarrow Mn^{2+}\text{-SOD} + O_2 \quad (8)$$

$$Mn^{2+}\text{-SOD} + O_2^{\bullet -} + 2H^+ \rightarrow M^{3+}\text{-SOD} + H_2O_2 \quad (9)$$

Glutathione peroxidise (GPx)

Glutathione peroxidase is the general name of an enzyme family, which consists of eight known human isoforms, whose main role is to protect the organism from oxidative damage. It is more versatile than catalase's action (as seen above) on lipid peroxides and in addition to hydrogen peroxide, is not limited to organelles, but its reaction speed (km) is much slower.

In order to detoxify peroxides it requires glutathione as a cofactor (eq. 9).

$$2GSH + H_2O_2 \rightarrow GSSG + 2H_2O \quad (10)$$

Since this process oxidize glutathione another enzyme is required to reduce the oxidize glutathine, via NADPH spending, the glutathione reductase. This process allows the glutathione to be used again by the peroxidase or another process (see Glutathione).

$$GS\text{–}SG + NADPH + H^+ \rightarrow 2\,GSH + NADP \quad (11)$$

Heme oxygenase

Human heme oxygenase-1 (hHO-1) is a stress protein linked to cytoprotection against oxidative stress. It catalyzes the reaction of heme to biliverdin, Fe^{2+} and carbon monoxide (CO). The carbon monoxide has pro- and antioxidant effects and also pro- or antiapoptotic effects that depend on dose (Piantadosi et al., 2006).

$$Heme + 3O_2 + 3\tfrac{1}{2}NADPH + 3\tfrac{1}{2}H^+ + 7e^- \rightarrow biliverdin + Fe^{2+} + CO + 3\tfrac{1}{2}NADP^+ + H_2O \quad (12)$$

The biliverdin reductase acts on biliverdin by reducing its double-bond between the pyrrole rings into a single-bond with $NADPH+H^+$ generating then, biliverdin and $NADP^+$. The biliverdin then takes on antioxidant properties by scavenging peroxyl radicals and limiting the peroxidation of membrane lipids and proteins.

1.2.2 Non-enzymatic

Glutathione

Glutathione (GSH) is a tripeptide, the most ubiquitous peptide found in cells. GSH can be obtained from the diet or can be synthesized *de novo* in the liver. It is the most abundant intracellular antioxidant. It works as a cofactor to GPx (as seen above) and also reacts, *in vitro*, with $HO^\bullet$, $ONOO^-$ among others species. It can also chelate copper, reducing its interaction with hydrogen peroxide, decreasing the Fenton reaction, and therefore reducing the formation of $HO^\bullet$. Its reaction with $ONOO^-$ leads to the formation of nitrosothiol (GSNO) which can be converted to $NO^\bullet$.

Ascorbic acid (vitamin C)

Ascorbic acid is an antioxidant produced by plants and some animals (e.g. rats, some birds) and one of its functions is to maintain redox homeostasis. The animals that do not synthesize ascorbic acid (including humans) must obtain ascorbic acid from the diet. They are unable to synthesize due to the lack of the enzyme gulonolactone oxidase, which catalyzes the final step in the synthesis of ascorbic acid (Yoshihara et al., 2010). Ascorbic acid has two oxidizable -OH groups. At physiological pH, it remains in the ionized form, ascorbate.

Among the many roles of vitamin C, we can highlight it acting as the scavenger of superoxide, hydroxyl, among others, also in the absorption of iron in the intestine (eq. 13) by reducing it from Fe^{3+} to Fe^{2+}, which works as a cofactor for several enzymes but also may be involved in Fenton reaction (see eq. 1) and regenerates the tocopheryl radical in tocopherol (very important).

$$Fe^{3+} + \text{ascorbate} \rightarrow Fe^{2+} + \text{ascorbyl} \qquad (13)$$

Lower vitamin C levels found in elderly people, diabetic patients and cigarette smokers are most likely due to increased oxidative stress. Some studies showed that vitamin C supplementation decreased the level of oxidative DNA damage in mononuclear blood cells and also increased the LDL oxidation in patients' hemodialysis, but failed to prevent steady-state levels of lipid peroxidation (Yoshihara et al., 2010). There are some encouraging data to support vitamin C as a protective factor against cardiovascular diseases, but as a matter of fact there are more discouraging data (Collins et al., 2002) on this topic.

Tocopherols (vitamin E)

Tocopherols are a fat-soluble antioxidants (vitamin E is a name used to design several tocopherols) and are the most important inhibitors of lipid peroxidation. It can reduce Fe^{3+} to Fe^{2+} and Cu^{2+} to Cu^{+}. This ability is the basis of colorimetric method for measuring tocopherols. At high concentrations, the tocopherols present pro-oxidant effects, promoting lipid peroxidation. It can also affect blood clotting by interfering with the action of vitamin K. Its supplementation in diet is not recommended (Yoshihara et al., 2010).

1.3 Iron homeostasis

Iron is by far the most abundant transition metal in the human body and essential element for life. It is crucial for DNA synthesis, respiration and key metabolic reactions. It is an important component of enzymes that are involved in oxidation or reduction of biologic substrates, due to its ability to exist in two redox states making it useful at the catalytic centre like in cytochomes. It is also an essential component of oxygen carriers hemoglobin and myoglobin; alternatively, iron can bind to enzymes in a form of non-heme moieties or iron-sulfur (Fe-S) motifs (several mitochondrial enzymes). When iron exceeds the metabolic needs of the cell it may form a low molecular weight pool, tentatively referred to as the labile iron pool, which converts normal by-products of cell respiration, like $O_2^{\bullet-}$ and H_2O_2, into highly damaging hydroxyl radicals or equally aggressive ferryl ions. The redox state that do this is ferrous iron and the reaction that produces $OH^{\bullet-}$ is called Fenton Reaction. Therefore, iron must be chelated in very specific ways that discourage redox cycling. However, iron can have benign or malign effects on the cell, depending on whether it is a micronutrient or a catalyst of free radical reactions. The average human adult contains approximately 4 g of iron, a little more than 2 g of which is in hemoglobin and 1g in body stores predominantly in the liver, the rest are in other iron-containing proteins, mainly in skeletal muscle (~300mg, most in myoglonbin) and macrophages (~600mg in total). Since total plasma iron turnover is some 35mg/day, iron deficiency can cause cellular growth arrest and death; iron excess can cause damage lipid membranes, proteins and nucleic acids. For example, iron deficiency represents the most common cause of anaemia worldwide and can cause development retardation in children as iron overload in hereditary hemochromatosis and thalassemias leads to potentially fatal liver or heart failure due, in the most part, to the amount of iron deposits.

Iron absorption needs to be tightly controlled due its activity redox which can also lead to the production of ROS. Its absorption occurs in the proximal small intestine and involves many key molecules. Iron absorption occurs in lumen of the duodenum and can be modulated by the size of the body's iron stores, by erythropoietic activity and by recent dietary iron intake. Iron can be absorbed from diet in two forms: as inorganic (non-heme) iron predominantly released from foods such as vegetables or cereals, or as heme iron from the breakdown of hemoglobin and myoglobin contained in red meat. Most iron in food is in ferric form [Fe (III) state], the most stable oxidation state for iron. Iron across is mediated by brush border iron transporter divalent metal transporter 1 (DMT1), which transports iron in the ferrous form [Fe (II))]. Hence, there are agents in gastric juice that solubilize and reduce Fe (III) in Fe (II), such as the ascorbate and hydrochloric acid (Frazer & Anderson, 2005), moreover, there are also in the epithelial surface apical ferric reductases. Heme (protoporphyrin ring that binds ferrous form) is more efficiently absorbed than inorganic iron and taken up by apical heme transporters after being released by proteolysis of hemeproteins in gut lumen is taken up and the iron removed from it in the mucosal cells by the action of heme oxygenase in ferrous form (Figure 1).

Inside the enterocytes, iron can be stored in ferritin in the cytoplasm, utilized in mitochondria or exported to plasma by ferroportin on the basolateral surface. Ferroportin cooperates with the multicopper ferroxidase hephaestin, which converts ferrous to ferric iron for uptake by plasma transferrin and regulated by hepcidin, an inhibitor of iron absorption and releases from macrophages and other cell types. The hepcidin causes ferroportin internalization and degradation, decreasing the transfer of iron to the body. Extracellular iron is bound with high affinity by the serum iron-transport protein transferrin and taken into the circulation (the labile iron pool). The majority of it is destined for nascent erythrocytes in the bone marrow. The cellular uptake of iron occurs through receptor-mediated endocytosis of transferrin (TfR). TfR containing transferrin binds on the cell membrane and is internalized by endocytosis. So, iron is used for cellular processes and excess iron is stored in ferritin (Dunn et al., 2007). It is important to know about these proteins because they have key roles in healthy processes and diseases in relation to iron homeostasis, for example, formation of atherosclerotic lesions, as will be discussed later. The excess of iron is lost by epithelial shedding in the gastrointestinal tract and the skin (approximately 1 to 2 g each day), through blood loss in menses of premenopausal women, in sweat and possibly a small amount excreted by lungs into mucus. The amount of iron absorbed can be affected by several mechanisms like inflammation, hypoxia, anaemia and iron overload. Iron can be recycled or stored as needed. Human erythrocytes undergo surface alterations that mark them to be phagocyted and digested by macrophages in the spleen and the liver. In macrophages, iron is recovered from heme by the action of heme oxygenase and stored in ferritin, but the major site of iron storage is the liver, into hepatocytes. The capacity of readily exchanging electrons makes iron not only essential for fundamental cell functions, but also a potential catalyst for chemical reactions involving free-radical formation and subsequent oxidative stress and cell damage. Therefore, iron levels are carefully regulated to minimize the pool of potentially toxic "free iron". The majority of proteins described above are posttranscriptional controlled by iron regulatory proteins (IRP-1 and IRP-2). Iron regulatory proteins recognize at the mRNA level non-coding sequences (the iron-responsive elements [IRE]) which have been found in genes that control the iron homeostasis like ferritin and TfR, being that the ferritin synthesis is increased to sequester excess iron and TfR is downregulated in order to stop iron uptake (Cairo & Pietrangelo, 2000).

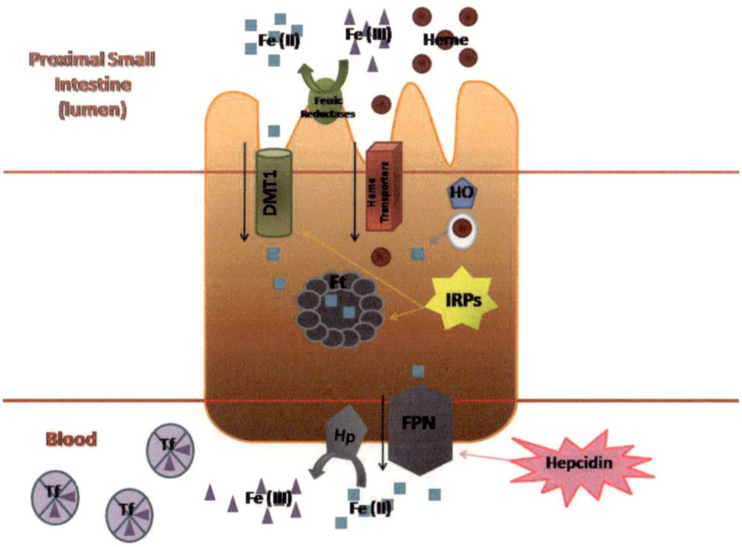

Fig. 1. Intestinal iron absorption. Iron absorption in the proximal small intestine mucosa of the gut requires transport across the apical and basolateral membranes of duodenal enterocytes. The dietary non-heme iron in the duodenal lumen is reduced by a ferric reductases and thus made available for divalent metal transporter 1 (DMT1), which transports ferrous iron across the apical brush border membrane and heme iron is transported by heme transporters. The amount of iron not retained by the cell inside the iron storage protein ferritin (Ft) is transferred to the bloodstream. The basolateral release of non-heme iron (which is also derived from heme catabolized by heme oxygenase [HO]) is mediated by ferroportin (FPN) which transports the metal across the membrane and hephaestin (Hp), which re-oxidizes iron as a necessary step for binding to the plasma carrier protein transferrin (Tf). The hepcidin causes ferroportin internalization and degradation, decreasing the transfer of iron to the body. The main proteins involved in iron absorption are controlled by iron regulatory proteins (IRPs), whose activity is regulated by the levels of the metal in the labile iron pool.

1.4 Oxidative damage

Oxidative stress describes the damage that occurs when oxidants overwhelm the antioxidants' defences; this can cause oxidative damage in macromolecules like DNA and proteins. The progressive and irreversible accumulation of oxidative damage may contribute to impaired physiological function and increased incidence of disease. Oxidative damage to lipids, proteins and DNA occurs primarily via the action of ROS. ROS can be generated by several mechanisms, but the principal source in aerobic cells is mitochondria. In an electron transport chain, oxygen can be reduced in superoxide ($O_2^{\bullet -}$). Superoxide itself does not appear to damage all macromolecules at physiologically relevant concentrations; redox reactions involving $O_2^{\bullet -}$, however, generate other reactive species that damage nucleic acids, proteins and lipids. This process generates the reactive intermediates encompassing a wide spectrum of oxygen-, carbon- or sulfur-centred radicals, originated from oxygen, hydrogen peroxide and lipid peroxides. Such damage is detectable under normal physiological conditions even in young animals, suggesting that endogenous protective mechanisms cannot suppress all oxidative damage even during basal levels of ROS generation (Halliwell & Gutteridge, 2007).

1.4.1 DNA damage

Damage to various macromolecules may not accumulate and therefore may not be critical. DNA, on the other hand, is the prime information molecule of the cell and nuclear DNA, in particular, must last the lifetime of the cell, therefore, DNA damage represents a critical threat to cell function. If DNA damage is severe or its accumulation exceeds its elimination by DNA repair mechanisms, cellular senescence or apoptosis will occur. Oxidative damage to nuclear DNA causes strand breakage that may lead to cell death. Additionally, oxidative damage to DNA causes mutations that can impair protein synthesis and lead to cell dysfunction. The hydroxyl radical ($OH^{\bullet}$) reacts with DNA by addition to double bonds of DNA bases and by hydrogen atom from abstraction the methyl group of thymine and each of the C-H bonds of 2′-deoxyribose. One of the DNA base products of interaction with reactive oxygen and other free radical species is 8-oxo-7,8-dihydro-2′-deoxuguanosine (8-OHdG). This is the oxidative lesion major and its level in DNA has, therefore, been consistently used as a measure of oxidative damage to DNA (Cooke et al., 2003). In addition, with $OH^{\bullet}$, it is important to note that hydrogen peroxide (H_2O_2) can cause massive acute DNA double-strand breaks and is involved in signalling cell stress (Chen et al., 2007).

1.4.2 Protein damage

Damage to proteins can occur by direct attack of reactive species or by secondary damage involving attack by end-products, like lipid peroxidation (Halliwell & Gutteridge, 2007). The importance of protein oxidation towards cellular homeostasis derives from the fact that proteins serve vital roles in regulating cell structure, cell signalling and the various enzymatic processes of the cell. Therefore, protein oxidation can rapidly contribute to oxidative stress by directly affecting cellular functions. Oxidation of proteins can lead to the formation of oxidized amino acids, such as dityrosine, 3-nitrotyrosine, 3-chlorotyrosine, oxohistidine and altered amino acid side-chains containing reactive carbonyls, and result in the loss of catalytic function, increased sensitivity to denaturation and increased susceptibility to proteolysis. One major pathway believed to generate protein carbonyls *in vivo* is the metal-catalyzed protein oxidation pathway. In addition, there are others modes of inducing protein oxidation, among them are oxidation induced cleavage, amino acid oxidation and the conjugation of lipid peroxidation products. It is important to know that the accumulation of oxidized proteins is often measured by the content of reactive carbonyls. Some protein damage is reversible, such as methionine sulphoxide formation and destruction of Fe-S clusters by $O_2^{\bullet -}$. Other damage, for example of side-chains to carbonyl residues, appears irreversible and the protein is destroyed and replaced. Several mechanisms are activated when a protein undergoes damage by reactive species. This is necessary because accumulation of proteins with incorrect conformation can lead to cell death. When oxidized proteins resist proteolytic attack, they form aggregates which decrease their toxicity by sequestering them in insoluble clumps (Halliwell & Gutteridge, 2007).

1.4.3 Lipid peroxidation

Lipid peroxidation is involved in various and numerous pathological states including inflammation, atherosclerosis, neurodegenerative diseases and cancer. It has been know that lipid peroxidation induces disturbance of fine structures, alteration of integrity, fluidity and permeability, causes functional loss of biomembranes, modifies low density lipoprotein (LDL) to proatherogenic and proinflammatory forms and generates potentially toxic products. However, recently products of lipid peroxidation have been shown to exert various biological functions *in vivo,* such as regulators of gene expression, signalling messengers, activators of receptors and nuclear transcription factors, and inducers of adaptive responses, as well as ROS and RNS. Initiation of lipid peroxidation can be caused by addition of reactive species or, more usually, by hydrogen atom abstraction from a methylene group by reactive species (Halliwell & Gutteridge, 2007). The process of lipid peroxidation occurs by three distinct mechanisms, that is, (1) free radical-mediated oxidation, (2) free radical-independent, non-enzymatic oxidation, and (3) enzymatic oxidation. There are specific antioxidants to inhibit each type of lipid peroxide formed by mechanisms. For example, in the first situation $O_2^{\bullet -}$ and $NO^{\bullet}$ do not activate per se lipid peroxidation directly, but they react quite rapidly at the diffusion-controlled rate to give peroxynitrite ($ONOO^-$), which may initiate lipid peroxidation chain reactions. Both molecules are important to control muscular contraction in endothelium. A non-enzymatic oxidation example is the lipid oxidation by singlet oxygen, which can cause deleterious damage, such as a disease porphyria on the skin for oxidizing unsaturated lipids mainly. The thirst mechanism is another important type. It has been shown that lipoxygenase and ciclooxigenase oxidize arachidonic acid to prostaglandins, prostacyclin, thromboxane and leukotrienes, moreover, lipoxygenase directly oxidizes phospholipids and cholesteryl esters in LDL particles. It is important to cite that cholesterol is oxidized by three mechanisms noted above (Niki, 2009). Various molecular weight aldehydes, such as acrolein, malondialdehyde (MDA) and 4-hydroxy-2-nonenal (HNE) are formed during lipid peroxidation as secondary or decomposition products, and they are highly reactive and readily react with proteins, DNA and phospholipids to cause deleterious effects. MDA and HNE are considered good biomarkers of lipid peroxidation *in vivo*. Lipid peroxide alters chemical characteristics and the physical organization of cellular membranes to induce functional loss and modifies lipoproteins to proatherogenic and proinflammatory forms. It is assumed to be pathogenic and contribute to the etiology of various diseases (Niki, 2009).

Carbon radicals often stabilize by molecular rearrangement to form conjugated dienes, but if two radicals collide within a membrane they cross-link the fatty acid side-chain. When the formation of peroxy radical (by O_2 action) occurs, this can abstract a hydrogen atom from an adjacent fatty-acid side-chain. Thus happen the propagation stage of lipid peroxidation, mainly in membranes.

2. Atherosclerosis

Cardiovascular diseases are the leading cause of death and disability in the Western world. The majority of cardiovascular diseases result from complications of atherosclerosis. Atherosclerosis is a progressive disease that is generally characterized by the accumulation of lipids, fibrous elements and inflammatory cells and molecules within the arterial wall. The lesions of atherosclerosis occur principally in large and medium-sized elastic and muscular arteries and can lead to ischemia of heart, brain or extremities, resulting in infarction.

2.1 Formation and progression

The initiation of atherosclerosis begins with endothelial injury or dysfunction that is characterized by enhanced endothelial permeability and LDL deposition in the intima. LDL is accumulated in the preferred sites for lesion formation and undergoes oxidative modification as a result of its interaction with ROS. The endothelial injury likely is caused by ox-LDL itself, as well as physical or chemical forces and infection. This lesion induces the expression of a number of proinflammatory molecules, like adhesion molecules such as P-selectin, chemotactic and growth factors. These lead to the tethering, activation and attachment of monocytes and T lymphocytes to the endothelial cells. Monocytes ingest lipoproteins and morph into macrophages; macrophages generate ROS, which convert ox-LDL into highly oxidized LDL, which is, in turn, taken up by macrophages to form foam cells. Foam cells combine with leukocytes to become the fatty streak and as the process continues foam cells secrete growth factors that induce smooth muscle cells' migration into the intima. Endothelial cells, macrophages and smooth muscle cells highly oxidize LDL by the action of ROS produced. The foam cells secrete more growth factors that induce smooth muscle cells' migration into the intima and proliferation forming the fibrous plaques. Later, calcification can occur and cause plaque stabilization. In plaques that are not calcified the fibrous plaques may rupture and form thrombi that may ultimately occlude vessels, for example in the case of acute coronary syndromes that lead to myocardial infarction. Possible causes of endothelial dysfunction leading to atherosclerosis include elevated and modified LDL; free radicals caused by cigarette smoking, hypertension and diabetes mellitus; genetic alterations; elevated plasma homocysteine concentrations (toxic to endothelium and prothrombotic); infections microorganisms; and combinations of these or other factors. The process of atherosclerosis occurs primarily in certain arteries, such as coronary and carotid arteries (Ross, 1999).

2.2 Oxidative stress and inflammation

Oxidative stress plays an important role in the formation of atherosclerosis plaque. The oxidation hypothesis suggests multiple mechanism(s) by which oxidation of LDL might promote atherosclerosis. LDL retained within the artery can be oxidized by a number of cell types present within arteries, including endothelial cells, smooth muscle cells, monocytes and macrophages, and lymphocytes. HDL can also be oxidized by endothelial cells and by chemical means. Oxidation of these lipoproteins can be blocked by antioxidants. Ox-LDL also has potentially atherogenic affects, inhibits the mobility of tissue macrophages, enhances production of chemotatic factors and adhesion molecules, induces smooth muscle cells' migration and both proliferation and apoptosis in endothelial cells, smooth muscle cells and macrophages (Schwenke, 1998). In the vasculature, production of reactive species occurs that are used to control physiological functions. Oxygen undergoes reduction to $O_2^{\bullet -}$ by means of enzymes, such as the nicotinamine adenine dinucleotide (phosphate) (NADH/NAD(P)H) oxidases and xantine oxidases (XO). The $O_2^{\bullet -}$ is used to promote vasoconstriction and can form H_2O_2 that can react with other radicals, such as transition metal Fe^{2+} to produce $OH^\bullet$ (Fenton reaction). Myeloperoxidase, a heme protein secreted by phagocytes, can amplify the oxidative potential of H_2O_2 by production of hypoclorous acid (HOCl) that can react with $O_2^{\bullet -}$ to produce $OH^\bullet$. Other sources of ROS in the vessel wall include mitochondria, ciclooxygenase (COX), lipoxygenase and uncoupled endothelial nitric oxide synthase (eNOS). This last, in normal conditions, generates nitric oxide ($NO^\bullet$), but if there is availability of precursors, eNOS become uncoupled generating $O_2^{\bullet -}$. Although $NO^\bullet$ is a reactive species, it is thought be antiatherosclerotic because it is a vasodilator potent and inhibits LDL peroxidation by scavenging peroxil radicals. These reactive species ($O_2^{\bullet -}$, H_2O_2 and $NO^\bullet$) cannot oxidize LDL, but form other reactive species that can do this, like $OH^\bullet$ and $ONOO^-$ (described above) (Madamanchi et al., 2005, Halliwell & Gutteridge, 2007). But how can free ferrous iron in the body be a catalyst for the formation of $OH^\bullet$, powerful pro-oxidants and promote lipid oxidation (increased formation of ox-LDL)? In 1981 Sullivan created The Iron Heart Hypothesis suggesting that increased body iron stores are a risk factor for coronary heart disease and thus that iron depletion though phlebotomy or other means can reduce risk (Sullivan, 1981). In addition to enhancing oxidative stress, increased iron stores are believed to adversely affect cardiovascular disease through other mechanisms, including alteration of endothelial function, decreased vascular reactivity and reperfusion injury by iron-induced free radicals (Hu, 2007). Furthermore, iron can contribute to the signalling in inflammatory pathways and hypoxia response. Atherosclerosis is an inflammatory disease and inflammatory mechanisms have emerged as playing a pivotal role in all stages of atherosclerotic plaque formation. Systemic inflammation occurs in the vasculature as a response to injury, lipid peroxidation and perhaps infection. A number of inflammatory mediators are released by cells involved in the lesion, including tumour necrosis factor α (TNFα) or interleukin 1 (IL-1), chemokines, such as IL-8 or monocyte chemoattractant protein-1 and adhesion molecules, such as intercellular adhesion molecule 1 (ICAM-1) or selectins. In particular, smooth muscle cells also release IL-6 which is the main hepatic stimulus for the acute phase reactant, C-reactive protein (CRP), which causes expression of adhesion molecules and also stimulates hepcidin. The ferritin also has synthesis regulated by cytokines, such as TNFα and IL-1, at various levels (transcriptional, posttranscriptional and translational) (You & Wang, 2005).

Abnormal ferritin levels or iron homeostasis have been linked to atherosclerosis. To prove the iron hypothesis, many epidemiological studies have been performed. Most studies testing the hypothesis of iron measured levels of ferritin. The ferritin level rises with iron loading and declines with depletion of tissue iron stores. Salonen et al. first reported a significant association between the serum ferritin levels and the risk of myocardial infarction of 1,931 middle-aged men during an average follow-up of three years (2.2 higher risk of myocardial infarction in men with higher serum ferritin levels) (Salonen et al., 1992). A study from our laboratory compared patients with coronary heart disease and sleep apnea (also inflammation disease) showing that serum ferritin levels increased in coronary heart disease patients and positively correlated with sleep apnea. These studies are supported by the evidences that show iron deposition in human atherosclerotic lesions, suggesting that iron may play a role in the development of atherosclerosis (Hower et al., 2009).

With regard to sleep apnea, studies have demonstrated sleep disordered breathing to be associated with cardiovascular disease, include coronary artery disease, heart failure, hypertension, cardiac arrhythmias and stroke, which further increase morbidity and mortality in the sleep disordered breathing population (Flemons et al., 1999). Hypoxia events, endothelial dysfunction, coagulopathy, impaired sympathetic drive, oxidative and inflammatory stress are the pathophysiological pathways suggested for the development of cardiovascular disease in sleep disordered breathing (Butt et al., 2010). Increase in ROS in endothelial cells exposed to hypoxia has been evidenced. Among the possible sources of ROS by hypoxia are the mitochondria, leukocytes (NADPH oxidase pathway) and epithelial tissue enzymes, such as xanthine oxidase, cyclooxygenase, lipooxygenase, NO-synthase and hemeoxygenases (Lavie, 2003). As discussed above, hepcidin is a peptide also involved in iron homeostasis and has impact in inflammatory hypoferrimia because inflammation is mediated by citokine-driven increase in hepcidin production, causing release and recycled iron from macrophages and and blocking the passage of iron from enterocytes to plasma. Hepcidin production is controlled by inflammatory citokines like ferritin. The main citokines are IL-6 and TNFα. In addition to cytokines, hepcidin is downregulated under hypoxia conditions and little is known of the involvement of ROS in this mechanism. A study suggested that ROS (produced by hypoxia) repress the hepcidin gene (Choi et al., 2007).

The same recent study in our lab that verified the serum ferritin levels in coronary heart disease (CHD) and sleep apnea patients also verified the serum prohepcidin levels (the precursor of hepcidin). The study was performed in 56 patients with stable coronary heart disease referred for angiography (male gender 54%). Exclusion criteria, to avoid potent oxidative stress factors, were: smoking, age older than 65 years, morbid obesity, diabetes. Patients underwent a portable polysomnography to verify the apnea-hypopnea index (AHI) and determination of hemoglobin, hematocrit, ferritin, prohepcidin and high-sensitivity C-reactive protein (hs-CRP) levels. Patients were divided into controls and cases at the median AHI, 28 controls with an AHI low and 28 cases with moderate to severe AHI. The mean ferritin levels are significantly higher in cases than the control and this is the first report of such findings in sleep apnea (170±140.1 vs. 285±194.5; $p < 0.05$). There were a significantly greater percentage of subjects with CHD in the group with moderate to severe sleep apnea (72%; p 0.001). The Pearson's correlation coefficients showed positive significance between ferritin and AHI ($r = 0.398$, $P = 0.002$), prohepcidin and ferritin ($r = 0.432$, $P = 0.001$) and iron and ferritin ($r = 0.346$; $P = 0.009$); between AHI and prohepicidin was $r = -0.15$ ($P = 0.3$) (figure 2). How hypoxia could be affecting the ferritin and hepcidin levels is not known. In a multivariate regression, however, controlling for age, sex, body mass index and coronary heart disease, the AHI and ferritin explain 30.4% of the variance of prohepcidin. Thus, it is suggested that hypoxia-reoxygenation in obstructive sleep apnea may influence prohepcidin in human and, consequently, iron homeostasis, aggravating oxidative stress and contributing to the emergence of coronary heart disease (increased ferritin levels).

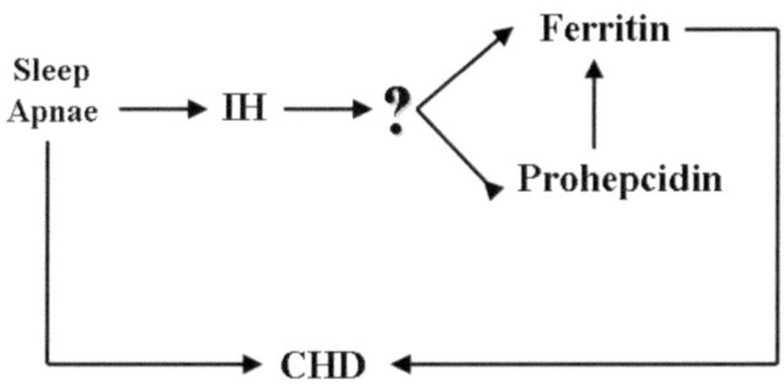

Fig. 2. Scheme of regressions and correlations found among studied parameters. The sleep apnea through intermittent hypoxia (IH) events activates some unknown route (?) generating decreased prohepcidin levels and increased ferritin levels. The hypoxia interferes positively in the ferritin levels and negatively in prohepcidin levels. Prohepcidin already induces the ferritin synthesis. It is suggested that the hypoxia induction by ferritin levels overlaps the prohepcidin inhibition by hypoxia, because there was increased ferritin levels, as well as increased AHI. A relationship was found between OSAS and CHD, as well as ferritin and CHD corroborating with literature data.

2.3 Oxidative stress biomarkers

Many experimental and observational studies showed the relationship between oxidative stress biomarkers and cardiovascular disease. Among the most used are ox-LDL, myeloperoxidase, lipid peroxidation products and protein oxidation. The ability of oxidative stress biomarkers to predict cardiovascular disease has yet to be established. Some of them have already been examined, now we will look in more detail at these and comment about new markers. As described above, ox-LDL is believed to play an intrinsic role within atherosclerosis plaque formation and progression of atherosclerosis. In the same study that showed a relationship between ferritin and hepcidin with coronary heart disease, the levels of ox-LDL and paraoxanase-1 (enzyme present in HDL that reduces ox-LDL accumulation) were also analyzed, indicating that they are important predictors of coronary heart disease (intern communication). Paraoxanase-1 possess antioxidant and anti-inflammatory properties and protect against atherogenesis, and for this, can be associated with the action of HDL (Jayakumari & Thejaseebai, 2009). The measurement of F_2-isoprostanes (a prostaglandin-like compound formed from radical catalyzed peroxidation of fatty acids, like arachidonic acid, without the direct action of enzymes) has emerged as one of most sensitive and reliable biomarkers of lipid peroxidation *in vivo* (Davies & Roberts, 2011). As previously indicated, damage to proteins by ROS produces carbonyls and other amino acid modifications. Some studies used protein oxidation as a predictor of cardiovascular disease endpoints (Strobel et al., 2011). For example, the study that analyzed the cardiovascular disease linked to sleep apnea verify that the carbonylation of erythrocytic proteins associated with sleep apnea is a predictor of cardiovascular disease (Klein et al., 2010).

The 8-OHdG is typical biomarker of oxidative stress. Increased 8-OHdG levels are frequently related to cardiovascular disease. The level of 8-OHdG has been demonstrated to be very high in aorta fragments taken at surgery from patients suffering from severe atherosclerosis lesion. An increase 8-OHdG levels in DNA isolated from lymphocytes are related to cardiovascular disease (Gackowski et al., 2001).

3. Hypercholesterolemia

Cardiovascular disease is a complex and multifactorial disease; there can be no doubt now that elevated plasma cholesterol levels play a dominant role. Hypercholesterolemia is associated with an increased risk of atherosclerosis. Fatty streaks can even be found in the foetus, to an extent increasing with maternal plasma cholesterol levels. There are genetic disorders that may have a relationship with hypercholesterolemia, such as a disease familial hypercholesterolemia, in which the LDL receptors are defective or absent, so that blood LDL (and hence cholesterol) levels become very high and these people have high atherosclerosis incidence (Halliwell & Gutteridge, 2007).

3.1 Hypercholesterolemia and oxidative stress

There are many possible factors involved in the atherosclerosis process; the oxidation hypothesis has been the central focus on the pathogenesis of atherosclerosis for almost 30 years. This hypothesis states that the oxidative modification of LDL, or other lipoproteins and polyunsaturated fatty acids, is central, if not obligatory to the atherogenic process. The important issue is that inhibition of such oxidation should reduce the progression of atherosclerosis, independent of reduction of other risk factors, such as elevated LDL levels. The interest in ox-LDL is based on the fact that ox-LDL is cytotoxic to endothelial and other cells, and thus, could directly cause damage to arterials cells and, in addition it can activate an immune and proinflammatory response. There are many potential mechanisms by which oxidized forms of LDL may influence atherogenesis, these include uptake of ox-LDL by macrophages leading to foam cell formation; ox-LDL products are chemotactic for monocytes and T-cells, they can inhibit the motility of tissue macrophages and induce apoptosis; ox-LDL or its products are mitogenic for smooth muscle cells and macrophages, for example, they can induce proinflammatory genes and macrophage scavenger receptors, thereby enhancing its own uptake; ox-LDL is immunogenic and elicits autoantibody formation and activated T-cells; ox-LDL may enhance procoagulant pathways (induction of tissue factor and platelet aggregation, and can adversely impact arterial vasomotor properties (Witztum & Steinberg, 2001). We already know that ox-LDL is proatherogenic, but how is it generated *in vivo*? There are lingering uncertainties about the mechanism of LDL oxidation *in vivo*. The LDL is not necessarily oxidized within the plasma compartment, the LDL could undergo oxidative modification on the artery wall or in fact in any extravascular, extracellular site and then return to the plasma compartment (Chisolm & Steinberg, 2000). Oxidation of LDL results in the generation of a variety of modifications to the lipid and protein moieties, including the covalent modification of apolipoprotein B (ApoB) with reactive products of the decomposition of oxidized lipids, yielding MDA and HNE. Remembering that core lipid particles are composed of cholesterol ester and triglyceride, an outer monolayer is composed of free cholesterol and phospholipid including phosphatidilcholine, and on molecule of ApoB surrounds LDL particles (Yoshida & Kisugi,

2010). In addition, the residual oxidized phospholipid containing aldehyde terminate fatty acids. These, and presumably many other changes, generate immunogenic neo-epitopes on the modified LDL and are important to the atherosclerotic process. A variety of oxidized lipids' products, with similar characteristics of ox-LDL, are found in human plasma, atherosclerotic tissue and urine. Although some of these may indeed arise from oxidation of LDL, they could equally derive from oxidation of lipids at other sites and that oxidation may or may not parallel the rate at which LDL itself is undergoing oxidative modification (Witztum & Steinberg, 2001). Some of these proatherogenic effects of ox-LDL could also be induced by organic phase extracts of ox-LDL, suggesting that oxidized lipids themselves were proatherogenics, in addition to oxidatively modified ApoB (Davies & Roberts, 2011).

Still addressing LDL, it can be oxidized non-enzymatically by transition metal ions, heme and other catalysis. On the other hand, there are many postulated mechanisms by which LDL could become oxidized via several enzymes within the artery wall. Transitions metals are important to lipid oxidation. Most cells present in the arterial intima can promote LDL oxidation by its enzymes that mediated LDL oxidation, but it arguably requires the presence of transitions metals, iron or copper microconcentration. Elevated levels of metal ions are present in the advanced atherosclerotic lesions. Tissue homogenates prepared from atherosclerotic lesions contain catalytically active metal ions, indicating that these metals may stimulate LDL oxidation in the artery wall. One mechanism that has now gained strong support is the enzimatic. Lypoxygenase is one intracellular enzyme that directly oxygenates polyunsaturated fatty acids. The enzyme initiates the seeding of LDL with hydroperoxides, leading to the subsequent initiation of lipid peroxidation. These lipid peroxides could be released from cells and might translocate to LDL. Leucocytes-released myeloperoxidase catalyzes the formation of reactive substance species (HOCl) and generates a series of secondary radical or non-radical oxidants that may provide lipid peroxidation, oxidized LDL, advanced glycation end products and nitrating species. Among the mechanisms protein glycation is included. The last mechanism cited refers to $NO^{\bullet}$ (which has already been mentioned here). Although $NO^{\bullet}$ is a stable radical that fails to oxidized LDL at physiological pH, it is rapidly inactivated by $O_2^{\bullet-}$ to form peroxynitrite, a potent oxidant, implicating in LDL oxidation. This mechanism should be important *in vivo* since endothelial cells, smooth muscle cells and macrophages generate $O_2^{\bullet-}$ (Yoshida & Kisugi, 2010). There are lipid peroxidation products in the vasculature that do not arise directly from LDL and could contribute to atherogenesis. These oxidation products create proinflammatory mediators that drive a chronic inflammatory state, such as isoprostanes. It is important to know that well-established risk factors as causes of cardiovascular disease may have lipid peroxidation as part of its mechanism, such as smoking and diabetes (Davies and Roberts, 2011). Therefore, the evidence shows us clearly that hypercholesterolemia plus other risk factors increase the disease process and progression.

The oxidant hypothesis makes us question whether or not administration of antioxidants significantly slows the formation of atherosclerotic lesion. In a large number of epidemiologic studies, the dietary intake or plasma levels of antioxidant nutrients correlates negatively with risk of clinical cardiovascular disease. The user in clinical trials is tocopherols and beta-carotene because they are naturally occurring nutrients which would pose no toxicological problems. The relevance of vitamin C is as a potent trap for singlet oxygen, but much less effective in terminating free radical chain reactions and the vitamin E is an excellent terminating free radical chain reaction. The protect effect against LDL oxidation is more effective with use of vitamin E than C. This difference may be because vitamin C is distributed exclusively in the aqueous phase, whereas vitamin E takes up residence predominantly in lipoprotein (Witztum and Steinberg, 2001).

HDL normally plays an anti-atherogenic role, unlike LDL. The protective capacity of HDL has been ascribed primarily to its ability to remove excess cholesterol from peripheral tissues in the reverse cholesterol transport pathway. However, recent studies have suggested more mechanisms. For example, HDL can inhibit LDL oxidation and this may contribute to inverse association between plasma HDL levels and risk of developing atherosclerosis. These protective effects of HDL have been attributed to the various proteins associated with HDL. Paraoxonase-1 is an enzyme associated with HDL in blood and has been reported to posse antioxidant and anti-inflammatory properties. This enzyme is able to hydrolyze oxidized phospholipids and to destroy the biologically active lipids in ox-LDL. There is growing evidence that reduced activity of HDL-associated paraoxonase-1 is predictive of vascular disease (Jayakumari & Thejaseebai, 2009).

4. Hypertension

Previous studies have indicated that hypertension and hypercholesterolemia frequently co-exist, causing what is known as "dyslipidemic hypertension". The combination of these factors more than additively increases the risk of cardiovascular disease events compared with the occurrence of one alone (Wong et al., 2006). The resultant oxidative stress is considered a unifying mechanism for hypertension and atherosclerosis.

Hypertension development is intrinsically linked with vascular function and structural changes, including endothelial dysfunction, altered contractility and vascular remodelling. One of the key characteristics of hypertension is increased peripheral resistance, due largely to a reduced lumen diameter of the resistance vessel, and a small change in diameter can significantly impact on vascular resistance. The small arteries and arterioles that determine peripheral resistance undergo both structural and functional changes in hypertension. Examples of these changes include endothelial function, vascular smooth muscle growth, extracellular matrix deposition and vascular inflammation, altering contractility and vascular remodelling (Paravicini & Touyz, 2006).

4.1 Hypertension and oxidative stress

Within the cardiovascular system the ROS have a key role including regulation of cell growth and differentiation, modulation of extracellular matrix production and breakdown, $NO^{\bullet}$ inactivation and stimulation of many kinases. Many of this effects are associated with pathological changes observed in hypertension (Madamanchi et al., 2005).

Patients with hypertension demonstrate increased levels of oxidative stress by-products together with decreased activity of endogenous antioxidants enzymes, oxidative DNA damage and higher levels of $O_2^{\bullet -}$ production. ROS are produced by all vascular types of cells and can be formed by numerous enzymes, such as xanthine oxidase, uncoupled endothelial NO synthase and NAD(P)H oxidase, that are the most relevant in vascular disease and hypertension. It is worth keeping in mind the function of this enzymes, the xanthine oxidase catalyses the oxidation of hypoxanthine and xanthine to form $O_2^{\bullet-}$, and is known to be present in vascular endothelium. Although xanthine oxidase-derived $O_2^{\bullet-}$ has been primarily studied in the context of ischemia-reperfusion injury and heart failure, there is also some evidence to suggest involvement in the endothelial dysfunction seen in hypertension. Nitric oxide synthase (NOS) can also contribute to ROS production, as all three NOS isoforms have been shown to be susceptible to the uncoupling that leads to the formation of $O_2^{\bullet-}$ (rather than $NO^{\bullet}$) under certain conditions. Many studies have shown that the major source of ROS in the vascular wall is nonphagocytic NAD(P)H oxidase, which utilizes NADH/NADPH as the electron donor to reduce molecular oxygen and produce $O_2^{\bullet-}$. Activation of this enzyme is regulated by many vasoactive hormones, growth factors and mechanical stimuli (shear stress and stretch) (Higashi et al., 2009).

The biomechanical forces influence the redox signalling. Two main forces acting on the blood vessel wall are shear stress (movement of blood) and stretch (luminal pressure). Shear stress and cyclic mechanical stretch influence vascular function and structure, in part, by stimulating production of $NO^{\bullet}$ and ROS. Summarizing, the biomechanical forces increase activation and expression of endothelial NOS and stimulate production of $O_2^{\bullet-}$ and H_2O_2 (Paravicini & Touyz, 2006). Again, remembering that $O_2^{\bullet-}$ and $NO^{\bullet}$ can form $ONOO^-$; increased vascular pressure in hypertension is associated with stretch of endothelial and vascular smooth muscle cells, which can directly activate NAD(P)H oxidase to generate ROS. This effect may be amplified by activation of the rennin-angiotensin system. Increased oxidative stress in response to stretch contributes to activation of pro-inflammatory transcription factors, activation of growth-promoting MAP kinases, upregulation of profibrogenic mediators and altered vascular tone, important processes contributing to the vascular phenotype associated with hypertension (Paravicini & Touyz, 2006).

As discussed before, the excessive ROS have a central common pathway by which disparate influences may induce and exacerbate hypertension. Furthermore, a significant number of epidemiological and clinical trial data suggest that diets known to contain significant concentrations of naturally occurring antioxidants appear to reduce blood pressure and may reduce cardiovascular risk. Because of this, there is much interest in identifying key, naturally occurring antioxidants to both prevent and treat hypertension (Madamanchi et al., 2005). As in hypercholesterolemia, the focus is on vitamins E and C, and also vitamin A. The interest in vitamin A derivates has turned to lycopene, a potent antioxidant found in tomatoes. One small study has shown a reduction in blood pressure with tomato extract-based intervention. Vitamin C antihypertensive efficacy has been evaluated in small studies, showing modest reductions in blood pressure in both normotensive and hypertensive populations. With regard to vitamin E, small studies show either no effect or a pressor effect from supplementation. It is important to take care with the use of higher doses of supplements, since there is the risk of an antioxidant becoming pro-oxidant when used at high doses, for example, the ascorbate increase the risk of forming oxalate renal calculi (Kizhakekuttu & Widlansky, 2010). The addition of vitamins, the L-arginine, flavonoids and mitochondria-targeted agents are part of a target group of studies. L-arginine is an amino acid and the main substrate for the production of $NO^{\bullet}$ from NOS, and reduced levels lead to uncoupling of NOS resulting in the generation $O_2^{\bullet-}$ (low levels could contribute to hypertension). L-arginine supplementation could reduce blood pressure allowing for a restoration of normal $NO^{\bullet}$ bioavailability. There are studies demonstrating that flavonoids can inhibit NADPH oxidase and increase NOS-specific $NO^{\bullet}$ production, but investigation into the antihypertensive effects of flavonoids are inconclusive. The mitochondria-target agents include mainly coenzyme Q10 (CoQ) and lipoic acid. CoQ levels have been shown to be lower in hypertensive patients. CoQ may reduce mitochondrial $O_2^{\bullet-}$ production and reduce lipid peroxidation in plasma; CoQ supplementation was also demonstrated to reduce blood pressure. The potential beneficial effects of lipoic acid supplementation is given because it may improve coupling of NOS and has anti-inflammatory actions (Kizhakekuttu & Widlansky, 2010).

5. Conclusion

Throughout this chapter we have seen the numerous connections between heart disease, associated diseases and oxidative. Therefore, we cannot talk of homeostasis or change it without talking about redox balance. Any event that alters the delicate balance between defences and ROS moves the scales and triggers oxidative stress. Luckily our bodies are adapted to these constant changes, but only to a limited extent. Minor damage accumulates over the years. The fittest survive and we must be aware that not escaping natural selection, it continues to act upon us.

An alert on the evaluation of data involving oxidative stress: strict criteria are needed. For example, studies of ascorbic acid supplementation in rats and mice should be evaluated very carefully since these species synthesize vitamin C, while humans do not. Extrapolation of this data type for the human species must be carefully evaluated if it is to have any value. In the case of human data it must not be forgotten that the effect of an antioxidant that shows promise for a patient group cannot be extrapolated to healthy humans for example. In addition, dietary supplements that may be beneficial for the chronically ill should not be recommended for healthy people. What may be an antioxidant to one group can be pro-oxidant to another. A simple explanation of why: chemical reactions are reversible. The direction of the reaction in one group may be different from the direction of the reaction in the other group. The inclusion of a reactant or product may mean the reactions favouring or inhibiting the reactions that follow.

As we have learned over the past years for various diseases that afflict humanity, coronary heart disease can be triggered by many environmental and genetic factors. The disease in itself can trigger numerous other changes altering the homeostasis of the organism. Where is oxidative stress involved? Is it a cause or consequence? These questions are difficult to answer as we cannot address this issue without being aware of the chemistry of reactive species; we only know them with a solid knowledge of basic chemistry, which leads us to basic biochemistry, a deep knowledge of cell biology, physiology and so on. Molecular biology and genetics will help us with information no less important. Therefore, we need many more research groups than in the past century and in the clinical area, multidisciplinary cooperation. Maybe this is the biggest challenge for the 21st century.

6. References

Arens, R. & Marcus, C. L. (2004). Pathophysiology of upper airway obstruction: a developmental perspective. *Sleep,* 27, 997-1019. ISSN 0161-8105

Bradley, T. D. & Floras, J. S. (2009). Obstructive sleep apnoea and its cardiovascular consequences. *Lancet,* 373, 82-93. ISSN 0140-6736

Butt, M., Dwivedi, G., Khair, O. & Lip, G. Y. H. (2010). Obstructive sleep apnea and cardiovascular disease. *International Journal of Cardiology,* 139, 7-16. ISSN 0167-5273

Cairo, G. & Pietrangelo, A. (2000). Iron regulatory proteins in pathobiology. *Biochemical Journal,* 352, 241-250. ISSN 0264-6021

Chisolm, G. M. & Steinberg, D. (2000). The oxidative modification hypothesis of atherogenesis: An overview. *Free Radical Biology and Medicine,* 28, 1815-1826. ISSN 0891-5849

Choi, S. O., Cho, Y. S., Kim, H. L. & Park, J. W. (2007). ROS mediate the hypoxic repression of the hepcidin gene by inhibiting C/EBP alpha and STAT-3. *Biochemical and Biophysical Research Communications,* 356, 312-317. ISSN 0006-291X

Christou, K., Moulas, A. N., Pastaka, C. & Gourgoulianis, K. I. (2003). Antioxidant capacity in obstructive sleep apnea patients. *Sleep Medicine,* 4, 225-228. ISSN 1389-9457

Collins, R., Armitage, J., Parish, S., Sleight, P., Peto, R. & Heart protection study, C. (2002). MRC/BHF Heart Protection Study of antioxidant vitamin supplementation in 20536 high-risk individuals: a randomised placebo-controlled trial. *Lancet,* 360, 23-33. ISSN 0140-6736

Cooke, M. S., Evans, M. D., Dizdaroglu, M. & Lunec, J. (2003). Oxidative DNA damage: mechanisms, mutation, and disease. *Faseb Journal,* 17, 1195-1214. ISSN 0892-6638

CousE, J. F. & Korach, K. S. (1999). Estrogen receptor null mice: What have we learned and where will they lead us? *Endocrine Reviews,* 20, 358-417. ISSN 0163-769X

Davies, S. S. & Roberts, L. J. (2011). F-2-isoprostanes as an indicator and risk factor for coronary heart disease. *Free Radical Biology and Medicine,* 50, 559-566. ISSN 0891-5849

Dunn, L. L., Rahmanto, Y. S. & Richardson, D. R. (2007). Iron uptake and metabolism in the new millennium. *Trends in Cell Biology,* 17, 93-100. ISSN 0962-8924

Fadini, G. P., Albiero, M., Cignarella, A., Bolego, C., Pinna, C., Boscaro, E., Pagnin, E., De toni, R., DE Kreutzenberg, S., Agostini, C. & Avogaro, A. (2009). Effects of androgens on endothelial progenitor cells in vitro and in vivo. *Clinical Science,* 117, 355-364. ISSN 0143-5221

Flemons, W. W., Buysse, D., Redline, S., Pack, A., Strohl, K., Wheatley, J., Young, T., Douglas, N., Levy, P., Mcnicholas, W., Fleetham, J., White, D., Schmidt-Nowarra, W., Carley, D., Romaniuk, J. & Amer acad sleep med task, F. (1999). Sleep-related breathing disorders in adults: Recommendations for syndrome definition and measurement techniques in clinical research. *Sleep,* 22, 667-689. ISSN 0161-8105

Flint, D. H., Tuminello, J. F. & Emptage, M. H. (1993). The inactivation of fe-s cluster containing hydro-lyases by superoxide. *Journal of Biological Chemistry,* 268, 22369-22376. ISSN 0021-9258

Frazer, D. M. & Anderson, G. J. (2005). Iron Imports. I. Intestinal iron absorption and its regulation. *American Journal of Physiology-Gastrointestinal and Liver Physiology,* 289, G631-G635. ISSN 0193-1857

Gackowski, D., Kruszewski, M., Jawien, A., Ciecierski, M. & Olinski, R. (2001). Further evidence that oxidative stress may be a risk factor responsible for the development of atherosclerosis. *Free Radical Biology and Medicine,* 31, 542-547.ISSN 0891-5849

Gourdy, P., Calippe, B., Laurel, H., Tremollieres, F., Douin-Echinard, V., Lenfant, F., Bayard, F., Gueryt, J. C. & Arnal, J. F. (2008). Role of inflammatory cytokines in the effect of estradiol on atheroma. *Clinical and Experimental Pharmacology and Physiology,* 35, 396-401 ISSN 0305-1870

Guo, S., Miyake, M., Liu, K. J. & Shi, H. (2009). Specific inhibition of hypoxia inducible factor 1 exaggerates cell injury induced by in vitro ischemia through deteriorating cellular redox environment. *Journal of Neurochemistry,* 108, 1309-1321. ISSN 0022-3042

Halliwell, B. & Gutteridge, J. M. C. (2007). *Free radicals in biology and medicine,* New York, Oxford University Press. ISBN 978-0-19-856868-1

Higashi, Y., Noma, K., Yoshizumi, M. & Kihara, Y. (2009). Endothelial Function and Oxidative Stress in Cardiovascular Diseases. *Circulation Journal,* 73, 411-418. ISSN 1346-9843

Hower, V., Mendes, P., Torti, F. M., Laubenbacher, R., Akman, S., Shulaev, V. & Torti, S. V. (2009). A general map of iron metabolism and tissue-specific subnetworks. *Molecular Biosystems,* 5, 422-443. ISSN 1742-206X

Hu, F. B. (2007). The iron-heart hypothesis - search for the ironclad evidence. *Jama-Journal of the American Medical Association,* 297, 639-641. ISSN 0098-7484

Ip, M. S. M., Lam, B., Chan, L. Y., Zheng, L., Tsang, K. W. T., Fung, P. C. W. & Lam, W. K. (2000). Circulating nitric oxide is suppressed in obstructive sleep apnea and is reversed by nasal continuous positive airway pressure. *American Journal of Respiratory and Critical Care Medicine,* 162, 2166-2171. ISSN 1073-449X

Jayakumari, N. & Thejaseebai, G. (2009). High Prevalence of Low Serum Paraoxonase-1 in Subjects with Coronary Artery Disease. *Journal of Clinical Biochemistry and Nutrition,* 45, 278-284. ISSN 0912-0009

Jordan, W., Cohrs, S., Degner, D., Meier, A., Rodenbeck, A., Mayer, G., Pilz, J., Ruther, E., Kornhuber, J. & Bleich, S. (2006). Evaluation of oxidative stress measurements in obstructive sleep apnea syndrome. *Journal of Neural Transmission,* 113, 239-254. ISSN 0300-9564

Kaushik, M., Sontineni, S. P. & Hunter, C. (2010). Cardiovascular disease and androgens: a review. *International Journal of Cardiology,* 142, 8-14. ISSN

Kirbas, G., Abakay, A., Topcu, F., Kaplan, A., Unlu, M. & Peker, Y. (2007). Obstructive sleep apnoea, cigarette smoking and serum testosterone levels in a male sleep clinic cohort. *Journal of International Medical Research,* 35, 38-45. ISSN 0300-0605

Kizhakekuttu, T. J. & Widlansky, M. E. (2010). Natural Antioxidants and Hypertension: Promise and Challenges. *Cardiovascular Therapeutics,* 28, e20-e32. ISSN 1755-5914

Klein, C., Martinez, D., Hackenhaar, F. S., Medeiros, T. M., Marcolin, M. L., Silveira, F. S., Wainstein, M. V., Goncalvez, S. C. & Benfato, M. S. (2010). Carbonyl groups: bridging the gap between sleep disordered breathing and coronary artery disease. *Free Radical Research,* 44, 907-912. ISSN 1071-5762

Kokturk, O., Ulukavak, T., Mollarecep, E. & Ciftci, B. (2005). Elevated C-reactive protein levels and increased cardiovascular risk in patients with obstructive sleep apnea syndrome. *International Heart Journal,* 46, 801-809.ISSN 1349-2365

Lavie, L. (2003). Obstructive sleep apnoea syndrome - an oxidative stress disorder. *Sleep Medicine Reviews,* 7, 35-51. ISSN 1087-0792

Lefter, R., Morency, C.-E. & Joseph, V. (2007). Progesterone increases hypoxic ventilatory response and reduces apneas in newborn rats. *Respiratory Physiology & Neurobiology,* 156, 9-16. ISSN 1569-9048

Madamanchi, N. R., Vendrov, A. & Runge, M. S. (2005). Oxidative stress and vascular disease. *Arteriosclerosis Thrombosis and Vascular Biology,* 25, 29-38. ISSN 1079-5642

Mendelsohn, M. E. (2000). Nongenomic, estrogen receptor-mediated activation of endothelial nitric oxide synthase - how does it work? What does it mean? *Circulation Research,* 87, 956-960. ISSN 0009-7330

MungruE, I. N., Stewart, D. J. & HUSAIN, M. (2003). The Janus faces of iNOS. *Circulation Research,* 93, E74-E74. ISSN 0009-7330

NikI, E.(2009). Lipid peroxidation: physiological levels and dual biological effects. *Free Radical Biology and Medicine,* 47, 469-484. ISSN 0891-5849

Paravicini, T. M. & Touyz, R. M. (2006). Redox signaling in hypertension. *Cardiovascular Research,* 71, 247-258. ISSN 0008-6363

Pedram, A., Razandi, M., Wallace, D. C. & Levin, E. R. (2006). Functional estrogen receptors in the mitochondria of breast cancer cells. *Molecular Biology of the Cell,* 17, 2125-2137. ISSN 1059-1524

Pendaries, C., Darblade, B., Rochaix, P., Krust, A., Chambon, P., Korach, K. S., Bayard, F. & Arnal, J. F. (2002). The AF-1 activation-function of ER alpha may be dispensable to mediate the effect of estradiol on endothelial NO production in mice. *Proceedings of the National Academy of Sciences of the United States of America,* 99, 2205-2210. ISSN 0027-8424

Piantadosi, C. A., Carraway, M. S. & Suliman, H. B. (2006). Carbon monoxide, oxidative stress and mitochondrial permeability pore transition. *Free Radical Biology and Medicine,* 40, 1332-1339. ISSN 0891-5849

Ramara, A., Duckles, S. P., Krause, D. N. & Procaccio, V. (2007). Estrogen suppresses brain mitochondrial oxidative stress in female and male rats. *Brain Research,* 1176, 71-81. ISSN 0006-8993

Salonen, J. T., Nyyssonen, K., Korpela, H., Tuomilehto, J., Seppanen, R. & Salonen, R. (1992). High stored iron levels are associated with excess risk of myocardial-infarction in eastern Finnish men. *Circulation,* 86, 803-811. ISSN 0009-7322

Schwenke, D. C. (1998). Antioxidants and atherogenesis. *Journal of Nutritional Biochemistry,* 9, 424-445. ISSN 0955-2863

Sullivan, J. L. (1981). Iron and the sex difference in heart-disease risk. *Lancet,* 1, 1293-1294. ISSN 1293-1294

Suzuki, Y. J., Jain, V., Park, A. M. & Day, R. M. (2006). Oxidative stress and oxidant signaling in obstructive sleep apnea and associated cardiovascular diseases. *Free Radical Biology and Medicine,* 40, 1683-1692. ISSN 0891-5849

Tan, K. C. B., Chow, W. S., Lam, J. C. M., Lam, B., Wong, W. K., Tam, S. & Ip, M. S. M. (2006). HDL dysfunction in obstructive sleep apnea. *Atherosclerosis,* 184, 377-382. ISSN 0021-9150

Titorenko, V. I. & Terlecky, S. R. (2011). Peroxisome Metabolism and Cellular Aging. *Traffic,* 12, 252-259. ISSN 1398-9219

Traish, A. M., Saad, F., Feeley, R. J. & Guay, A. (2009). The Dark Side of Testosterone Deficiency: III. Cardiovascular Disease. *Journal of Andrology,* 30, 477-494.

Vanhoutte, P. M. (2009). Endothelial Dysfunction - The First Step Toward Coronary Arteriosclerosis. *Circulation Journal,* 73, 595-601. ISSN 0027-8424

Vina, J., Borras, C., Gambini, J., Sastre, J. & Pallardo, F. V. (2005). Why females live longer than males? Importance of the upregulation of longevity-associated genes by oestrogenic compounds. *Febs Letters,* 579, 2541-2545. ISSN 2541-2545

Wang, M., Crisostomo, P. R., Markel, T., Wang, Y., Lillemoe, K. D. & Meldrum, D. R. (2008). Estrogen receptor beta mediates acute myocardial protection following ischemia. *Surgery,* 144, 233-238. ISSN 0039-6060

Wong, N. D., Lopez, V., Tang, S. & Williams, G. R. (2006). Prevalence, treatment and control of combined hypertension and hypercholesterolemia in the United States. *American Journal of Cardiology,* 98, 204-208. ISSN 0002-9149

Yamauchi, M. & Kimura, H. (2008). Oxidative stress in obstructive sleep apnea: putative pathways to the cardiovascular complications. *Antioxidants & Redox Signaling,* 10, 755-768. ISSN

Yamauchi, M., Nakano, H., Maekawa, J., Okamoto, Y., Ohnishi, Y., Suzuki, T. & Kimura, H. (2005). Oxidative stress in obstructive sleep apnea. *Chest,* 127, 1674-1679. ISSN 0012-3692

Yamazaki, H., Haji, A., Ohi, Y. & Takeda, R.(2005). Effects of progesterone on apneic events during behaviorally defined sleep in male rats. *Life Sciences,* 78, 383-388. ISSN 0024-3205

Yoshida, H. & Kisugi, R. (2010). Mechanisms of LDL oxidation. *Clinica Chimica Acta,* 411, 1875-1882. ISSN 0009-8981

Yoshihara, D., Fujiwara, N. & Suzuki, K. (2010). Antioxidants: benefits and risks for long-term health. *Maturitas,* 67, 103-107. ISSN 0378-5122

You, S. A. & Wang, Q. (2005). Ferritin in atherosclerosis. *Clinica Chimica Acta,* 357, 1-16. ISSN 0009-8981

2

Prediction of Coronary Heart Disease Risk in a South European Population: A Case-Control Study

Maria Isabel Mendonça[1], Roberto Palma Reis[2] and António Brehm[3]
[1]*Funchal Hospital Centre (Research Unit),*
[2]*New University of Lisbon,*
[3]*Madeira University,*
Portugal

1. Introduction

1.1 Coronary heart disease etiology

Coronary heart disease (CHD) is the most common cause of death in the industrialized countries. Although the past two decades have brought considerable advances in its detection and treatment, it remains a leading cause of death and disability in Western countries (Mackay & Mensah, 2004). CHD is a complex disease, whose primary cause is atherosclerosis. It is a progressive chronic disease process with contributions from environment, lifestyle and genetic factors. This complex disease clusters in families, suggesting a substantial genetic predisposition (Marenberg et al., 1994) and we know that its susceptibility can be mediated by both genetic and environmental factors (Talmud, 2007).

The influence of a family history of CHD, particularly of early onset, while universally recognized as important, has proved difficult to clarify fully. Habits and behaviors tend to persist in families, and familial aspects of the disease are partially explained by associations of behavioral risk factors and others in which behavior is important, including obesity, smoking, hypertension, dyslipidemia and diabetes. Having a parent with a history of myocardial infarction (MI) nearly doubles a person´s own risk of future MI, and the risk increases if both parents have a history risk of MI (Chow, 2011).

Furthermore, family history is a significant risk factor for atherosclerosis, and the contribution of family history cannot be fully accounted for by known cardiac risk factors (Colditz et al., 1986; Slack & Evans, 1966; Snowden et al., 1982). Genetic factors also contribute significantly to most of the major risk factors for CHD [diabetes, hypertension, elevated plasma levels of low-density lipoprotein cholesterol (LDL-C) and low levels of plasma high-density lipoprotein cholesterol (HDL)], and yet the contribution of family history is not fully explained by known cardiac risk factors, suggesting that other yet-to-be-determined genetic factors also contribute to cardiovascular risk (Cohen, 2006; Slack et al.,1966).

However no common major genetic alterations have been found that can explain CHD, and the scientific evidence accumulated over recent years on the pathophisiology and genetics of this complex disease indicates that there is unlikely to be a single gene that is responsible for its genetic component. Genetic predisposition for cardiovascular disease appears to be the result of the cumulative effects of various genetic polymorphisms and allele combinations, which in isolation would only confer moderately elevated risk, but the risk can be increased by various gene-gene and gene-environment interactions. (Lanktree & Hegele, 2009). Despite extensive exploration of many genes, strong evidence of a molecular genetics association with coronary artery disease or myocardial infarction remains to be obtained. The existence of these multiple predisposing genes with modest individual effect, gene–gene and gene–environment interactions, and interpopulation heterogeneity of both genetic and environmental disease have made its molecular detection and replication very difficult (Hunter, 2005).

Interactions between genes belonging to different physiological and enzyme systems have been investigated in recent years, involving adipocyte differentiation, lipid metabolism and glucose homeostasis, all of which affect the development of atherosclerosis and CHD. One of these studies (Peng et al., 2004) suggests that the association of the ε4 allele of the apolipoprotein E (apo E) gene and the 151C/T variant of the peroxisome proliferator-activated receptor gamma (PPARγ) gene reduces CHD risk. The ε4 carrier's had significant higher LDL-C levels than other apo E carriers and this tendency could be modified by PPAR gamma C/T genotype. In the Peng study, the ε 4 allele was an independent risk factor for CHD (OR=4.29, 95%CI: 1.6-11.48, P=0.004). A significant interaction between ε 4 allele and PPAR gamma C/T variant, was detected on CHD risk (P=0.045), and the interaction effect of the two genes on serum cholesterol level, attenuated de risk of CHD.

The concept of gene-gene interaction can thus be extended to the existence of protective and/or suppressive genetic variants, which when identified could make an important contribution to preventing further development of CHD or improving its clinical course.

Gene-environment interaction implies that, in combination, the effect of the genotype and the environmental factor is greater than the additive effect of each. At the molecular level the environment modifies the molecular function of the gene product, because in the population there is a range of genetic risk profiles under the influence of the environmental spectrum of risk and lifestyle choices they made (e.g. smoking). Smoking alone is known to approximately double the life time risk of CHD (1.94; 1.25-3.01), but the male smoker´s with the ε4 genotype had a hazard ratio of 3.17; 1.82-5.50, even after adjusting for the traditional risk factors (including plasma lipids) the risk remained high at 2.79 (1.59-4.91) (Humphries & Donati, 2002; Humphries et al., 2007).

Diseases such as CHD may be thought of as resulting from failure of adequate homeostasis within a physiological system. This may occur as a result of failure at the genetic level (gene transcription), due to an environmental exposure (smoking, alcohol, diet, etc.) or due to an imbalance between the two [Stephans & Humphries, 2003].

Therefore, CHD is the terminal manifestation of multiple intermediate disease processes, which have genetic, environmental determinants and their interactions (Hunter, 2005; Manolio et al., 2006).

1.2 Personalized medicine and possibility to predict coronary heart disease risk

Although there has been considerable success in identifying genetic variants that influence well-known risk factors, such as cholesterol levels, the progress done in new genes which might influence the early occurrence of CHD, has been slow. Recent genetic approaches involving genomic associations in large scale (GWA) can identify novel susceptibility genes and genetic variants involved in the pathophysilogy of CHD (vasculogenesis, inflammation, immunity, new apolipoprotein and some genes with pathophysiological role still unknown (Watkins & Farrall, 2006). It is also expected that genetic profiling, that is, the simultaneous testing of multiple genetic variants, can eventually be used to predict CHD risk in individuals. This may lead to personalized medicine in which preventive and therapeutic interventions will be targeted at genetic profiles rather than at conventional risk factors (Van der Net et al., 2009).

One of the major promises is that this advance will lead to personalized medicine, in which preventive and therapeutic interventions for complex diseases are tailored to individuals based on their genetic profiles (Shiffman et al., 2006). Personalized medicine already exists for monogenetic disorders such as hereditary forms of cancer, in which genetic testing is the basis for informing individuals about their future health status and for deciding upon specific, often radical interventions. Because the etiology of complex diseases is essentially different from that of monogenic diseases, new emerging genomic knowledge that may be applied to primary care and public health will be one of the major challenges for the next decades (Janssens & Van Duijn, 2008). The existence of a predictive test or a prediction model that can discriminate between individuals who will develop coronary disease and those who will not is important for personalized medicine. However, current risk assessment protocols are imperfect, particularly in assessing the risk of early onset CHD (Akosah, 2003).

Data from Framingham study population enabled prediction of CHD during a follow-up interval of several years, based on blood pressure, smoking history, total cholesterol and HDL-cholesterol levels, diabetes, and left ventricular hypertrophy on the ECG. These prediction algorithms have been adapted to simplify score sheets that allow physicians to estimate multivariable CHD risk in middle-aged patients (Wilson et al., 1998).

Diamond and Forester understood that different results, obtained from different tests with substantial imperfections, must be integrated into a diagnostic about the probability for coronary disease, in a given patient. This approach estimates the pretest likelihood of coronary disease (defined by age, sex and symptoms) and the sensitivity and specificity of four diagnostic tests: stress electrocardiography, cardiokymography, thallium scintigraphy and cardiac fluoroscopy. The probability for coronary artery disease was estimated by Bayes´ theorem from each patient´s age, sex and symptoms classification, and from the observed test responses (Diamond & Forester, 1979).

For estimating the likelihood of severe coronary heart disease, investigators from Duke University elaborated a risk score based on clinical symptomatic variables (Pryor et al., 1983, 1991, from Duke University). A similar score also based in the patient´s history was investigated by the Stanford University (Sox et al., 1990).

Another score denominated ARIC score following the study with the same name, Atherosclerosis Risk in Communities (ARIC) (Chambless et al., 2003), was also developed. At European level, the Score risk algorithm led by Ian Graham, based on a European population of 250,000 people, allows prediction of the risk of atherosclerotic manifestations other than cardiovascular diseases, such as stroke and peripheral vascular disease, according to age sex, smoking habit, systolic blood pressure and total cholesterol level (Graham, 2004).

However, these protocols may be improved by the inclusion of genetic information which is independent of traditional risk factors (Zdravkovic et al., 2002). Recent studies have attempted to assess whether the addition of new emerging risk factors, such as C reactive protein, homocysteine and genetic polymorphisms, can improve CHD risk prediction in addition to traditional risk factors (Folsom et al., 2006; Koenig et al, 2004; Morrison et al., 2007; Humphries et al., 2007) This is the goal to achieve through the new millennium genetic epidemiology: the development of tests, based on DNA, to determine the genetic predisposition to CHD. However, the contribution of an isolated genetic variant is small considering the polygenic nature of the disease. Several genetic markers, relevant in the pathophisiology of CHD, have been studied, such as the candidate genes variants involving several enzymatic pro-atherosclerotic systems, anti-oxidants, inflammatory, pro thrombotic and other involving the lipid and carbohydrates metabolism. More recently research has centered on genetic variants with strong associations with CHD, identified through genome wide association studies (GWA), some with pathophysiological roles that are still unknown, such as the single nucleotide polymorphism (SNP), situated at the 9p21 genetic locus (McPherson et al., 2007; Ripatti et al., 2010).

To validate, in our population setting (Madeira Island), the risk conferred by these recently discovered genetic factors and to improve assessment information about the magnitude of CHD risk associated to traditional risk factors, biochemical risk marker and genetic factors, we aimed to obtain a new model of risk score useful in the discrimination of total coronary disease risk in this population.

We therefore performed an epidemiological study, based on 7 genetic variants, some of them with a consistent association with CHD. These variants had already been investigated in previous works by our research group (Mendonça et al., 2004a, 2004b, 2008a, 2008b).

2. Combined model of risk score, including genetic and environmental information for CHD risk prediction (case-control study)

2.1 Methodology

2.1.1 Study design and population

Case-control study with a total of 1406 Caucasian subjects, average 53.5±9.7 years, 77.0% male, native and resident in Madeira Island (Portugal).

The cases (n=723), mean age 53.7±8.9 years and 79.9% male, were selected consecutively following hospital discharge from patients admitted with myocardial infarction or coronary artery disease confirmed by coronary angiography showing at least 75% obstruction of at least one coronary artery. Myocardial infarction was defined by a positive troponin blood test in the setting of symptoms and electrocardiogram changes (both ST-segment elevation and non–ST-segment elevation changes) consistent with MI (*Joint European Society of Cardiology/American College of Cardiology Committee criteria, 2000*). The control group was comprised of 683 healthy volunteers, mean age 53.3±10.5 years and 73.9% male, selected randomly from the electoral register from individuals with no history or suggestion of CHD.

The use of the electoral register to select the controls was intended to ensure that they did not differ significantly from the cases in terms of gender and age. For each control, a clinical observation with reference to the classical risk factors and ECG was registered, but in doubtful cases complementary exams such as a stress test, and echocardiogram or an angiography, were requested. After the subject's inclusion, the clinical history of each one was recorded, with reference to demographic and other data including age, place of birth and residence, family history of CHD, personal history of hypertension or diabetes, smoking and alcohol habits, dyslipidemia and quantity and type of physical exercise. Their weight, height, waist and hip circumference, heart rate, blood pressure were measured. Subjects were considered to have a family history of CHD if it had been diagnosed in their father or a brother before the age of 50 or mother or a sister before the age of 60 (Sesso et al., 2001). Subjects were classified as having hypertension if they reported the fact, were taking antihypertensive medication or had systolic BP of ≥140 mmHg and/or diastolic BP of ≥90 mmHg, based on the mean of three measurements (Chobanian et al., 2003). They were classified as having diabetes if they were taking oral anti-diabetic medication or insulin or if their fasting plasma glucose was higher than 7.0 mmol/l or 126 mg/dl (Report of the Expert Committee on the Diagnosis and Classification of Diabetes Mellitus, 1997). Waist measurements were taken at the level of the umbilicus and we classified men as having a large waist if it was greater than 102 cm (40 inches) and women as having a large waist if it was greater than 88cm (Xavier F. Pi-Sunyer, 1998). Body mass index (BMI) was calculated as weight in kilograms divided by height in meters squared, with obesity defined as a BMI of >30 (Veja, 2002; Pi-Sunyer, 1998). Subjects were considered to be smokers if they smoked or had ceased less than five years previously. Dyslipidemia was defined as total fasting cholesterol of >5.2 mmol/l or 200 mg/dl, or LDL cholesterol of ≥3.4 mmol/l or 130 mg/dl, HDL ≤ 40 mg/dL, triglycerides ≥ 1.5 mmol/L or 150 mg/dL, as well as being considered present in individuals taking lipid-lowering medication (NCEP, 2001)). We evaluated physical activity by asking subjects if they exercise or play sports in their leisure time and their responses were classified as either never/seldom, sometimes, or often/very often (Mainous et al., 2007).

Blood samples were collected from cases and controls for biochemical and genetic analysis.

The study protocol was approved by the hospital's Ethics Committee and all participants gave their informed consent.

2.1.2 Biochemical and genetic analysis

The blood for routine tests, biochemical risk markers: Apo B 100, Homocysteine, Total Cholesterol, HDL, LDL, Triglycerides, Lipoprotein (a), CRP (hs) and genetic analysis, were collected in all subjects.

Biochemical analysis: To determine serum glucose, total, HDL and LDL cholesterol and triglycerides, blood samples were extracted after 14-16 hours' fasting, placed in dry tubes and centrifuged half an hour later at 3500 g. Serum levels of total, LDL, HDL cholesterol and triglycerides were quantified by an enzymatic technique using a Hitachi 911 auto-analyser. A direct enzymatic technique was used for HDL and LDL cholesterol. Biochemical risk markers lipoprotein (a), apolipoprotein B100, and high-sensitivity C-reactive protein (hs-

CRP) were quantified by nephelometry using a Behring BN 100 automatic system. Homocysteine was measured by fluorescence polarized immunoassay using an Abbot IMX automatic device. To measure fibrinogen, samples were also collected with the patient fasting and placed in a tube containing sodium citrate, and measurements were taken with a Behring BSC automatic analyser.

Genetic analysis: For both patients and controls, genomic DNA was extracted from an 80 μL aliquot of whole blood collected in tubes containing EDTA using standard phenol/chloroform methodologies with ethanol precipitation. The genotypes chosen for this study, were screened for their association with CHD, already investigated in previous studies (ACE I/D, AGT 235 M/T, ATIR 1166 A/C, MTHFR 677 C/T, PON 192 Q/R, Apo E (ε4), rs1333049 G/C).

The genotypic analysis was effectuated using probes oligonucleotydes marked with specific fluorescence for each one of the alleles in a test that combines the stipulated PCR technique and TaqMan (7300 SDS Software, Applied Biosystems).

2.1.3 Statistical analysis

Allele frequencies were deduced from the genotype distribution. To test deviation of the Hardy Weinberg Equilibrium (HWE), was performed by Pearson's χ^2 tests, using the observed genotype frequencies and the expected genotype frequencies. The student T test and *one way* ANOVA procedures were used for means comparison between groups. Multiple comparisons were performed by the adequate post hoc (Tukey). Genotypes distributions and allele frequencies were compared between the cases and the controls using a χ^2 test. Strength of the association was expressed by odds ratio (OR) as well as their 95% confidence intervals (CI).

We constructed a Genetic Risk Score (GRS) using a coding value of "0" for original non risk homozygote, "1" for heterozygote and "2" for mutated risk homozygote, and summing these values for each single nucleotide polymorphism (SNP). The obtained score was divided into five quintiles (0-4; 4-5; 5-6; 6-7; ≥7) and these was compared in patient and control population (using independent T-Student test) and odds ratio and 95% Confidence Intervals, were determined. To investigate independent variables associated with coronary heart disease, a multivariate logistic regression model (forward Wald), containing the traditional risk factors, the biochemical markers and GRS), was constructed. Finally, a receiver operating characteristic (ROC) curve, based on sensitivity and specificity of the multivariable model, was computed, to estimate CHD susceptibility and Hosmer-Lemeshow goodness-of-fit test, estimated the model calibration.

3. Results

3.1 Basal characteristics of the population

As expected, the cases were more likely to be smokers, diabetics and hypertensives. They had a higher alcohol intake, higher values for glycemia, triglycerides, dyslipidemia, body mass index, high-sensitivity C-reactive protein (hs-CRP), lipoprotein (a) and lower values for HDL cholesterol (Table 1).

	Total (n=1406)	Cases (n=723)	Controls (n=683)	p-value
Age (Years)	53.5 ± 9.7	53.7 ± 8.9	53.3 ± 10.5	0.387
Sex M (%)	1083(77.0%)	578 (79.9%)	505 (73.9%)	0.007
Hypertension (%)	704 (50.1%)	416 (57.5%)	288 (42.2%)	<0.0001
Diabetes (%)	324 (23.0%)	240 (33.2%)	324 (23.0%)	<0.0001
Obesity (%)	397(28.2%)	231(32.0%)	166 (24.3%)	<0.0001
Smoking (%)	484 (34.4%)	325 (45.0%)	159 (23.3%)	<0.0001
Alcohol gr/ day	0.8	1.6	0.0	<0.0001
Dyslipidemia (%)	1246 (88.6%)	694 (96.0%)	552 (80.8%)	<0.0001
Glycemia mg/dl	102.0	107.0	98.0	<0.0001
Triglycerides mg/dl	132.0	152.0	115.0	<0.0001
HDL mg/dl	44.6 ± 14.6	38.5 ± 10.3	51.2 ± 15.7	<0.0001
Systolic BP (mm Hg)	135.5 ± 20.4	136.4 ± 20.2	134.4 ± 20.6	0.040
Diastolic BP (mm Hg)	81.2 ± 11.3	81.7 ± 11.2	80.8 ± 11.5	0.206
Fibrinogen (mm Hg)	348.9 ± 94.1	344.9 ± 96.6	341.1 ± 96.7	0.397
Lp(a (mg/dl))	16.5	20.8	15.2	0.010
(hs) CRP mg/dl	2.0	3.0	1.6	<0.0001
Genetic Risk Score	5.03 ± 1.84	5.4 ± 1.7	4.6 ± 1.9	<0.0001

Table 1. Basal characteristics of the population.

3.2 Selection of the used polymorphisms and genetic risk score

The genotypes chosen for this study, were screened for their association with CHD, already investigated in previous studies (ACE I/D, AGT 235 M/T, ATIR 1166 A/C, MTHFR 677 C/T, PON 192 Q/R, Apo E (ε4) and rs1333049 G/C).

The genetic risk score based on 7 SNPs variants (ACE I/D, AGT 235 M/T, ATIR 1166 A/C, MTHFR 677 C/T, PON 192 Q/R, Apo E (ε4), rs1333049 G/C), was calculated for 1406 individuals and ranged from 11 and 0 in the whole population. The GRS average was 5.03±1.84 in the whole population. CHD patients had higher GRS than control population (5.41±1.73 vs. 4.63±1.87, $p<0.0001$).

In the last GRS quintile (score ≥7) including more than a quarter of the patients, the CHD risk was three times higher than in the reference group.

3.3 Independent variable associated with CHD and risk prediction models of CHD

The association of the GRS with CHD was tested in a multivariate analysis containing the traditional risk factors and comprising the GRS. After logistic regression model the GRS stayed in the equation as an independent risk marker associated with increased risk of CHD; (OR=1.333; $p<0.0001$). Diabetes type 2, dyslipidemia, arterial hypertension and alcohol, also remained in the equation as independent risk factors of CHD (Table 3).

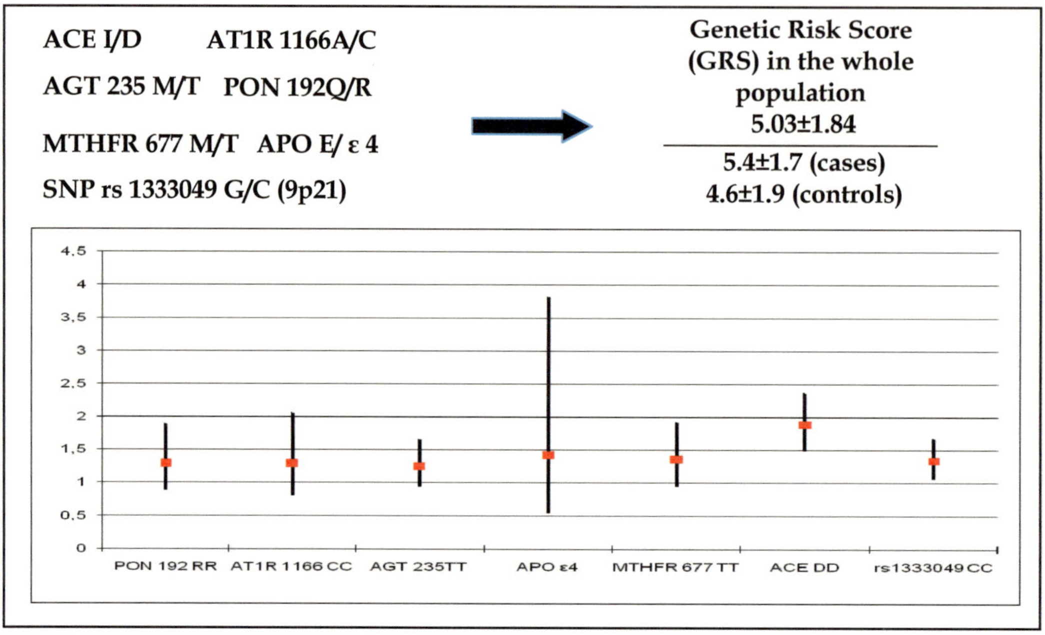

Fig. 1. CHD genetic risk (OR) conferred by each isolated polymorphism and the GRS obtained by the addition of all the 7 risk alleles of the studied variants.

GRS by Quintiles	Cases (n=723)	Controls (n=682)	Odds ratio (CI 95%)	P value
1º - [0-4[	90 (12.4%)	184 (27.0%)	Reference	-------
2º - [4-5[	127 (17.6%)	118 (17.3%)	2.20 (1.52 – 3.19)	<0.0001
3º - [5-6[	172 (23.8%)	151 (22.1%)	2.33 (1.65 – 3.30)	<0.0001
4º - [6-7[	151 (20.9%)	121 (17.7%)	2.55 (1.78 – 3.67)	<0.0001
5º - ≥7	183 (25.3%)	108 (15.8%)	3.46 (2.41 – 4.98)	<0.0001

Table 2. Association between the *SGR* by quintiles and CHD risk (OR) in the studied population.

Variables	**B**	**S.E.**	**Wald**	**df**	**Odds Ratio (IC 95%)**	**Valor-p**
Diabetes 2	1.072	0.153	49.310	1	2.922 (2.166-3.941)	<0.0001
Dyslipidemia	1.713	0.231	54.946	1	5.545 (3.526-8.723)	<0.0001
AHT	0.265	0.123	4.652	1	1.304 (1.025-1.659)	0.031
Alcohol	0.010	0.002	40.435	1	1.010 (1.007-1.014)	<0.0001
GRS	0.287	0.034	70.725	1	1.333 (1.246-1.425)	<0.0001
Constant	-3.499	0.301	135.090	1	0.030	<0.0001

Table 3. Independent variables associated with coronary heart disease risk.

Afterwards, two predictive models of CHD risk were constructed and the area under the receiver operating characteristic (AUC) curves for the constructed model which included both genetic and traditional risk factors was compared with the AUC for the model, which included only the traditional risk factors. The top chart including the GRS increased the AUC over the bottom chart which was only based on traditional risk factors (Figure 2 and 3).

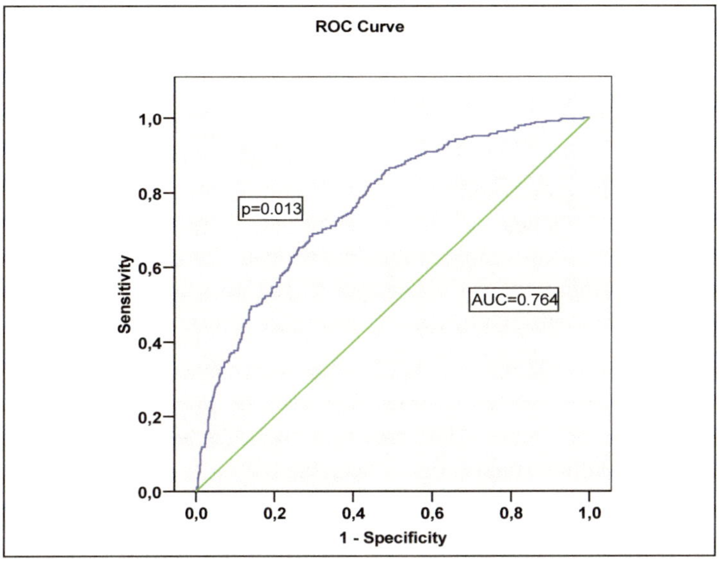

Fig. 2. ROC curve, based on sensitivity and specificity of the multivariable model, with traditional risk factors and GRS.

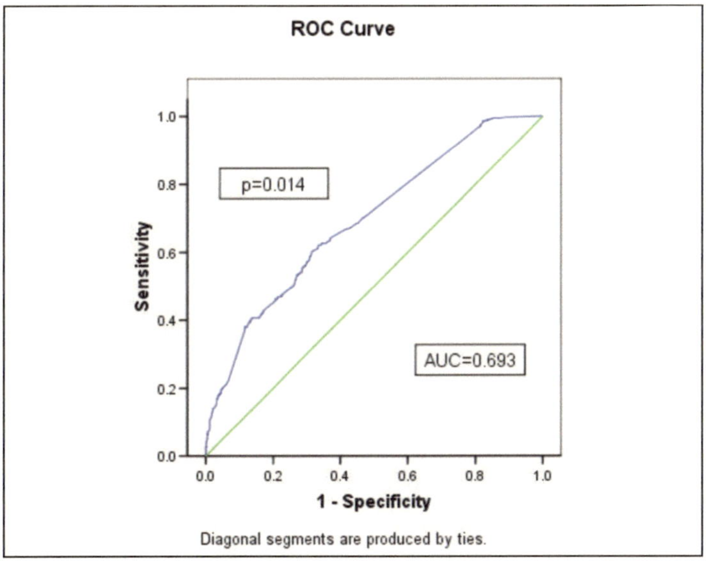

Fig. 3. ROC curve, based on sensitivity and specificity of the multivariable model, with traditional risk factors and without GRS.

In the model with GRS (Figure 2), the AUC was 75%, indicating good CHD discrimination and the goodness-of-fit statistic test value was 6.186; p=0.626, indicating a good calibration of the model. In the model without the GRS (Figure 3) the AUC was 69.3%.

4. Discussion

Risk prediction is an important part of cardiovascular disease prevention and the ability to identify high risk individuals who do not present with the traditional risk factors enable clinicians to personalize strategies for prevention and treatment.

Risk prediction is based on the knowledge of the conventional risk factors (high blood pressure, smoking, blood cholesterol level) and in the family history. However the fact that some individuals with coronary disease are of low risk when considering the classic risk factors forced the scientific community to go further in the predictive models. The GRS used in this work comprises SNPs selected from candidate genes and others identified through large-scale genomic association studies, and introduced the concept that the addition of a GRS can improve the prediction of CHD beyond that supplied by traditional risk factors, especially in the population fringe with few classic risk factors.

It was based essentially in variants which had shown association with coronary disease not only in the published literature in general but also in previous studies in our Funchal research group, already mentioned. The fact that these genes have shown, an association with CHD in our population makes them of great value in CHD risk prediction, in our population.

In the present work the risk associated with each single polymorphism is small with the exception of angiotensin convertion enzyme (ACE DD) and the SNP rs1333049, (OR=1.8 $p<0.0001$ and 1.4 $p<0.0001$, respectively). However, although the risk associated to each isolated variant was modest, the sum of the risk alleles, represented by GRS, was associated with a significant elevation of the risk. To illustrate this finding when the GRS, was codified in quintiles, the highest quintile (6 or more risk alleles) presented a 3.5 times higher risk than the reference group (OR=3.46 [2.41-4.98]; $p<0.0001$).

The availability of clinical genetic testing for cardiovascular disease has only recently emerged. In large part, this has stemmed from technological advances in molecular sequencing, which have substantially decreased testing costs. While a decade ago the sequencing of a single gene might have cost tens of thousands of Euros and taken months of effort, the same result can now be obtained with much less time and cost. Sequencing technology is now undergoing a period of extremely rapid development that portends revolutionary advances in the field. When validated and implemented in clinical testing, these advancements could greatly improve our ability to provide genetic diagnoses for many conditions.

In our Human Genetic Laboratory the genotypic analysis was done using oligonucleotides probes marked with specific fluorescence for each one of the alleles in a test that combines the stipulated PCR technique and TacMan (Applied Biosystems).

The genotypes were determined by 7300 System SDS Software (Applied Biosystems). The calculated material cost is 1.1 Euros by individual sample and by each SNP. This value includes all required material and reagents to perform the whole analysis.

To establish an appropriate coronary risk score, with reduced costs, in spite of the large sample size, we used only SNPs that already had shown functional impact in coronary pathophisiology and large prevalence in our population.

Outsourcing might seem another way to reduce costs and these operating processes are gaining acceptance in many hospitals.

Genome-wide association studies suggest that common genetic variants explain only a modest fraction of heritable risk for common diseases, raising the question of whether rare variants account for a significant fraction of unexplained heritability. Although DNA sequencing costs have fallen markedly, they remain far from what is necessary for rare and novel variants to be routinely identified at a genome-wide scale in large cohorts (Sarah Ng et al., 2009).

Meanwhile, if we are evaluating not a single SNP, but a group of SNPs, creating a genetic score based on a small number of genes with reasonable costs, if this score can improve our prediction of the coronary artery disease risk, this genetic score could potentially be useful in the clinical practice.

In an epidemiologic study conducted in 2004, with the use of new risk prediction models which included genetic information, Khoury et al predicted that the prevention measures aiming at a small fraction (about 15%) of the high risk population with few classical risk factors, will be performed with the resources currently dedicated to the prevention, used in a more judicious way, but will also allow to significantly reduce the global load of coronary disease (Khoury et al., 2004).

The success of a model including a GRS should be measured by its ability to help individuals and physicians in making decisions regarding lifestyle advice or pharmacological treatment in order to decrease CHD risk and disability.

In this study, after multivariate logistic regression, the independent predictors of CHD were dyslipidemia, type 2 diabetes, hypertension, daily intake of alcohol and GRS. Although after multivariate logistic regression the risk of CHD determined by the GRS did not exceed that of conventional risk factors, this independent predictor based on genetic risk variants has some advantages.

The genetic analysis is easy to perform and is highly reliable in respect to certain biomarkers, most of which require lengthy methods for their determination, more prone to biological variation and error.

One of its greatest benefits will be its usefulness in identifying the 15% of high risk individuals who are masked as borderline or apparently low risk and that would not be identified in clinical surveys based on current protocols (Framingham, National Cholesterol Education Program Adult Treatment Panel III guidelines). In 2003, Akosah et al reported that among individuals who have suffered premature myocardial infarction (age <55 years male and <65 years female) 70% were considered to be of low risk, and of these 87% had not been eligible for treatment with statins (Akosah et al., 2003).

In the present study the inclusion of the genetic profile represented by GRS greatly increased the predictive capacity of the model over the observed in the model which included the traditional risk factors only (69.3% to 74.6%), showing the value of the genetic profile in the prediction of coronary heart disease risk. It introduces the concept of a GRS that aggregates information from multiple genetic variants into a single score and indicates that a GRS can improve the ability to predict incident CHD beyond that afforded by traditional non genetic risk factors (Morrison et al., 2007).

A potential advantage of genetic profiling over conventional risk factors in the prediction of CHD risk is that genetic information is already present at birth. Therefore, genetic profiles could theoretically predict CHD risk before conventional risk factors become deleterious (Van der Net et al., 2009).

However, the dream of personalized medicine and predictive indexes may yet be achieved, but it seems that will take far more than these first steps on the road to gene discovery. This is a topic that surely should be revisited once efforts toward gene discovery, identification of functional variants and pathways, and searches for less common variants allowing for heterogeneity have progressed (Ioannidis, 2009).

5. Conclusions

The result of this study has demonstrated that a GRS, based on the presence of some susceptibility gene variants for coronary heart disease, allow the identification of sub-groups with a significantly higher risk of coronary disease.

The risk model that includes the GRS, the classical risk factors and some new risk markers, increases the GRS predictive power and provides a good estimation of the CHD risk. It introduces the concept that a risk model that aggregates information from several genetic variants (GRS), the traditional risk factors and some new risk markers, can improve the ability to predict incident CHD beyond that supplied by the classical risk factors.

The proposed model can become a simple and useful tool in the CHD risk stratification, giving us an early estimate of the disease susceptibility and prevention.

Key message

- Coronary Heart Disease is a complex multifactorial disease.
- Genetic profile, lifestyle and environmental factors play an important role in its development.
- Its genetic predisposition appears to be the result of the cumulative effects of various genetic polymorphisms or allelic combinations that in isolation would only confer a light or moderate risk. However, this risk will be modulated (increased or decreased) by various gene-gene and gene-environment interactions.
- Risk prediction of incident CHD is based on the knowledge of the conventional risk factors (high blood pressure, smoking, blood cholesterol level) and in the genetic profile, which can improve the prediction of incident CHD beyond that supplied by traditional risk factors, especially in the population fringe with few classical risk factors.
- The GRS aggregates information from some genetic variants into a single score and the present work indicates that the addition of this GRS to the information obtained by the classical risk factors can improve the ability to predict CHD risk
- With these mixed risk assessment tools, we can identify patients at high risk who would get the most benefit from the correction of modifiable risk factors through lifestyle interventions or specific medications.
- In the future, these new technologies and risk algorithms may change the strategies followed nowadays by Health Systems, and will permit to significantly reduce the load and the global burden of coronary disease.

6. Summary

Coronary heart disease (CHD) is the most common cause of death in the industrialized countries. As these populations are aging, the prevalence of CHD is arising, and it is expected that this tendency will increase, in the future, due to the obesity epidemic that is rising all over the world and this will place a considerable burden on healthcare systems. The knowledge of new risk models, can improve the diagnosis capacity and prevention as well as the early treatment of this condition.

The aim of this chapter is to obtain a risk model, which includes the classical risk factors and the genetic profile through the genetic risk score (GRS), in which the risk of CHD was estimated in a South European population. For that purpose a total of 1406 individuals, 723 consecutive patients with documented CHD in the coronary angiogram (53.7±8.9 years, 79.9% male) and 683 controls without any clinical manifestation of CHD (53.3±10.5 years, 73.9% male), randomly selected from electoral rolls, were evaluated. Cases and controls were selected with no significantly difference in terms of sex and age. Seven genetic polymorphisms, ACE I/D, AGT 235T/M , AT1R1166 A/C, PON Q192R, MTHFR M677C/T, Apo E (ε2, ε3, ε4) and 9p21 locus (rs1333049), were determined, using the combined PCR stipulated technique with TaqMan (Applied Biosystems). A genetic risk score (GRS) was obtained, for each individual, using a coding value of 0 for the original non mutated homozygote, 1 for the heterozygote, and 2 for the mutated homozygote. The GRS was created by summing these values for each individual. The obtained score was divided into five quintiles (0 and 4; 4 and 5; 5-6; 6-7; ≥7) and was compared in patient and control population, using independent T-Student test. Case control Odds ratios and 95% Cornfield Confidence Intervals were determined. A forward Wald logistic regression model was constructed, adjusted for age and gender, having entered all conventional risk factors. Finally, a ROC curve was computed, to evaluate the capacity of this model to predict coronary disease susceptibility and *Hosmer Lemeshow goodness-of-fit* test estimated model calibration.

The mean GRS was 5.03±1.84, in the total population (maximum 11 and minimum 0). CHD patients had higher GRS than the control population (5.41±1.73 vs. 4.63±1.87, $p<0.0001$). In the last GRS quintile (score≥7) including more than a quarter of the patients, the CHD risk was three times higher than in the reference group. After logistic regression the GRS stayed in the equation as an independent risk marker associated with increased risk of CHD; (OR=1.333; $p<0.0001$). Diabetes type 2, dyslipidemia, arterial hypertension and alcohol intake, also remained in the equation as independent risk factors of CHD.

Two receiver operating characteristic (ROC) curve models were constructed and the model including both genetic and traditional risk factors was compared with the model which included only the traditional risk factors. The first presented increased AUC (75%) over that observed when the receiver operating characteristic curve was based only on traditional risk factors (69.3%).

Conclusion: This risk model including the GRS, the classic risk factors and the new risk markers, provided a good estimation of the CHD risk. It introduces the concept that a GRS that aggregates information from multiple genetic variants can improve the ability to predict incident CHD beyond that afforded by traditional non genetic risk factors. The proposed model can become a simple and useful tool in the CHD risk stratification, supplying us with an early estimation of disease susceptibility and prevention.

7. Acknowledgment

This work was supported by "Operational Program to Revaluate the Economic Potential and Territorial Cohesion of the Autonomic Region of Madeira (Intervir + for an increasingly European Region).

8. References

Akosah, K.O., Schaper, A., Cogbill, C. & Schoenfeld, P. (2003). Preventing Myocardial Infarction in the Young Adults in the first place: How do the National Cholesterol Education Panel III Guidelines perform?. *J Am Coll Cardiol*, Vol. 41, No.9 (2003) pp.1475-1479

Chambless, L.; Folsom, A.; Sharrett, A., et al. (2003). Coronary heart disease prediction in the Atherosclerosis Risk in Communities (ARIC) Study. 2003. *J Clin Epidemiol* Vol. 56 (2003) pp. 880–90.

Chobanian, A.V. et al. (2003).The Seventh Report of the Joint National Committee on Prevention, Detection, Evaluation and Treatment of High Blood Pressure (JNC 7). 2003. *JAMA*, (May 21, 2003) Vol. 289 pp. 2560-2572.

Chow, C.K. (2011). Parental history and myocardial infarction risk across the world: the INTERHEART Study. (2011). *J Am Coll Cardiol* (2011) Vol. 57 pp. 619-27

Cohen, J.C. (2006). Genetic Approaches to Coronary Heart Disease. *J. Am. Coll. Cardiol* (2006) Vol. 48 pp. A10-A14.

Colditz, G.A., Stampfer, M.J., Willett, W.C. et al. (1986). A prospective study of parental history of myocardial infarction and coronary heart disease in women. *Am J Epidemiol* (1986) Vol. 123 pp. 48–58

Diamond G., A., & Forrester J., S. (1979). Analysis of Probability as an Aid in the Clinical Diagnosis of Coronary-Artery Disease. *N Engl J Med* (1986) Vol. 300 pp.1350-1358

Expert Panel on Detection, Evaluation and Treatment of High Blood Cholesterol I Adults.

Executive summary of the third report of the National Cholesterol Education Program (NCEP) expert panel on detection, evaluation and treatment of high blood cholesterol in adults (Adult Treatment Panel III). 2001. *JAMA* (2001) Vol. 285 pp. 2486–2497

Folsom, A.R., Chambless, L.E., Ballantyne, C.M. et al. (2006). An assessment of incremental coronary risk prediction using C-reactive protein and other novel risk markers: the Atherosclerosis Risk in Communities study. *Arch Intern Med* (2006) Vol.166 pp.1368–73.

Graham I. (2004). Principles of prevention of cardiovascular disease: Reply. *Eur Heart J* Vol.25 No. 5 pp. 446

Humphries, S.E. & Donati, M.B. (2002). Analyse of gene environment interaction in coronary artery disease. *Ital Heart J* (2002) Vol. 3 pp. 3-5

Humphries, S.E.; Cooper, J.A.; Talmud, P.J. & Miller, G.J. (2007). Candidate Gene Genotypes, Along with Conventional Risk Factor Assessment, Improve Estimation of Coronary Heart Disease Risk in Healthy UK Men. *Clinical Chemistry* (2007) Vol. 53 No.1 pp. 8-16

Hunter, D.J. (2005). Gene-environment interactions in human diseases. *Nat Rev Genet* (2005) Vol. 6 No. 4 pp 287-298

Ioannidis, J.P.A. (2009). Prediction of cardiovascular disease outcomes and established cardiovascular risk factors by genome-wide association markers. *Circ Cardiovasc Genet.* (2009) Vol. 2 pp. 7–15.

Janssens C.,J.,W., & van Duijn C.,M. (2008). Genome-based prediction of common diseases: advances and prospects. *Human Molecular Genetics (2008)* Vol. 17 No. 2 pp.R166-R173

Joint ESC / ACC Committee. (2000). *Eur Heart J 2000* Vol. 21pp.1502-13, *JACC* 2000 Vol. 36 pp.959-69.

Koenig, W., Lowel, H., Baumert, J. et al. (2004). C-reactive protein modulates risk prediction based on the Framingham Score. Implications for future risk assessment: results from a large cohort study in southern Germany. *Circulation* (2004) Vol. 109 pp.1349–53.

Khoury M.,J., Davis R., Gwinn M., Lindegren M.,l., & Yoon P. Do We Need Genomic Research for the Prevention of Common Diseases with Environmental Causes? 2005. *Am. J. Epidemiol.* (1 May 2005) Vol. 161 No. 9 pp 799-805.

Lanktree, M.B. & Hegele, R.A. (2009). Gene-gene and gene-environment interactions: new insights into the prevention, detection and management of coronary artery disease. *Genome Medicine* Vol.1 pp. 28

Mackay, J. & Mensah, G. (2004). *The Atlas of Heart Disease and Stroke,* Word Health Organization, Geneva 27, Switzerland.

Mainous, A.G., Koopman, R.J.,Everett, C.J., Wilson, PW.F. & Tilley,B.C. A. (2007). Coronary Heart Disease Risk Score Based on Patient Reported Information *Am J Cardiol.* (May 1, 2007) Vol. 99 No. 9 pp.1236–1241.

Manolio, T.A., Bailey-Wilson, J.E. & Collins, F.S. (2006). Genes, environment and the value of prospective cohort studies. *Nat Rev Genet (2006)* Vol. 7 pp. 812-820

Marenberg, M.E., Risch, N., Berkman, L.F., Floderus, B., de Faire, U. (1994). Genetic susceptibility to death from coronary heart disease in a study of twins. *N Engl J Med* (1994) vol. 330 pp 1041-6.

McPherson, R.; Pertsemlidis, A.; Kavaslar, N., Stewart, A., Roberts, R., Cox, D.R., Hobbs, H. & Cohen, J.C. (2007). A Common Allele on Chromosome 9 Associated with Coronary Heart Disease. *Science* (2007) Vol. 316 pp.1488-1491

Mendonça, I.; Freitas, A.I., Sousa, A.C., Gomes, S., Faria, P., Drumond, A., Silva, G.,Araújo, J.J., Freitas, S., Ornelas, I., Andrade, G., Coelho, P., Marques, S.,P., Cardoso, A.A., Brehm, A. & Palma dos Reis, R. (2004). O polimorfismo do gene da ECA está associado com a gravidade e extensão da doença coronária. *Rev Port Cardiol* 2004 Vol. 23 pp 1605-1611

Mendonça, I.; Freitas, A.I.; Sousa, A.C.; Gomes, S.; Faria, P.; Drumond, A.; Silva, G.; Araújo, J.J.; Freitas, s.; Ornelas, I.; Andrade, G.; Coelho, P.; Marques, S.P.; Cardoso, A.A.; Brehm, A. & Palma dos Reis, R. (2004). Polimorfismos do gene da ECA e sisco de Doença coronária numa população Portuguesa. *Rev Port Cardiol 2004 Vol.*23 pp.1593-1601

Mendonça, M.I., Palma dos Reis, R., Freitas, A.I., Sousa, A.C., Pereira, A., Faria, P., Gomes, S., Silva, B., Santos, N., Serrão, M., Ornelas I., Freitas, S., Araújo, J.J., Brehm, A., Almada Cardoso, A. (2008). Polimorfismos do Gene da Paraoxonase Humana e Risco de Doença Coronária, *Rev Port Cardiol* 2008 Vol. 27 No. 12 pp. 1539-1555

Mendonça, M.I., Palma dos Reis, R., Freitas, A.I., Sousa, A.C., Pereira, A., Faria, P., Gomes, S., Silva, B., Santos, N., Serrão, M., Ornelas, I., Freitas, S., Araújo, J.J., Brehm, A., Almada Cardoso, A. (2008). A Interacção Gene Gene Afecta o Risco de DC. *Rev Port Cardiol* 2008; 28 No. 4 pp. 397-415

Morrison, A.C., Bare, L.A., Chambless, L.E., Ellis, S.G., Malloy, M., Kane, J.P., Pankow, J.S., Devlin, J., Willerson, J.T. & Boerwinkle, E. (2007). Prediction of Coronary Heart Disease Risk using a Genetic Risk Score: The Atherosclerosis Risk in Communities Study. *Am J Epidemiol* 2007 Vol.166 pp. 28–35

Ng., Sarah., B. et al. Targeted capture and massively parallel sequencing of 12 human *exomes.* (2009) *Nature* Vol.461 pp.272-276

Peng, D.Q., Zhao, S.P., Nie, S. & Li, J. (2003). Gene-gene interaction of PPAR gamma and ApoE affects coronary heart disease risk. *Int J Cardiol* (2003) Vol. 92 No. 2-3 pp 257-63.

Pi-Sunyer, X.F. (1998). NHLBI. Obesity Education Initiative, Expert Panel on the Identification, Evaluation, and Treatment of Overweight and Obesity in Adults. Clinical guidelines on the identification, evaluation and treatment of overweight and obesity, in adults. North American Association for the study of obesity (NAASO).

Pryor D.,B. et al (from Duke University). (1983) Estimating the likelihood of significant coronary artery disease. *Am J Med* 1983 Vol.75 pp.771-80

Pryor D.,B. et al. Estimating the likelihood of severe coronary artery disease. (1991) The *American Journal of Medicine.* 1991 Vol. 90 No.1 pp. 553-562

Report of the Expert Committee on the Diagnosis and Classification of Diabetes Mellitus. *Diabetes Care* 1997 pp. 1183-1197.

Ripatti, S., Tikkanen, E., Orho-Melander, M., Havulinna, A.S., Silandera, K., Sharma, A., Guiducci, C., Perola, M., Jula, A., Sinisalo, J., Lokkif, L-M., Nieminen, M.S., Melander, O., Salomaa, V., Peltonen, L. & Kathiresan, S.A. (2010). Multilocus genetic risk score for coronary heart disease: case-control and prospective cohort analyses. *Lancet*, 23 October, 2010 Vol. 376 No 9750 pp. 1393–1400.

Sesso, H.D., Lee, I.M., Gaziano, J.M., Rexrode, K.M., Glynn, R.J. & Buring, J.E. (2001). Maternal and paternal history of myocardial infarction and risk of cardiovascular disease in men and women. *Circulation* (2001) Vol.104 pp.393–398.

Shiffman, D., Rowland, C.M., Sninsky J.J. & Devlin, JJ. (2006). Popymorphisms associated with coronary heart disease: Better by the score. *Current Opinion in Molecular therapeutics (*2006*) Vol.* 8 No 6 pp. 493-499.

Slack, J. & Evans, K.A. (1966). The increased risk of death from ischaemic heart disease in first degree relatives of 121 men and 96 women with ischaemic heart disease. *J Med Gene (1966)* Vol.3 No. 4 pp. 239-57.

Snowden, C.B., McNamara, P.M., Garrison, R.J., Feinleib, M., Kannel, W.B. & Epstein, F.H. (1982). Predicting coronary heart disease in siblings—a multivariate assessment: the Framingham Heart Study. *Am J Epidemiol (1982) Vol.* 115 pp. 217–22.

Sox H.,C., Jr, Hickam D.,H., Marton K.,I., Moses L., Skeff K.,M., Sox C.,H., Neal E.,A. Using the patient's history to estimate the probability of coronary artery disease: a comparison of primary care and referral practices. (1990) Am J Med. 1990 Vol.89 No.1 pp.7-14

Stephens, J.W. & Humphries, S.E. (2003). The molecular genetics of cardiovascular disease: clinical implications. *Journal of Internal Medicine (*2003) *Vol.*253 pp 120–127

Talmud, PJ. (2007). Gene-environment interaction and its impact on coronary heart disease risk. *Nutr Metab Cardiovasc Dis.* (Feb 2007) Vol.17 No. 2 pp.148-52

Van der Net J.B., Janssens C.J.W., Sijbrands E. J.G. & Steyerberg, E.W. (2009). Value of genetic profiling for the prediction of coronary heart disease *.Am Heart J* 2009 Vol. 158 pp.105-10.

Veja, G.L. *(2002).* Cardiovascular Outcomes for Obesity and Metabolic Syndrome. *Obesity Research*; Vol. 10 pp 27S–32S; doi: 10.1038/oby.2002.186

Watkins H. & Farrall M. (2006). Genetic susceptibility to coronary artery disease: from promise to progress. *Nature Reviews Genetics (March* 2006*) Vol.* 7 pp 163-173

Wilson, P.W.F., D'Agostino, R., Levy, D., Belanger, A.M., Silbershatz, H. & Kannel, W.B. (1998). Prediction of Coronary Heart Disease Using Risk Factor Categories. *Circulation (1998) Vol.* 97 pp 1837-1847.

Zdravkovic, S., Wienke, A., Pedersen, N. L., Marenberg, M. E., Yashin, A. I., & de Faire, U. (2002). Heritability of death from coronary heart disease: A 36-year follow-up of 20 966 Swedish twins. *Journal of Internal Medicine.* (2002) Vol. 252 pp 247–254.

Part 2

Coronary Artery Disease: Diagnostic Features

3

Magnetocardiography in Unshielded Setting: Heart Electrical Image Based on 2-D and 3-D Data in Comparison with Perfusion Image Based on PET Results – Clinical Cases

Illya Chaikovsky[1], Michael Primin[2],
Igor Nedayvoda[2] and Mykola Budnyk[2]
[1]*International Research and Training Centre for Informational Technologies and Systems of NAS of Ukraine,*
[2]*Institute for Cybernetics of NAS of Ukraine,*
Ukraine

1. Introduction

Worldwide, coronary artery disease (CAD) is becoming pandemic (Omran, 1979). Mortality from CAD is predicted to reach 23.4 million in 2030. Now days, chronic CAD s estimated to affect 16.8 million people in the United States; and 2.65 million people in the UK. CAD was the single most frequent cause of death in USA and Western Europe (about 1 in every 5 deaths).The estimated direct and indirect economic cost of CAD in the United States for 2009 is $165.4 billion. Moreover, in the developing world, particularly in Ukraine, prevalence of CAD is even higher and there is the tendency tends to affect people at a younger age and thus could negatively affect the workforce and economic productivity. The morbidity, mortality, and socioeconomic importance of CAD make its diagnosis and management fundamental for all practicing physicians (Cassar et al., 2009).

Non-invasive, rapid and reliable diagnosis of coronary artery disease (CAD) and patients with chest pain remains a clinical challenge.

Methods of detecting the presence and assessing the extent of CAD have become increasingly important in informing therapies aimed at reducing mortality and morbidity. Coronary angiography (CA) is considered to be the 'gold standard' for defining the site and severity of coronary artery lesions. However, routine use of CA without prior non-invasive testing is not advisable, except in those with a high pre-test probability of significant disease, partly due to the high cost, but also because of the associated morbidity and mortality. The most serious complications of CA are death (0.1–0.2%), non-fatal MI (0.1%) and cerebrovascular accidents (0.1%).

Functional (non-invasive) testing is used as a gateway to angiography for management of coronary artery disease. Among those the most important are the following methods: stress (usually treadmill or bicycle exercise) electrocardiography, Stress-Echo, MRI myocardial perfusion, nuclear perfusion.

All existing methods have certain merits and disadvantages. Stress–ECG is widely used for non-invasive detection of CAD owing to its availability and low cost. However, a normal EET does not exclude CAD and EET is a poor diagnostic test in low-risk populations (such as women) owing to its low positive predictive value in a population with a low prevalence of the disease. Deaths occur rarely, in <0.05% of tests. Echo is one of the most frequently used tools for the investigation of a wide range of cardiological problems. The portability and relative affordability of the equipment have led to a very rapid acceptance of the technique by the general medical community. The sensitivity, specificity and accuracy of stress-echo is in the range 80–85% with the highest sensitivity (>90%) for three-vessel disease and the lowest (75%) for single-vessel disease. There are limitations inherent to the stress echo technique. Chief among these is the problem of reliably obtaining good images and reproducible tomographic slices as the heart rate goes up with increasing rate of dobutamine infusion. Furthermore, there may be significant inter-observer variability in image interpretation due to the subjective nature of wall motion assessment.

MRI is a relatively new tool for the examination of the heart compared with the other non-invasive modalities and clinical value of this method is still doubtful.

Nuclear perfusion has an extensive pedigree extending back over a quarter of a century, with hundreds of thousands of scans performed worldwide each year. Recent guidelines have suggested that the technique could be even more widely employed in the future (Sharples et al, 2007). Positron emission tomography (PET) is probably the most sensitive method to analyze myocardial perfusion and to detect myocardial ischemia. It is actually regarded the non-invasive "gold standard". Major disadvantages of PET-technique are high expenses, attenuation artifacts, use of ionising radiation, radiation and availability in specialist centers only.

Thus there is a need for low-cost, accurate, noninvasive diagnostic tools, more convenient and less complicated for both the diagnostics and screening of coronary artery disease. Magnetocardiography (MCG) is known as a completely non-invasive and risk- free method of measuring cardiac activity. Recent studies has shown significant potential of MCG in diagnosis of myocardial ischemia, although analysis of MCG-generated data is not standardized yet (Hailer et al, 2005; Kwon et al, 2010; Chaikovsky et al, 2011).

MCG technology closely related to modern methods of data processing. There is a variety of methods and indicators for medical analysis available in the current stage of MCG development. MCG analysis can be expressed at several levels of increasing complexity of MCG signal transformation (Chaikovsky et al, 2007).

- Level 1. The first level of analysis is similar to routine morphological analysis of the 12–lead ECG.
- Level 2. Spectrotemporal analysis. The relative power of a cardiac signal for various frequency bands and their spectral variability and time-domain analysis (such as QRS duration) of the MCG can be provided at specific measurement points.
- Level 3. 36 measurement points of the MCG-7 are summarized in an averaged curve. Such an approach provides a more generalized representation of myocardial excitation. For exam-ple, the areas under the P-wave or the QRS-complex reflect overall "electrical energy" generated due to excitation of atria and ventricles.

- Level 4. Magnetic field mapping. This requires the construction of maps showing the distribution of the magnetic field obtained at specific measurement points and precise moments of the cardiac cycle. These maps are constructed along the principles of geographical or meteorological maps. Areas with identical value of given parameter are color filled. There are variety of quantitative and semi-quantitative indicators to estimate such maps.
- Level 5. The representation of all electrical sources as one equivalent dipole. Here it is assumed that all electrical activity of the heart originates from one point.

The **sixth,** highest level of MCG software development are based on an inverse problem solution. This approach allow 2D reconstruction of distributed electrical cardiac sources and first steps have been made for 3-D reconstruction. This promising technical progress allow to utilize magnetocardiography routinely in the next future, e.g. in patients with "normal" or uncertain results of standard testing , especially in patients with high or intermediate pre-test probability of CAD.

This study intended to compare MCG-images of "difficult-to-diagnose" patients with normal left ventricular function and clinical suspicion of ischemic heart disease with perfusion images obtained by the PET-technique.

2. Method

The study includes 3 patients (2 female, 1 male, mean age 58 years) and one healthy volunteer (male, 47 year). All patients underwent resting and stress ECG, echocardiography, PET and coronaroangiography. The healthy volunteer had no history of any cardiovascular disease, normal ECG at rest and stress as well as a normal echocardiogram.

Coronary angiograms were documented in multiple projections according to standard clinical practice (Judkins-technique). *PET* was performed with adenosine to recruite coronary reserve. Resting and stress recordings were made using N-13-ammonium as tracer. MCG was performed in an unshielded setting using a 7-channel SQUID-magnetometer. Single MCG recordings were taken from 36 positions within a 20 by 20 cm rectangular grid with a 4 cm pitch over the precordial area. The sensor was positioned as close to the chest as possible, directly over the heart using the jugulum as landmark. The examination table with the patient resting in constant the same position was then moved systematically to each of the 36 predetermined positions under the SQUID detector. Data were recorded at each registration point for 30 seconds with simultaneous registration of lead II of the surface ECG and stored on hard disk for further evaluation. The analysis was based on the "inverse problem solution", i.e reconstruction of the intracardiac sources that originated the magnetic field measured.

3. Inverse problem solution

3.1 Description of the problem and definition

The "inverse problem solution" is based on the following physical considerations. Magnetocardiographic measurements are made with a sensor moving over a planar grid above the body surface. The distance from this planar grid to a signal source inside the heart differs from patient to patient. As the magnetic field parameters vary with the source-to-plane distance in a nonlinear way, magnetic field maps generated may also vary significantly in one and the same patient. To the technical set up with the analysis of the biomagnetic field source distribution, directly corresponding with the field registered, this problem can be overcome. Therefore magnetocardiographic information transformation should led to the inverse problem solution.

The full definition of inverse solution is following : inverse task solution in electrodynamics (magnetostatics) implies finding of special magnetic sources distribution from the known (registered) magnetic field parameters.

3.2 Steps of solution

Inverse problems may could be solved in different ways, using simple or more complex models of biomagnetic sources. There are the following steps in modeling and representation of bioelectrical sources in the heart.

3.2.1 Localization of the dipole magnetic field source (Primin & Nedayvoda, 1997)

We use a model of the magnetic dipole as the source of biomagnetic signal in contrast to common approaches using the electric dipole as a source. Based on this approach the more precise analytical solution of the inverse task could be obtained. The background for the analytical solution is to use the properties of the spatial derivatives of the magnetic induction vector $\boldsymbol{B}$ matrix in a homogeneous nonmagnetic and nonconductive medium (in points of measurements div$\boldsymbol{B}$=0, curl$\boldsymbol{B}$=0). In this case, matrices of the first (D_1) and second (D_{2i}, $i=x,y,z$) spatial derivatives of the $\boldsymbol{B}$ vector are symmetrical and possess several properties providing analytical solution of the inverse task to be fulfilled first in a new (own) and afterwards by reverse transition in a set-point coordinate systems. It is important that independent solutions can be obtained for every point in a plane of measurement. As a result "effective " dipole (i.e dipole which creates the magnetic field with parameters corresponding with high degree of accuracy to those of the field registered in the plane of measurement) could be localized. It means that three coordinates r_z, rx , ry and magnetic moment of these dipoles could be determined.

3.2.2 Reconstruction of currents distribution in the layer

(Gumenyuk-Sychevskii et al, 1993). Distribution of the current density vectors has been defined using double integral Fourier transform for the plane arranged at a distance equal to r_z coordinate of the "effective" source and parallel to the thorax and to the plane of measurements.

3.2.3 Reconstruction of 3-D magnetic dipole density (Primin & Nedayvoda, 2009)

Method is based on analytical method of inverse solution. Source of biomagnetic signal can be represented in the form of N elementary magnetic dipoles. Algorithm allows to make a solution on the determination of coordinates and magnetic moment vector for every dipole, homogenization of the source and finally representation of the "effective" biomagnetic signal source as a 3-D "clouds" of magnetic dipole density. That is way the most suitable model for solving of inverse problem in this class of patients is a system of currents, distributed in the plane or (what is the best) in the volume.

3.2.4 Tomographical (layer-to-layer) reconstruction (Primin et al, 2003; Primin et al, 2010)

Knowing density, coordinates and magnetic moments of all elementary magnetic dipoles currents distribution as a current density vectors maps could be obtained for any r_z coordinate i.e for any distance (layer) from the measurement plane. The layer with the highest current density values corresponds to the layer possessing maximum number of elementary sources. The specificity of our approach is that every further , more advanced step of inverse solution based on the results of the preceding step which allows us to approach reliable 3-D solution. The results of current distribution in the layer, reconstruction of 3-D magnetic dipole density and layer-to-layer reconstruction were used for further medical analysis. From all patients 32 CDV maps were generated on equal distance within the ST-T interval starting with the J-point.

3.2.5 Reconstruction of 3-D image of electrical activity in the heart

This reconstruction have been done for single time moment in the middle of ST-T interval. Two approaches for 3-D data representation have been used. One of them represents reconstruction of the 2-D CDV maps on the different distance from the probe, in other words this reconstruction of electrical activity on layers (methodologically similar to tomographical approach in other imaging methods). Other approach represents a 3-D distribution of magnetic dipoles density. "Cloud" of these dipoles represent the exited zones of myocardium

4. Results

Healthy volunteer	male, 47 years
Complaints	none
Resting ECG	normal
Echo	normal
Magnetocardiography	The 2-D CDV maps within ST-T interval show a highly homogeneous distribution of currents with only one main current area in each map. Main current density vectors are located at the center part of the maps and are directed left-to-downwards (Fig. 1a). The maps remain stabile over the ST-T interval. " Tomographical " representation is shown on Figure 1b. Homogeneous current distribution with similar structure of maps at each layer could be seen. The layer with maximal density is located on the middle distance from the measurements plane. "Cloud" of magnetic dipole density (Figure 1c) is very compact, spherical and located on the center of the cube of sources reconstruction

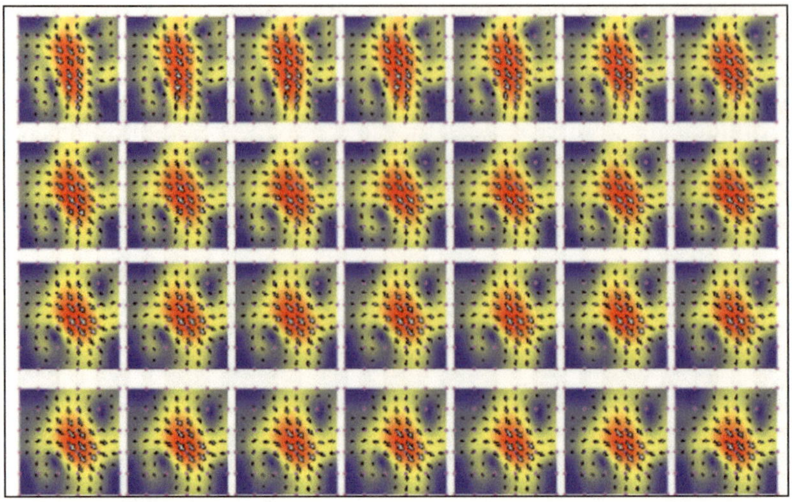

Fig. 1a. Example of reconstruction of several current density vector maps in the course of the ST-T interval of volunteer M.O.

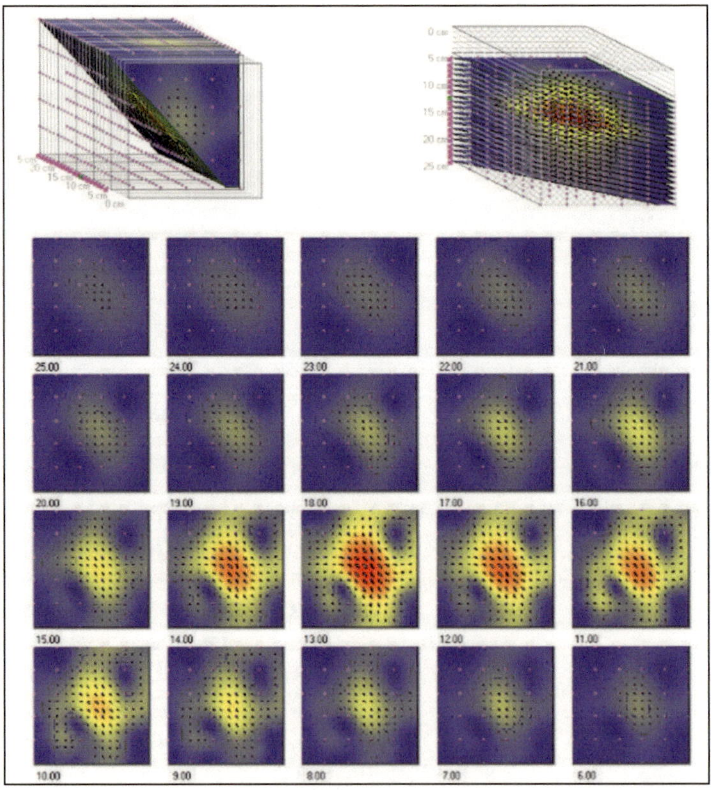

Fig. 1b. 3D current reconstruction at the middle of ST-T interval of volunteer M.O. Upper row: axonometric projection of cube of current reconstruction - frontal view (left) and sagittal view (right), Low rows : Current density vectors maps on different distance from plane of measurement (from 6 to 25 cm).

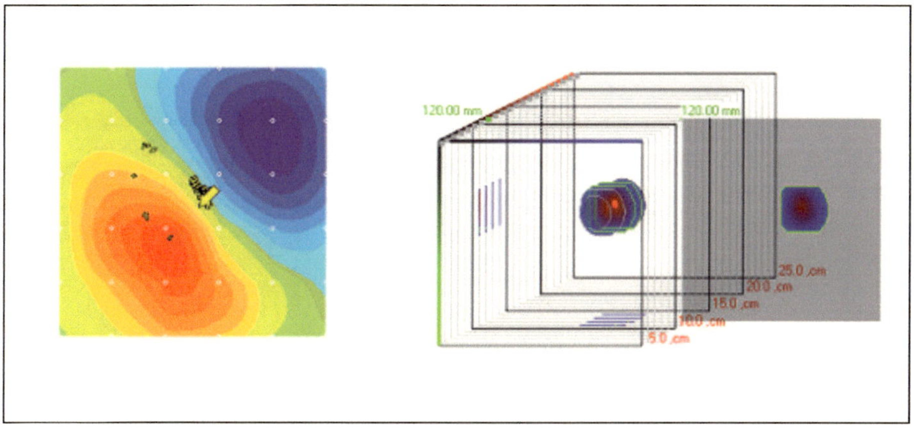

Fig. 1c. 3-D dipoles density reconstruction at the middle of ST-T interval of volunteer M.O. Axonometric projection of cube of current reconstruction with "cloud" of dipoles density. Layer with maximal density is marked.

Patient J	male, 72 years
Complaints	Typical chest pain
Resting ECG	unchanged
Echo	mild LV hypertrophy, otherwise - normal echocardiogramm
Coronaroangiography	1-vesel disease, stenosis (75 %) of proximal-to-mild LAD.
LV-angio	mild LV hypertrophy, otherwise - normal result
PET	reduced myocardial perfusion in the all walls in particular in septoapical area
Magnetocardiography	2-D CDV maps within ST-T interval are presented in Figure 2a. Maps are not homogenious, absence of dipole structure are seen within the hole ST-T interval. "Tomographical" representation (Figure 2b) clearly shows two area of activity: one of them is located on the anterior part of the cube of reconstraction with maximal intensity on the layer of 12cm, another is shifted left- backwards with maximal activity on 18 cm. "Cloud" of magnetic dipoles (Figure 2c) generally shifted downwards and also clearly divided on two areas

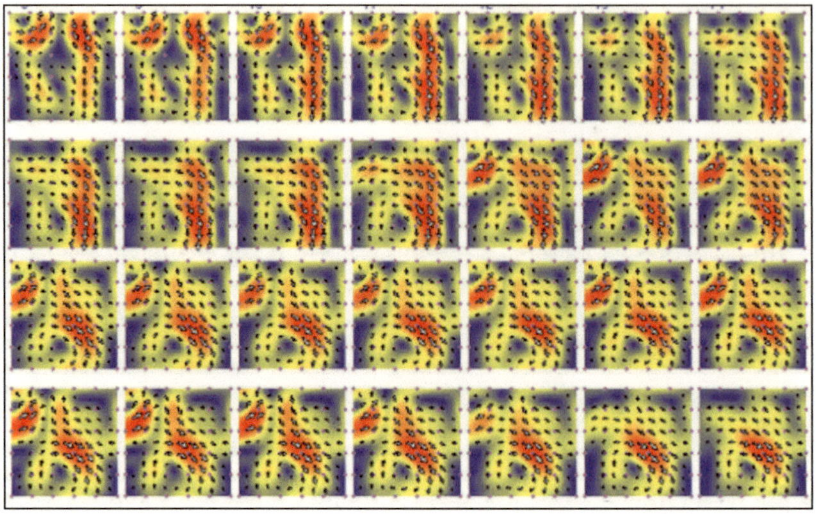

Fig. 2a. Example of reconstruction of several current density vector maps in the course of the ST-T interval of patient J.

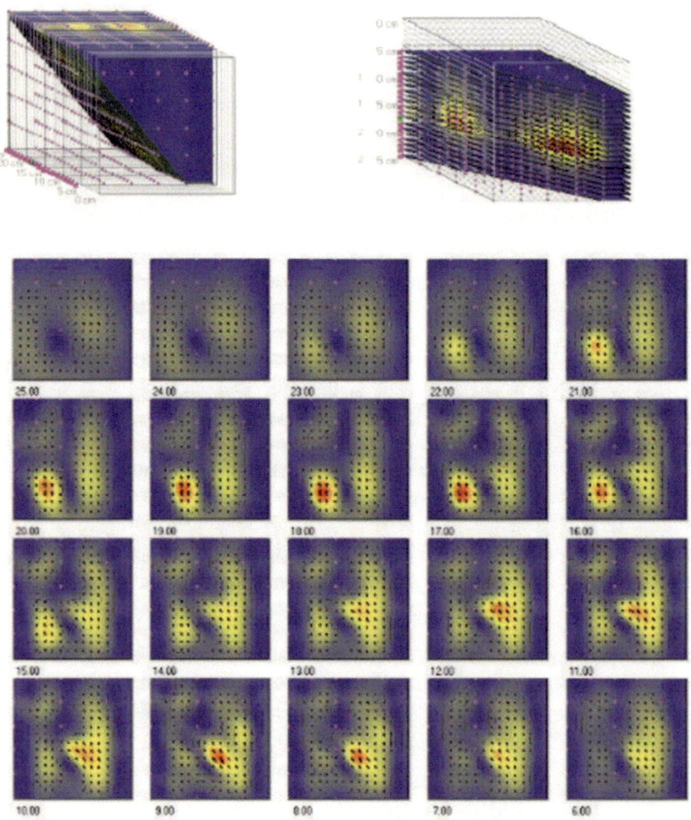

Fig. 2b. 3D current reconstruction at the middle of ST-T interval of patient J.

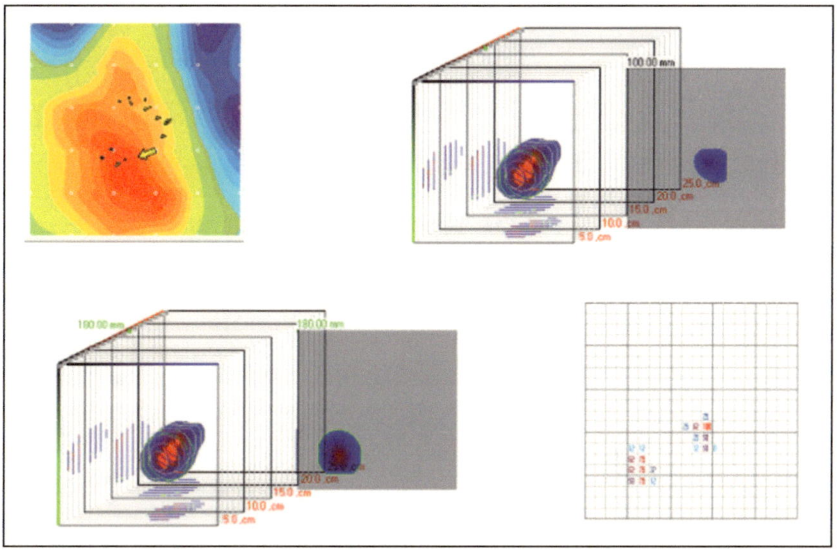

Fig. 2c. 3D dipoles density reconstruction at the middle of ST-T interval of patient J. Axonometric projection of cube of current reconstruction with "cloud" of dipoles density. Layers with maximal density of upper currents area (right) and lower currents area are marked.

Patient L.	male, 74 years
Complaints	Atypical chest pain
Resting ECG	unchanged
Ergometry	125 WT, end point criteria - targeting heart rate achieved
Echo	marginal local contractility disturbances in the anterior wall, otherwise - normal echocardiogram
Coronaroangiography	1-vesel disease, stenosis (50 %) of proximal-to -mild LAD.
LV-angio	marginal local contractility disturbances in the anteriolateral wall and septoapical area
PET	reduced myocardial perfusion in the apical, septoapical and suproapical areas
Magnetocardiography	2-D CDV maps within ST-T interval are presented in Figure 3a. Maps are not homogein, non-dipole especially at the beginning and at the and of ST-T interval, there are additional current areas at the upper and lower part of maps. "Tomographical" representation (Figure 3b) clearly shows two area of activity which are located approximately on one depth - 11-12 cm. "Cloud " of magnetic dipoles (Figure 3c) like in previous case generally shifted downwards and also clearly divided on two areas, one of them is shifted rather up backwards

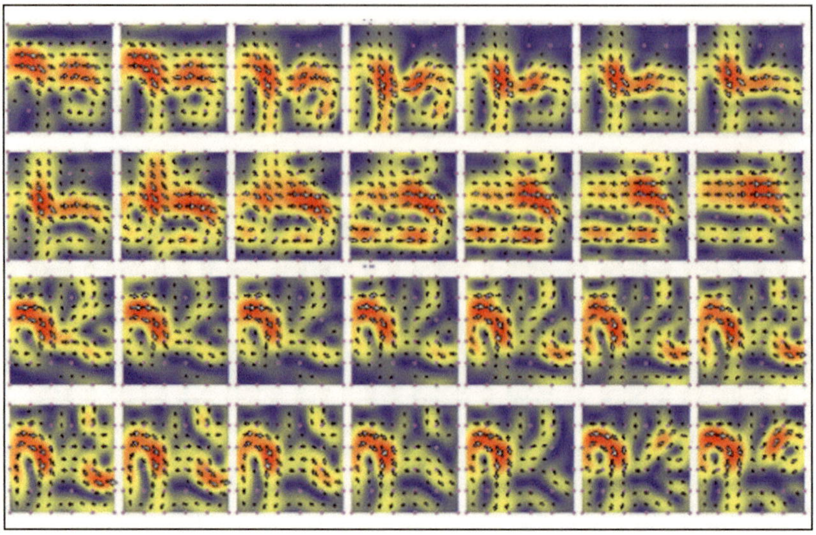

Fig. 3a. Example of reconstruction of several current density vector maps in the course of the ST-T interval of patient L.

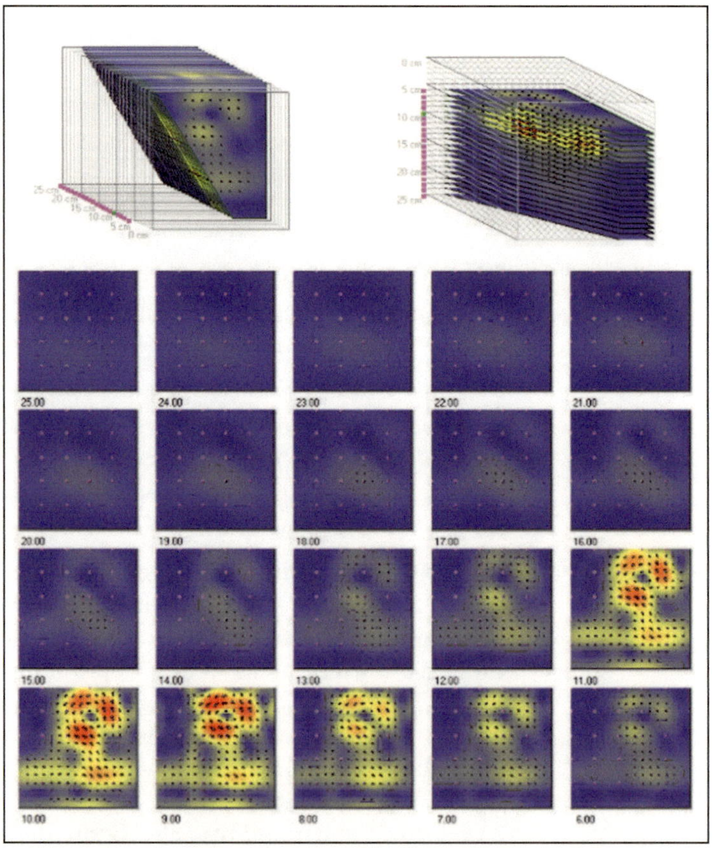

Fig. 3b. 3D current reconstruction at the middle of ST-T interval of patient L.

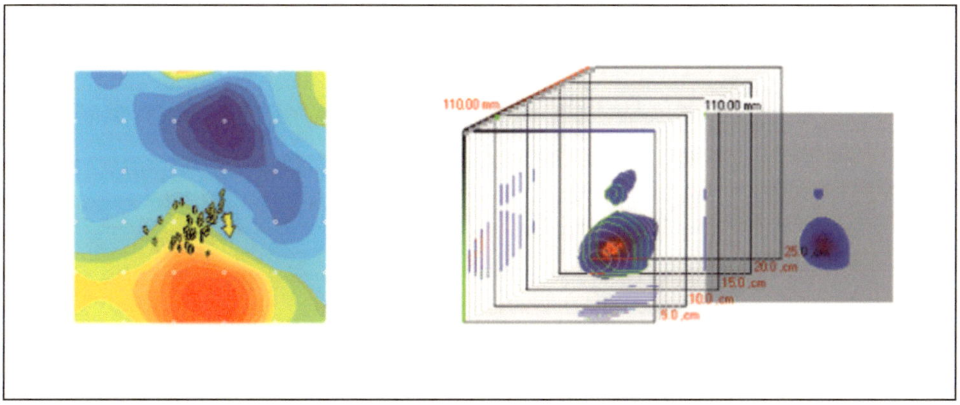

Fig. 3c. 3-D dipoles density reconstruction at the middle of ST-T interval of patient L. Axonometric projection of cube of current reconstruction with "cloud" of dipoles density. Layer with maximal density is marked.

Patient T	female, 42 years
Complaints	Atypical chest pain
Resting ECG	absolute arrhythmia due to atrial fibrillation, otherwise-unchanged ECG
Ergometry	125 WT, end point criteria – targeting heart rate achieved
Echo	normal echocardiogram
Coronaroangiography	Coronarosclerosis, macroangiopathy formally excluded.
LV-angio	Marginal hypokinesia of apical are, otherwise - normal results.
PET	Small local reducing of myocardial perfusion in the inferioapical area
Magnetocardiography	2-D CDV maps within ST-T interval are presented in Figure 4a. Maps are not homogein, absence of dipole structure are seen within the hole ST-T interval. "Tomographical" representation (Figure 4b) shows one but non-compact, distributed are of activity with fuzzy contours. "Cloud" of magnetic dipoles (Figure 4c) located approximately on the central part of the cube of source reconstruction but also non-compact and non-spherical

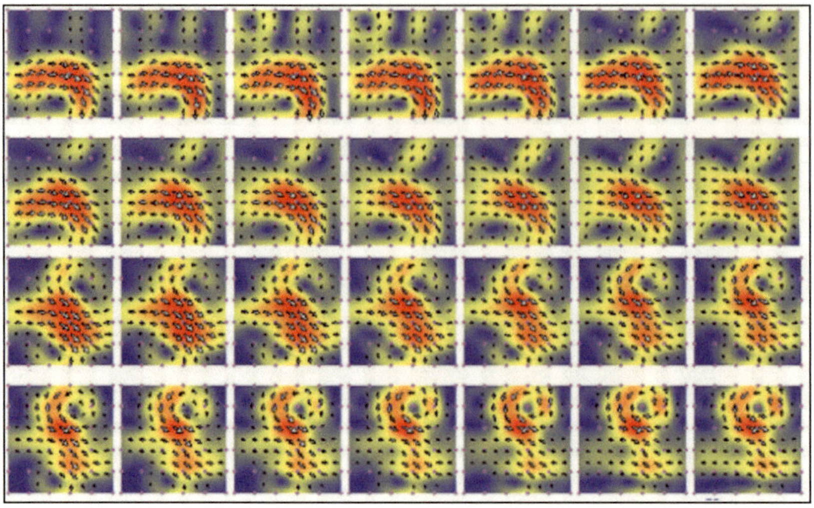

Fig. 4a. Example of reconstruction of several current density vector maps in the course of the ST-T interval of patient T.

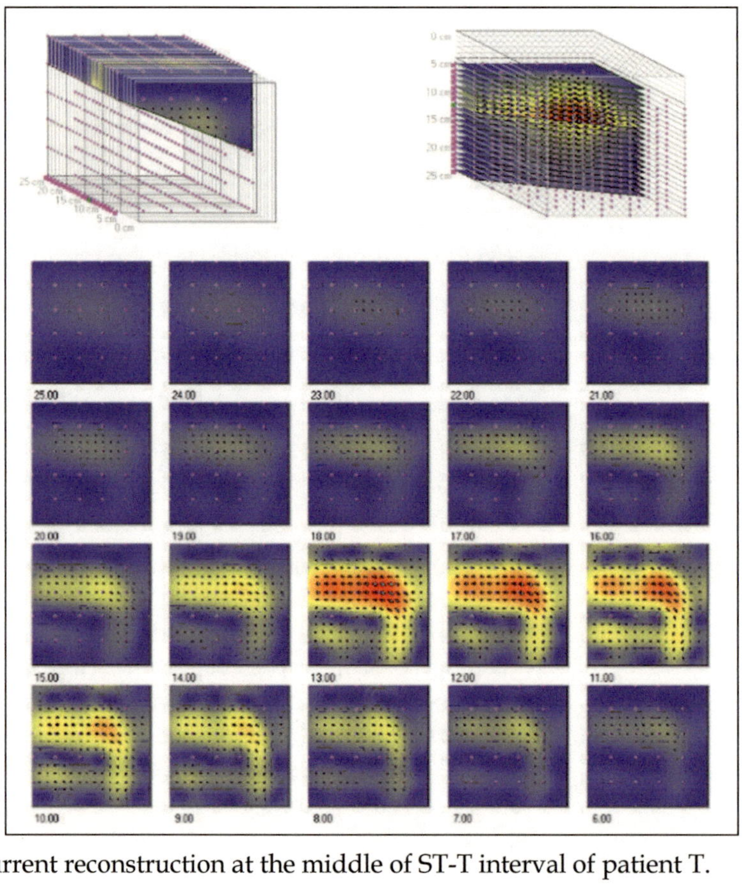

Fig. 4b. 3D current reconstruction at the middle of ST-T interval of patient T.

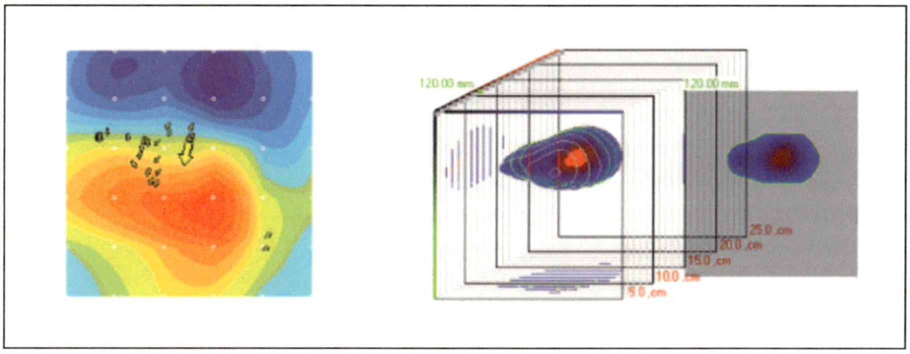

Fig. 4c. 3-D dipoles density reconstruction at the middle of ST-T interval of patient T.

Axonometric projection of cube of current reconstruction with "cloud" of dipoles density. Layer with maximal density is marked.

5. Discussion

Methods of MCG-data analysis based on inverse solution are able to give the most valuable information. However some methodological aspects should be taken into consideration for optimal using of this approach.

It is well known that the inverse solution in classical setting up has no unambiguous solution. The task is simplified and can acquire the uniqueness with definition of the "functional relationships" between magnetic field measured and sources reconstructed. In other words, definition of the field source models (point dipole, current layer distributed in a plane, current distributed in a volume) determines the relationships between field sources and magnetic field values and distribution in the plane of measurement.

It is rather complex to choose the field source model. This choice of the source model is determined on the one hand by the excitation area dimensions, distance from the sensor (registration point), diameter of the magnetic flux transformation coil and on the other hand by physiological characteristic of the process under investigation. In other words to substantiate the model of the biomagnetic signal source, the volume of the active heart tissue where the source is distributed should be considered in relationship with field parameters registered in points of the plane of measurements. For instant „ point dipole" model is correct in the cases of small, focal sources in a heart muscle stipulated by excitation of the Gis-Purkinje conducting system and arrhythmogenic focuses. In contrast, perfusion insufficiency, first of all because of CAD, is resulting in electrophysiological changes of more extended zones of myocardium. Therefore the most suitable model for solving of inverse problem in this class of patients is a system of currents, distributed in the plane or, what is the best, in the volume.

This is especially true when ventricular repolarisation period is analysed. Repolarisation is a diffuse process i.e. large zones of the whole myocardium are excited simultaneously in the case of normal ventricular myocardium. Pathological processes will led to the asynchronisation of the repolarisation process in the normal and affected zones of myocardium. In other words we could say that different zones of myocardium are in the different electrical stage due to the difference in the conduction velocity.

That is why the concept of clinical analysis of electrical images obtained is based on of homogeneity, "electromagnetic symmetry" evaluation. Highly homogeneous type of electrical currents within the whole ST-T interval in 2-d mode and at the middle of ST-T interval in the 3-D mode we could see in the healthy volunteer maps. In the framework of our concept we could assume that this maps reflect absence of myocardial zones with different electrical properties. The most non–homogeneous structure of current maps we could see in patient J. This is especially clear when 3-D image is analysed - two zones of activity located on two different levels of cube of reconstruction - more upwards and more downwards. This patient shown the most pronounced coronary stenosis and the most severe perfusion insufficiency by PET.

The maps of patient L. also not homogeneous especially at the beginning of ventricular repolarisation. 3-D image also shows two zones, both located on one level - a little bit upwards. Perfusion insufficiency was found in the apical and suproapical areas.

2-d maps and 3-d reconstruction of patient T could be settled on the intermediate position between maps of healthy volunteers and maps of patients with CAD in the sense of inhomogeneity of electrical images. At the same time only minor perfusion insufficiency (probably due to microangiopathy) in the apical was found. From pathophysiological point of view this inhomogeneity could be explained by the the presence of myocardial ischemia at rest. Indeed the absence of ischemia under resting conditions is generally accepted to be the explanation for a normal ECG at rest in CAD patients. Keeping in mind that ischemia is a dynamic process with an important temporal continuum starting with changes on molecular basis followed by some unspecific changes in the 12 lead standard ECG progressing, leading to wall motion disturbances, and angina as a last step, it could be possible that this new method is able to detect signs of ischemia in a very early phase of such a dynamic process.

Perfusion insufficiency proved based on PET results confirms presence of myocardial ischemia regardless to normal results of ECG and other routine tests. In what way insufficiently perused myocardial zones could represent themselves on 3-d current images. Generally two variants could be supposed : In the case of affected but viable myocardium areas of additional pathological electrical activity could overlap these zones or be located near by, representing so-called " currents of injury". In the case of non-viable myocardium, loosing electrical properties completely, electrical "defect" could be seen on 3-d electrical images.

To find a correlation between 3-d electrical images these areas and myocardial segments in pathological conditions (different stage of perfusion insufficiency, hibernation stunning and so on) will be the main subject of further studies. It is also important from methodological point of view to present digital information in "absolute terms" like it is achieved already in other diagnostic methods. "Absolute terms " for magnetocardiography, analyzing homogeneity of electrical properties of myocardium, is dispersion of conduction velocity within certain physiological periods of cardio cycle, first of all within ventricular repolarization.

In the near future such software, directly representing zones of hypo-, hyper- and normal conduction as well as diagnostic indicators might be developed to show a complete 3-D electrical image of the heart. The fact that CAD patients, presumably with ischemia but with a normal results of the routine tests, might be identified on the basis of a completely noninvasive method is of great clinical interest.

The original results of earlier studies with a multichannel MCG system inside a shielded setting, were always limited by the expensive costs of the system itself and by the lack of patient e.g. c.q. physician acceptance. The present data show the results of a much less expensive system not requiring a shielded room. A further confirmation of these results in a greater population would be an important step towards the aim to restrict invasive procedures like coronary angiography to those patients in whom the diagnosis of CAD is confirmed prior to the procedure and in whom interventional therapy appears to be indicated.

A main limitation of this study is small number of cases analyzed. Then, the analysis of 3-D magnetocardiographic images is rather subjective. As long as the score system depends to some degree on the experience of the observers, with the need for a training procedure, the implementation of an automatic process following the described criteria should improve this aspect.

Conclusion: presented cases shows a certain clinical potential of joint analysis of heart electrical images based on MCG and perfusion images based on PET. Further investigation will be done to make this diagnostical approach useful in a clinical routine.

6. Acknowledgements

This work was partly supported by the State Agency on science, innovation and informatization of Ukraine (project DZ/466-2011).

7. References

Cassar A, Holmes DR,Jr, Rihal CS, Gersh BJ. Chronic coronary artery disease: diagnosis and management. Mayo Clin Proc. 2009;84(12):1130-1146.

Chaikovsky I., Primin N., Hugenholtz P., Nedayvoda I., Horstkotte D., Berndt C., Korfer J., Hailer B., Budnyk M. Approaches and methods for the clinical interpretation of the magnetocardiogram // USIM, 2006:2: 33-43.

Chaikovsky I., Boychak M., Sosnytskyy V., Mjasnikov G., Sosnytskaja T., Ryschlik K., Frolov Yu., Budnyk V. Magnetocardiography in unshielded location : technologies of data analysis. Likarska sprava, 2011;3-4:54-64 (in Russian).

Gumenyuk-Sychevskii Vitalij I., Primin Michael A., Nedayvoda Igor V. Mathematical model and data processing algorithms for spatial analysis of weak magnetic fields. Engineering Simulation. 1993; Vol.11, 1 : 140-150.

Hailer B., Chaikovsky I., Van Leeuven P, Auth-Eisernitz S.. The value of MCG in pts with and without relevant stenoses of the coronary arteries using an unshielded system. PACE, 2005; 28:8-16.

Omran AR. Changing patterns of health and disease during the process of national development. In: Albrecht GL, Higgins PC, eds. Health, Illness and Medicine: A Reader in Medical Sociology. Chicago, IL: Rand McNally; 1979.

Kwon H, Kim K, Lee YH, Kim JM, Yu KK, Chung N, Ko YG. Non-invasive magnetocardiography for the early diagnosis of coronary artery disease in patients presenting with acute chest pain. Circ J. 2010 Jul;74(7):1424-30.

Primin Michael A., Nedayvoda Igor V., A mathematical model and measurement algorithms for a dipole source location. Int.J. of Applied Electromagnetics and Mechanics. 1997; vol. 8: 119 – 131.

Primin Michael, Chaikovsky Illya, Berndt Caroline, Nedayvoda Igor, Korfer Jan, Layer-to-layer heart electrical image based on magnetocardiography data in comparison with perfusion image based on PET, Int.J.of Biolectromagnetism. 2003;Vol. 5, 1 :27-28

Primin Michael A., Nedayvoda Igor V., Inverse problem solution algorithms in magnetocardiography: new analytical approach and some results. International Journal of Applied Electromagnetics and Mechanics. 2009; vol. 29, 2 :65-81.

Primin Michael A., Nedayvoda Igor V., Masslennikov Yuri V., Gulyaev Yuri V., Software for the magnetocardiographic complex for the early diagnostics and monitoring of heart deseases, Journal of Comunications Technology and Electronics.2010; vol. 55, 10: 1250-1269

Sharples L., Hughes., Crean A., Dyer M., Buxton M., Goldsmith K, Stone D. Cost-effectiveness of functional cardiac testing in the diagnosis and management of coronary artery disease: a randomised controlled trial. The CECaT trial. Health Technology Assessment 2007; Vol. 11: No. 49 :1-86.

4

Quantitative Functional Assessment of Ischemic Patients by Cardiopulmonary Exercise and Recovery Indices

Eliezer Klainman, Alex Yarmolovsky and Gershon Fink
Exercise Physiology Unit, Pulmonary Institute, Kaplan MC, Rehovot & "Gefen"- Cardiac Health Center, Givatayim
Israel

1. Introduction

Exercise stress testing is commonly used for assessing the presence and severity of coronary ischemia including heart rate (HR) and blood pressure (BP) responses as well as exertional symptoms estimation (Vivekananthan et al., 2000). Cardiopulmonary exercise test (CPET) indices, obtained by direct measurement of exercise respiratory gas exchange, may provide additional important clinical information for further and more quantitative evaluation of the ischemic response. Among these indices are the ventilatory anaerobic threshold (VAT), oxygen consumption (VO_2) and the oxygen pulse (O_2-P) measured during exercise. These indices mainly reflect cardiac problems (Milani et al., 1995, 2006). However, recovery cardiopulmonary indices have been found to be an important tool for assessing the overall exercise capacity in patients with chronic heart failure (CHF). These indices differ significantly from healthy subjects. The kinetics of post exercise VO_2 has been demonstrated to be delayed in relation to the severity of the disease and to be closely related to exercise capacity (Koike et al., 1998). Patients with severe CHF or dilated cardiomyopathy, demonstrated a prolonged recovery period to the baseline levels of VO_2 (Pavia et al., 1999; De Groot et al., 1999). Similar results were found in patients with mitral stenosis (Lim et al., 1998). This chapter is based on our five studies, and concerns a quantitative functional assessment of ischemic response in patients with documented coronary artery disease (CAD). The ischemic response was tested using various classic and novel cardiopulmonary indices. The first study demonstrates four O_2-P curve variables, achieved during exercise, which correlate well with different degrees of ischemic response. In the second study, the functional results following percutaneous transluminal coronary angioplasty (PTCA) were assessed in chronic CAD patients. In the third study there is a similar assessment of the effect of controlled exercise training in chronic CAD patients. In the fourth study the means by which ischemia can be improved, as a result of regular exercise training is explained. The most recent study deals with recovery indices of VO_2 kinetics and their contribution to quantitatively assessing varying degrees of CAD.

2. Assessment of the relationship between ischemic response by exercise multigated radionuclide test and the O2-P curve characteristics of the CPET

Four defined variable O_2-P curves were observed during CPET in different degrees of ischemic response in order to compare them with left ventricular ejection fraction (LVEF) [rest] - [exercise] response, as measured by multigated equilibrium 99mTc radionuclide cineangiography (MUGA) in ischemic patients. The hypothesis here was based on the direct relationship between the O_2-P and the stroke volume (SV) according to the Fick formula:

$$VO_2 = CO \times (a\text{-}v)\ O_2\ \text{content} \rightarrow O_2\text{-}P = SV \times (a\text{-}v)\ O_2\ \text{content}$$

$$\text{As } VO_2/HR = O_2\text{-}P;\ \text{and } CO/HR = SV$$

The O_2-P response during exercise, represented by its curve, is expected to increase till its peak in healthy subjects. In patients with varying degrees of CAD, different quantitative ischemic responses may variate the curve shape accordingly. In the case of left ventricular (LV) dysfunction, a flat curve response is expected.

2.1 Methods

46 patients, 39 men and 7 women, mean age 59.2+/-11 years, with no hypertrophic, valvular or pericardial disease participated in this study. MUGA exercise tests were performed in all patients and followed by a CPET within 2-3 weeks under the same medical regimen while stopping medications like beta-blockers, calcium channel blockers or nitrates 24 hours prior to all tests.

2.1.1 MUGA test

Muga was performed to determine LV ejection fraction (EF) at rest and at peak exercise, using a supine bicycle ergometer with increments of 25W every 2 min. Patients were asked to continue until the predefined endpoint such as appearance of symptoms, volitional fatigue, significant ST changes on ECG or attainment of target HR. 10 mg of stannous pyrophosphate was injected prior to the study, followed 15 min later by 20-25 mCi of 99mTc. Data were recorded with a small-field-of-view scintillation camera and a digital processor. The camera was interfaced to an inter-technique cine data system (Apex-SP409; Elcint, Haifa, Israel). The detector was located at 45 degrees left anterior oblique projection. The cardiac cycle was divided into 24 frames yielding an average time per frame of 20-30 mins. Calibration was set to 4,000 kilo-counts for rest and exercise for all frames. 2,000 kilo-counts were used at exercise. After rest, the study was repeated during supine exercise until peak load was reached. The work load was then immediately decreased by 50% to allow the patient's upper body to remain as immobile as possible, with a stable uniform R-R interval on ECG. Following this, ventricular scintigraphy was started. This procedure was based on the assumption that if an ischemic response is observed during exercise, recovery is not expected within such a short time after peak exercise. According to the ischemic response degree, the patients were classified into four groups: Group 1 (n=10, control), normal findings, defined as LVEF>55% and LVEFexercise–LVEFrest $\geq$ 5%; Group 2 (n=10), mild ischemia, LVEF>55% and 0%<LVEFexercise–LVEFrest<5%; Group 3 (n=9), LV dysfunction, LVEF$\leq$35% at rest, and group 4 (n=17), significant ischemia, LVEF>55%, LVEFexercise–LVEFrest<0.

2.1.2 CPET

An upright symptom-limited test was performed on an electronically-braked cycle ergometer (Ergoline-800). After two minutes of free pedaling, exercise was initiated at 20W followed by increased stepwise of 10-20W every minute until a predefined end-point was reached (i.e., symptoms, volitional fatigue or attainment of target HR). Cardiopulmonary data were collected by an on-line metabolic chart (CPX Medical Graphics, Minn., USA). Patients breathed through a low-resistance, two-way valve (Hans-Rudolph, Mo., USA) connected to the expiratory limb. The breath-by-breath signals were integrated by a computer to yield 30-second averages of HR, minute ventilation (Ve), VO_2, carbon dioxide output (VCO_2) and O_2-P (=VO_2/HR). Peak- VO_2 and peak- O_2-P were related to normal predicted values (Wasserman et al., 1987). VAT was defined as the point at which the ventilatory equivalent of oxygen (Ve/VO_2) increases in the absence of such an increase of ventilatory equivalent of carbon dioxide (Ve/VCO_2); or as described for the V-slope method, which uses regression analysis to present the inflection point on a plot of VCO_2 vs. VO_2 (Beaver et al., 1986). BP was measured with a cuff sphygmomanometer at the test beginning, and at least twice during exercise and peak exercise. 12-lead ECGs were recorded at each one-minute interval throughout the test.

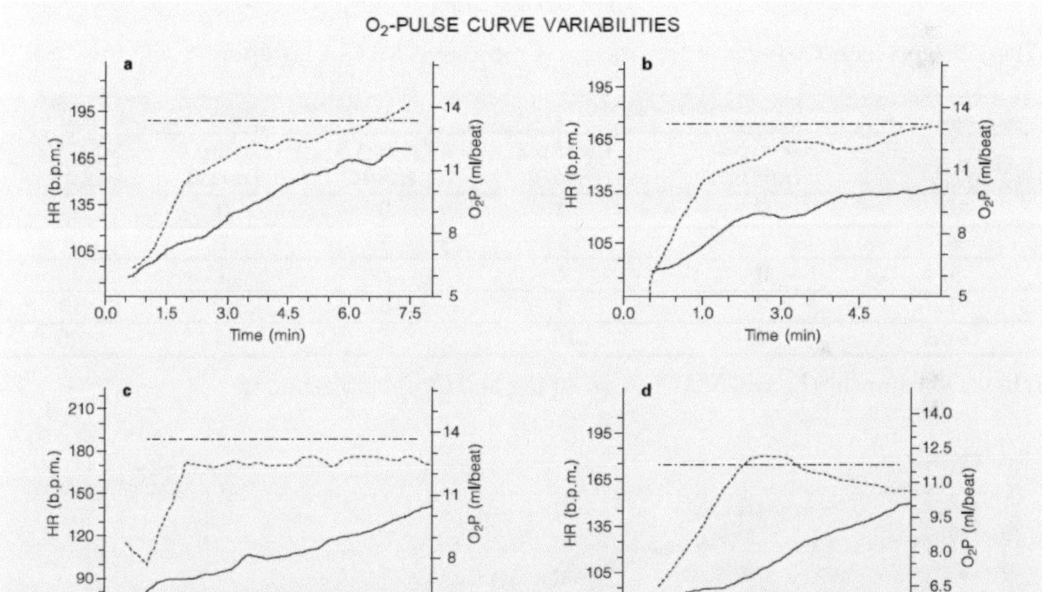

Fig. 1. The four O_2-P curve variables. Type A (top left): normal curve, 10 points; Type B (top right): normal curve, lower values, 8 points; Type C (bottom left): flat curve, low values, 5 points; Type D (bottom right): descending curve, 3 points. Dashed curve refers to O_2-P response. Continuous curve refers to the HR response. The dash-dot horizontal line refers to predicted O_2-P values.

The O_2-P curve appearance was scored on a 10-point scale as follows: Type A, a normal curve (10 points); Type B, a normal ascending curve with relatively low values, not reaching the predicted value at peak exercise (8 points); Type C, an ascending curve reaching a low peak, then flattening through the remainder of exercise on a lower level than the predicted one (5 points), and type D, an ascending curve which may reach the predicted level briefly, then decreases towards the end of the exercise (3 points). These four curves are shown in Figure 1. The hypothesis was, as mentioned above, that type B correlates with mild to moderate ischemic response, curve D correlates with significant ischemia while curve C tends to correlate with LV dysfunction, since these curves reflect the SV dynamics during exercise.

2.2 Results

The peak-HR achieved was similar for both tests in all four groups. Since the supine MUGA was the first test done, in which patients usually achieve a lower sub-maximal HR, the CPET was limited to this peak-HR as well. A significant relationship between the MUGA grouping according to exercise response vs. the O_2-P-curve scoring were demonstrated (Table 1; $p<0.001$). Figure 2 shows the linear regression between these two factors, defined by the equation:

$$Y = -2.1X + 11.85$$

Where Y represents O_2-P-curve scoring and X represents MUGA grouping.

O_2-P-C Scores	MUGA Grouping				Total
	Group 1 (n=10)	Group 2 (n=10)	Group 3 (n=9)	Group 4 (n=17)	
10	9	2	0	0	11
8	1	6	1	1	9
5	0	2	8	3	13
3	0	0	0	13	13
Total	10	10	9	17	46

Table 1. Relationship between MUGA grouping and O_2-P-curve scoring

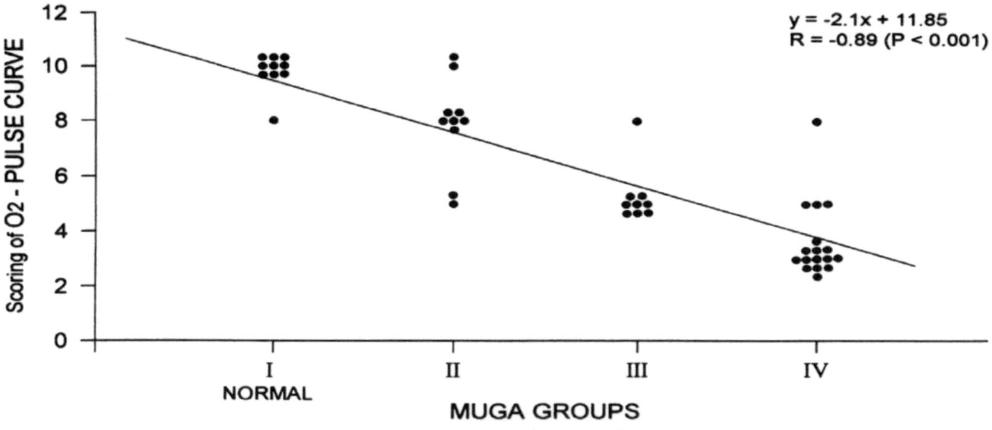

Fig. 2. Correlation between the MUGA grouping (X-axis) and the O_2-P-C score (Y-axis).

2.3 Conclusions

The present study demonstrates the physiological meaning of the O_2-P curve scoring which showed a significant correlation with the MUGA response during exercise. Thus, the exercise O_2-P-C and its scoring, which reflect the SV response during exercise, may serve as a good noninvasive, physiologically-based, parameter for quantitative assessment of ischemic patients and to distinguish between good or impaired LV function. This parameter was used in some of the following studies presented herein, among other indices, for further quantitative evaluation of ischemic patients.

3. Quantitative assessment of functional results after percutaneous transluminal coronary angioplasty by cardiopulmonary exercise indices

PTCA offers a means of improving the angiographic appearance of coronary arterial stenosis. Although a functional change is expected, owing to the augmented capacity of the dilated coronary artery to deliver blood to the previously ischemic myocardium, restenosis of the dilated vessel may occur. Thus, a recurrence of angina pectoris after successful PTCA is of major concern for both the patient and the clinician. Exercise stress testing has become a valuable clinical tool to assess myocardial efficacy and patient's prognosis following PTCA (Kent et al., 1982). As a result, traditional modalities are used before and after the PTCA procedure, including bicycle ergometer or treadmill exercise test, sequential isotopes myocardial perfusion or stress echocardiography (Fioretti et al., 1992), to assess persistence (dilated) or recurrence (stenosis) of the ischemic response. The success of PTCA may be manifested in global and regional cardiovascular function indices like reduced chest pain, increased ejection fraction, reduced abnormal ST segment morphology as well as improved wall motion and perfusion defects. Bengston et al., 1990 reported that since 20% of patients with restenosis following PTCA had neither recurrent angina nor exercise-induced ischemia, then regular exercise testing should be supplemented with more definite indices. This study was designed to investigate the potential importance of the CPET indices, such as VO_2, VAT, O_2-P and its curve appearance, on PTCA follow-up, while assessing the functional results of this procedure.

3.1 Methods

29 patients, candidates for PTCA, 26 men and 3 women aged 41-78 years (mean 63.24+/- 9) participated. All patients demonstrated good LV function by echo-Doppler tests, although 2 patients had suffered a recent non-Q-wave anterior wall myocardial infarction. All patients underwent a coronary angiography for further evaluation of ischemic heart disease (IHD) before the first CPET. The coronary angiography results are summarized in Table 2. The first CPET was performed within 1-2 weeks before PTCA and the second CPET within 2-4 weeks following PTCA. The same medication regimen was used on both tests, while stopping medications such as beta-blockers, calcium channel blockers and digitalis 24h before each test began. It was intended that similar peak-HRs would be achieved for each individual in both tests. The PTCA results are summarized in Table 3.

3.1.1 CPET protocol

The CPET protocol was performed as described in paragraph 2.1.2. Prior to PTCA, the CPET end-point of the patients was the appearance of angina or significant ST-segment depression, fatigue or target HR. After the PTCA, the CPET was terminated at a similar peak-HR as in the first test, even in the absence of the above pre-PTCA end-points, in order to compare the CPET indices under similar conditions.

3.1.2 PTCA

PTCA was performed within 1-2 weeks after the first CPET if the coronary lesions showed a stenosis of > 70% diameter and were responsible for myocardial ischemia. Successful PTCA was defined as a reduction in stenosis to < 50%

Patient No.	Sex	Age years	Coronary angiography	
			diseased vessel(s)	respective stenosis diameter, %
1	m	78	LAD, CX, M1	90, 100, 80
2	m	64	RCA	100
3	f	69	SEPT, D1, CX, RCA	75, 85, 80, 95
4	f	64	D1, D2, PL	95, 85, 80
5	m	67	LAD, D2, RCA	85, 50, 60
6	m	67	CX, RCA	90, 100
7	m	72	RCA	99
8	m	70	LM, LAD, CX, LPD, M1	60, 100, 85, 70, 95
9	m	71	LAD, CX, RCA	100, 75, 70
10	m	60	LAD, D2, RAM	60, 100, 95
11	m	75	CX, LAD	80, 40
12	m	55	LAD (+ recent MI)	70
13	m	66	CX, M1, M2	50, 90, 99
14	m	62	LAD, CX, RCA	70, 75, 100
15	m	62	CX, RCA	75, 100
16	m	59	RCA (mid)	100
17	m	45	LAD, D2	80, 70
18	m	71	M3, RCA	100, 70
19	m	54	LAD, D1, D2, M1, RPD, PL	70, 90, 95, 90, 99, 90
20	m	76	LAD, CX, M1, Inter.	95, 50, 60, 90
21	m	57	LAD (+ recent MI)	95
22	f	75	RCA, LAD, CX	90, 100, 60
23	m	41	LAD	95
24	m	60	LAD	90
25	m	52	CX, LAD	95, 90
26	m	54	LAD, D1, D2, RPD, PL	70, 90, 95, 99, 90
27	m	61	LAD, M1, M2, RCA	90, 100, 90, 40
28	m	69	D1	95
29	m	61	M1	85

LAD = Left anterior descending; CX = circumflex; M1 = 1st marginal; M2 = 2nd marginal; SEPT = septal; MI = myocardial infarction; D1 = 1st diagonal; D2 = 2nd diagonal; PL = posterior lateral branch; LM = left main; RAM = ramus intermediate; RCA = right coronary artery; RPD = right posterior descending; LPD = left posterior descending.

Table 2. Patient basic data and coronary angiography findings prior to PTCA (n=29).

Patient No.	Vessel(s) subjected to PTCA	Stenosis of vessels, %	
		before PTCA	after PTCA
1	CX	100	100
2	RCA	100	100
3	RCA	95	20
4	D2	85	0
5	LAD	85	0
6	CX	90	10
7	RCA	99	10
8	CX	85	0
9	LAD	100	20
10	RAM	95	0
11	CX	80	0
12	LAD (+ recent MI)	70	20
13	CX, M1, M2	50, 90, 99	0, 0, 0
14	LAD	70	0
15	CX	75	10
16	RCA(mid)	100	0
17	LAD	80	10
18	RCA	70	0
19	M1	90	0
20	LAD	95	0
21	LAD (+ recent MI)	95	0
22	RCA	90	0
23	LAD	95	0
24	LAD	90	0
25	CX	95	0
26	LAD, RPD	70, 99	0, 0
27	M2, LAD	90, 90	20, 0
28	D1	95	35
29	M1	85	10

LAD = Left anterior descending; CX = circumflex; M1 = 1st marginal; M2 = 2nd marginal; D1 = 1st diagonal; D2 = 2nd diagonal; RAM = ramus intermediate; MI = myocardial infarction; RCA = right coronary artery; RPD = right posterior descending.

Table 3. PTCA results in all patients, individually (n=29).

Variables	**Before PTCA**	**After PTCA**	**p value**
Peak-HR, b.p.m.	128.7±16.9	132.0±17.2	NS
Peak-VO_2, ml/min	1,526.8±470	1,686.2±390.1	<0.0001
Peak-O_2-P , ml/beat	12.40±2.73	13.44±2.9	<0.0005
O_2-P -Curve, points	7.62±1.92	8.85±1.26	<0.001
VAT, ml/min	993.1±177.6	1,089.8±150.9	<0.0005

Table 4. Summarized CPET results before and after successful PTCA (n=27)

Patient No.	peak-HR, b.p.m		peak-VO_2, ml/min		Peak-O_2-P, ml/beat		O_2-P-C, points		VAT, ml/min	
	before PTCA	after PTCA	before PTCA	after PTCA	before PTCA	after PTCA	before PTCA	after PTCA	before PTCA	after PTCA
1	115	112	1,490	1,431	13	13	8	8	984	960
2	115	116	1,443	1,369	13	12	8	8	1,013	1,027
3	116	120	1,376	1,585	12	13.5	8	8	899	991
4	126	130	1,054	1,106	8	9	5	8	778	871
5	130	140	1,558	1,597	11	11	5	8	879	961
6	105	110	1,102	1,558	11	14	8	10	873	1,192
7	125	122	1,374	1,520	12	14	8	10	875	1,008
8	140	150	1,975	1,985	13	13	10	10	870	1,067
9	105	107	1,048	1,050	10	10	8	8	724	883
10	120	130	1,486	1,543	11	12	8	8	986	1,012
11	115	125	1,480	1,754	13	14	10	10	968	1,081
12	125	135	1,652	1,693	14	14	5	8	1,210	1,185
13	100	100	1,320	1,569	13	15	8	10	780	1,008
14	130	135	1,724	1,887	13	15	5	8	1,168	1,222
15	135	135	1,885	2,080	15	17	8	10	1,224	1,230
16	160	150	2,659	2,580	18	18	10	10	1,161	1,128
17	180	180	1,476	1,647	9	10	8	8	856	910
18	130	120	1,751	1,680	14	14	10	10	885	966
19	133	135	2,076	2,251	15	17	8	10	1,310	1,365
20	116	125	1,675	1,702	15	14	10	10	1,108	1,319
21	140	160	1,680	1,615	12	11	5	5	980	1,061
22	122	122	974	1,004	8	9	8	8	726	810
23	150	155	1,298	1,472	9	10	5	8	925	1,093
24	121	124	956	1,179	11	13	5	8	925	990
25	124	130	1,336	1,770	12	14	5	8	1,080	1,190
26	135	137	2,251	2,412	17	18.5	10	10	1,365	1,407
27	145	146	1,623	1,695	11	12	8	10	959	1,093
28	130	128	1,317	1,363	10	11	8	10	1,082	1,176
29	118	115	2,120	2,232	18	20	10	10	1,219	1,208

In patients 1 and 2, PTCA was unsuccessful.

Table 5. Individual cardiopulmonary indices before and after PTCA (n=29).

3.2 Conclusions

After successful PTCA, patients generally showed improvement or absence of perfusion defects and thus achieved higher levels of exercise. The major findings of the present study, as summarized in tables 4 & 5, support this observation: 1) There was a significant functional aerobic improvement following a successful PTCA, as demonstrated by the CPET indices 2-4 weeks after the procedure and 2) This functional improvement occurred with similar peak-HRs in both CPETs, inferring that an increase in O_2-P is responsible, since VO_2 = HR x O_2-P. It is concluded that CPET carried out following PTCA is an effective, short-term, noninvasive method for quantitative functional assessment of the PTCA results. Further studies are required to determine the long-term effects and prognostic-predicting value for restenosis or for acute coronary events.

4. Quantitative assessment of functional results following a controlled exercise training program in CAD patients by cardiopulmonary exercise indices

Aerobic exercise training is widely used in patients with CAD, with and without LV dysfunction. It is intended to improve physiological fitness, exercise threshold and anginal symptoms. As a result of exercise training, the maximal VO_2 may increase by 10-30% or more (Clausen & Trap-Jenaen, 1970; Redwood et al., 1972; & Sullivan et al., 1988a). However, not all patients experience improved exercise tolerance and for some there is a negative impact (O'Callaghan et al., 1984; Froelicher et al., 1984; & Grodzinski et al., 1987). One of the most challenging aspects of designing exercise programs for patients with CAD is the prescription of appropriate exercise intensity. It must be effective (not too low) yet not too intense as to be a cardiovascular risk (American College of Sports Medicine, 1990; Kohl et al., 1992). It has been shown that the HR at the VAT level is an optimal target HR for exercise (Gordon & Scott, 1995). This study evaluated the effect of an exercise program, prescribed on the basis of HR at the VAT, in patients with varying degrees of CAD, with good or impaired LV function, by CPET indices.

4.1 Methods

Over a 36-month period, 52 male patients, aged 38-75 years, with CAD, completed a 6-9 month supervised, telemetry-monitored, exercise training program. In all patients the CAD was chronic, without any recent coronary events. LV function (expressed by LVEF) was determined by a resting MUGA test. Good LV function was defined when LVEF>45% (32 patients), and LV dysfunction, when LVEF<35% (20 patients). The patients were divided into four groups on the basis of a coronary angiogram and the MUGA test. Groups 1-3 included those with a good LV function as follows: Group 1, 10 patients with single-vessel disease (excluding proximal LAD coronary artery obstruction); Group 2, 12 patients with two-vessel disease, and Group 3, 10 patients with 3-vessel disease. Group 4 included 20 patients with LV dysfunction. The CAD extent was determined by the number of vessels with >50% occlusion. All participants underwent a CPET before and after the exercise training program. The CPET protocol was as described above (paragraph 2.1.2) using the modified Balke treadmill protocol (Froelicher et al., 1974) instead of the bicycle.

4.1.1 Exercise training protocol

All participants completed the exercise program. Each participant was assigned two to three, 30- to 40-min sessions a week of continuous treadmill and bicycle exercise. The training HR was maintained at the VAT level as calculated from the CPET data. Each session was preceded and followed by warm-up and cool-down periods. During exercise, the patients were electrocardiographically monitored by single-lead telemetry (Nihon-Kohden; Life Scope 6).

4.2 Results

The variables at baseline and for the four groups are summarized in Table 6. There were no significant differences concerning age or LVEF among groups 1-3. Although the HR for group 3 (three-vessel disease) was lower than in the other groups, it was still relative to the VAT level. The CPET indices before and after the exercise program are summarized in Table 7. In groups 1 and 2, no significant changes occurred in the standard exercise variables; testing time, peak-HR, maximal ST segment depression and recovery time. Nevertheless, there were significant improvements in the cardiopulmonary indices; peak-VO_2, peak- O_2-P, O_2-P curve levels, and VAT levels. By contrast, group 3 showed significant changes only in the O_2-P curve, while group 4 (LV dysfunction), showed significant improvements in all cardiopulmonary indices except the standard exercise test variables (as did groups 1 and 2).

Variable	Group 1 *(1-vessel disease)*	Group 2 *(2-vessel disease)*	Group 3 *(3-vessel disease)*	Group 4 *(LV dysfunction)*
Number of cases	10	12	10	20
Age, years	53±10	57±8	58±7.5	60±6
Mean LVEF at rest, %	56±9	54±7	53±8	29±6
Mean training HR , beats/min	104	101	92	102
Training HR/peak-HR,%	60	63	59	65
Training HR/HR-max.-predicted,%	57	58	54	59

Table 6. Baseline variables and data from the exercise training program of the four groups

4.3 Conclusions

A 6-9 month exercise training program, determined by HR at the VAT, significantly improves the overall circulatory and cardiac function, as assessed by CPET indices, in CAD patients with one- or two-vessel disease as well as in patients with LV dysfunction, most probably by a peripheral circulatory mechanism in the latter ones. Such improvements were not achieved in patients with three-vessel disease and may be explained by the limitation of significant ischemia which occurred even at this relatively low intensity of exercise. Once again, the CPET was shown to be a sensitive and effective tool for quantitative assessment of exercise training results in CAD patients, in contrast to the routine exercise test variables. It appears, as the PTCA results also demonstrated, that patients with one- or two-vessel disease benefit from an exercise program. This leads us to the next study in which the functional cardiopulmonary indices are evaluated and compared in trained versus untrained CAD patients seeking further explanation of the beneficial effects of exercise for chronic CAD patients.

Index	Before training	After training	p
Group 1: One-vessel disease (n=10)			
ETT, min	7.6±1.3	8.1±1.1	NS
Peak-HR, beats/min	168±22	169±17	NS
Max ST ↓, mm	1.15±1.3	0.9±1.2	NS
Rec. time, min	3.1±4.1	3.2±4.2	NS
Max. load, W	148±37	180±36	<0.005
Peak-VO_2, ml/min/kg	20.5±3.9	25.7±4.6	<0.0001
Peak-O_2 pulse, ml/min/beat	12.4±2.1	15.9±2.5	<0.0005
O_2 pulse curve, points	7.2±2	9.3±1.6	<0.01
VAT, % of VO_2 max	40.3±6	51±11	<0.01
Group 2: Two-vessel disease (n=12)			
ETT, min	6.54±1.9	6.8±1.5	NS
Peak-HR, beats/min	157±20	153±21	NS
Max ST ↓, mm	1.92±1.1	1.5±1.1	<0.1(borderline)
Rec. time, min	7.9±3	8.3±5	NS
Max. load, W	109±35	127±29	<0.025
Peak-VO_2, ml/min/kg	16±5	19±4	<0.025
Peak-O_2 pulse, ml/min/beat	11.3±3.6	14.3±3.1	<0.0005
O_2 pulse curve, points	7.25±2.4	9.25±1.5	<0.005
VAT, % of VO_2 max	43±9.3	48±7	<0.1(borderline)
Group 3: Three-vessel disease (n=10)			
ETT, min	5.5±1.6	6.35±1.5	<0.1(borderline)
Peak-HR, beats/min	152±24	153±22	NS
Max ST ↓, mm	2.35±1	2.2±0.8	NS
Rec. time, min	10.3±4	9.7±3	NS
Max. load, W	110±28	103±22	NS
Peak-VO_2, ml/min/kg	16.7±2.4	15.9±2.2	NS
Peak-O_2 pulse, ml/min/beat	12.3±2.2	12.6±2.2	NS
O_2 pulse curve, points	5.4±1.5	8.2±1.9	0.005
VAT, % of VO_2 max	43±4.7	39±9.5	NS
Group 4: LV dysfunction CAD (n=20)			
ETT, min	7.4±3	8±2.2	NS
Peak-HR, beats/min	152±20	154±17	NS
Max ST ↓, mm	1±1.2	1.2±1.4	NS
Rec. time, min	2.5±3	2.7±2.8	NS
Max. load, W	131±27	155±40	<0.005
Peak-VO_2, ml/min/kg	19±3	22.5±5	<0.001
Peak-O_2 pulse, ml/min/beat	12.2±2.1	14±2.5	<0.0005
O_2 pulse curve, points	7.2±2.5	8.5±2.4	<0.05
VAT, % of VO_2 max	41±8	49±7	<0.05

ETT = exercise treadmill time; max HR = maximal heart rate; max ST ↓ = maximal ST segment depression; rec. time = time of recovery of ST changes; NS = non significant, statistically

Table 7. CPET indices before and after the exercise training program in the four groups.

5. Quantitative functional assessment and comparison of trained versus untrained CAD patients by combined CPET and 99mTC-Sestamibi myocardial imaging

Several studies, amongst many, have confirmed the overall benefit of exercise training in reducing the risk of CAD (Sesso et al., 2000; Blair et al., 1993). Additional studies have shown specific benefits of exercise training in CAD patients: Improved endothelial function with CHF (Hambrecht et al., 1998) or without CHF (Walther et al., 2004; Hambrecht et al., 2000); improved C-reactive protein values (Church et al, 2002); and increased cytokine- activity (Goldhammer et al., 2005). It has been established that exercising at the HR of the VAT level has a favorable effect (Gordon & Scott, 1995). However, the means by which exercise achieves this remains unclear. Does it enhance the development of collateral coronary blood supply to the ischemic myocardium? Or can the improvement in cardiopulmonary function be readily explained by other mechanisms such as a more "cost-effective" metabolic-physiologic demand-supply balance. According to the Fick formula (paragraph 2), O_2-P, which is simply VO_2 divided by HR, is directly related to SV. If O_2-P is significantly increased with exercise, it follows that exercise improves SV. Theoretically this could be induced by improved myocardial perfusion (e.g., by augmented collateral circulation). However, until now there is a lack of evidence to show that exercise training indeed, exerts such a beneficial effect on myocardial oxygen supply. Alternatively, the increase in SV, especially if accompanied by a decrease in HR at VAT level, could simply reflect an improved and a more effective myocardial VO_2 as a result of exercising, which may be accompanied by an objective evidence of reduced myocardial ischemia. This could occur simply as a result of a significant decrease in HR during exercise. In this study, an assessment and comparison of the functional CPET indices in trained vs. untrained CAD patients was carried out. The CPET was followed by evaluation of the degree of ischemia in every patient by ^{99m}TC sestamibi myocardial perfusion imaging (MIBI-SPECT), while using the same exercise testing for both studies. It was assumed that a decrease in myocardial oxygen demand could explain the improved functional capacity observed after exercise training in chronic CAD patients, irrespective of its possible effects on collateral blood flow.

5.1 Methods

44 men aged 40-83, a mean 62+/-12 years, with a recent coronary angiogram participated. They were divided into three age-coordinated groups: Group I, nine patients with normal coronary arteries at the coronary angiography (control group); Group II, 20 patients with significant 1-3 vessel disease who did not participate in any exercise training program (untrained group), and Group III, 15 patients also with significant 1-3 vessel disease, yet who completed a 3-6 month supervised, telemetry-monitored exercise training program prescribed by the HR at the VAT (trained group). All 35 CAD participants had chronic CAD, without any previous acute coronary events. All had normal LV function (LVEF>50%), documented by multigated acquisition angiography (MUGA) or LV angiography. All 44 participants underwent a CPET together with a MIBI-SPECT study using standardized techniques. A single exercise test was used for both studies. Beta-blockers and calcium channel antagonists were stopped 24 hours prior to testing.

5.1.1 CPET protocol

This test was performed as described in paragraph 2.1.1.

5.1.2 MIBI-SPECT protocol

MIBI myocardial perfusion tomography was performed with a same-day "rest-stress" imaging protocol (Tailefer, 1990). The first myocardial perfusion imaging was done at rest, one hour after the injection of MIBI 7-8 mc. The second imaging was done 1-2 hours later, after exercise and additional injection of MIBI 21-22 mc at peak-exercise. Tomographic imaging acquisition was performed over a 180-degree arc, from the -45-degree right anterior oblique to the +135-degree left posterior oblique with an S-P-4x digital camera (Elscint Ltd, Haifa, Israel) fitted with an all-purpose collimator. The degree of ischemia was scored on a 4-point scale as follows: 0-no ischemia; 1-mild; 2-moderate, and 3-severe ischemia. Only stress-imaging defects that showed partial or complete resolution on corresponding rest images were considered as "reversible ischemia".

5.2 Results

The basic data and summary of results for all three groups are shown in Table 8, and the extent of disease in the trained and untrained patients is shown in Table 9. There was an almost equal distribution of 1-, 2- and 3-vessel disease within groups II and III with no significant difference in the extent of disease between the groups (Table 9). Nevertheless, significantly less ischemia was observed in the trained patients (group III) in comparison to the untrained patients (group II) (0.8±0.65 vs. 1.79±0.95; $p<0.001$), as also demonstrated in Figure 3, along with a significantly greater peak-VO_2 (1989±422 vs. 1608±296 ml/min; $p<0.001$). Since peak-VO_2 equals peak-O_2-P x HR, and a highly significant increase in peak-O_2-P was observed in the trained vs. the untrained group (139±29% vs. 94±11% of predicted values; $p<0.001$) concomitantly with a significantly lower peak-HR (70±11% vs. 84±9% of predicted values; $p<0.001$), it indicates that the increase of peak-O_2-P contributes more to the increase of peak-VO_2 than the reduction of peak-HR deletes from its level. The Peak-VO_2 and O_2-P were not significantly different in the trained group (group III) vs. the control group (group I). The relationship between the peak-VO_2, peak-O_2-P and peak-HR within the three groups is demonstrated in Figure 4.

	Group I (n=9) (no disease)	Group II (n=20) (untrained)	Group III (n=15) (trained)
Age(yrs)	64±7	61±8	64±9
No. of occluded vessels	0	1.95±.83	1.93±.85
Ischemic degree (score)	0	1.79±.95‡	0.8±.65
Peak-VO_2 (ml/min)	2171±536†	1608±296‡	1989±422
Peak- O_2-P (%pred.)	125±24*	94±11‡	139±29
Peak-HR (%pred.)	89±7†	84±9‡	70±11

*$p<0.05$ group I vs. group II; † $p<0.01$ group I vs. group III; ‡ $p<0.001$ group II vs. group III.

Table 8. Basic data and summary of results.

	Group II (untrained)	Group III (trained)
1-vessel disease	7(35%)	6(40%)
2-vessel disease	7(35%)	4(27%)
3-vessel disease	6(30%)	5(33%)
Total	20(100%)	15(100%)

Table 9. Extent of coronary disease on angiography in trained and untrained patients.

5.3 Exercise training in chronic and stable CAD

Exercise training is a highly valuable non-pharmacological treatment for patients with chronic stable angina. It reduces myocardial ischemia and, on the clinical level, reduces the frequency of anginal attacks while also improving functional capacity and long-term outcomes (Nigam & Tardif, 2008). As regular exercise has been shown to improve myocardial perfusion and to retard disease progression in patients with stable CAD and even with ischemic cardiomyopathy (Belardinelli et al., 1998), a randomized study was conducted (Hambrecht et al., 2004) to compare the effects of exercise versus percutaneous coronary intervention with stenting on clinical symptoms, angina-free exercise capacity, myocardial perfusion and cost-effectiveness. It was concluded that a 12-month program of regular physical exercise in patients with stable CAD resulted in superior event-free survival and exercise capacity at a lower cost, due to reduced re-hospitalizations and repeated revascularizations. What is the contribution of our study?

What is not clear from previous studies is the dominant mechanism that underlies the cardiovascular improvement induced by an exercise program. Is the improvement mainly dominated by enhanced myocardial blood flow (by increased coronary collateralization for example, as well as by augmentation in endothelial function) or is it due to decreased myocardial oxygen demand and improved metabolic cost effect balance? (The improved ischemic burden evidenced by perfusion studies is compatible with either one of these possibilities). This study does not deny the former possibility of increased myocardial perfusion, since it does not address this issue. However, it does show that the reduced ischemic burden seen in perfusion studies can be attributed substantially, if not completely, to the improved metabolic-physiologic state of the myocardium that accrues from exercise training. It is shown here that SV (as indicated by O_2-P) is significantly higher in the CAD patients after a 3-6 month training program (group III) than in group II patients, who were not subjected to training yet had similar severity of CAD, and also similar to SV levels of subjects without CAD (group I, control). Furthermore, peak-VO_2 is also significantly higher in the trained group than in the untrained one, indicating an improvement in functional capacity. Simultaneously, peak-HR is also significantly lower in the trained group at a higher degree of exercise, as expressed by higher peak VO_2, than in the untrained group (Figure 4). This peak-HR decrease indicates that exercise training decreases myocardial oxygen demand, and the combination of this with the cardio-pulmonary data suggests that the beneficial effect of regular exercise is mediated, at least substantially, by a significant decrease in peak-HR along with the significant increase in peak-O_2-P (related to SV) and peak-VO_2 (functional capacity). This metabolic-physiological advantage to the myocardium is expressed by the significant improvement of ischemia demonstrated by MIBI-SPECT imaging at the peak-HR that was simultaneously reached during the CPET. Thus, there is no need to invoke an improvement in myocardial blood flow to explain the beneficial effect of exercise training in chronic CAD. The results of this study need to be further validated by more extensive study.

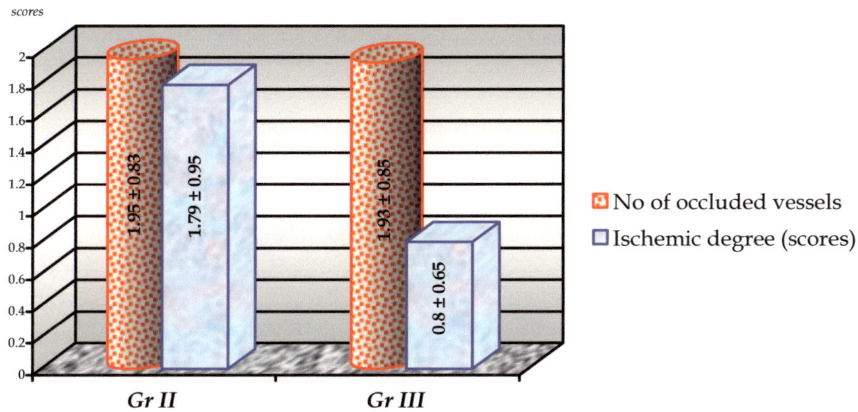

Fig. 3. Comparison of number of occluded coronary vessels and scoring of ischemic degree (Tecnetium-Sestamibi test) between groups II (untrained) and III (trained).

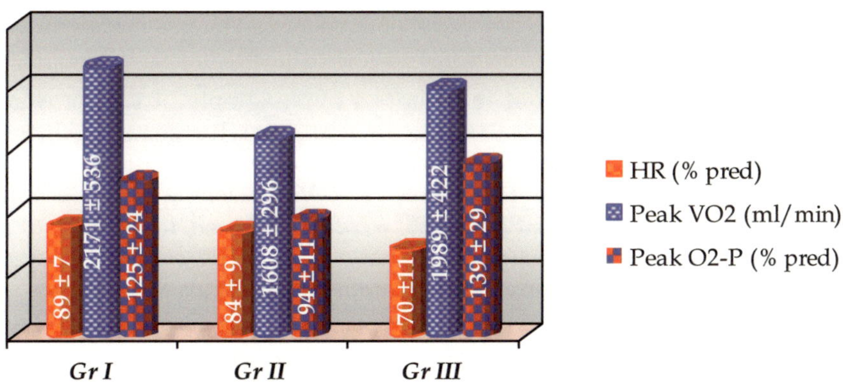

Fig. 4. Comparison of the relationship among peak- VO_2, peak- O_2-P and peak-HR within groups I (control), II (untrained) and III (trained).

6. Quantitative assessment of patients with varying degrees of coronary artery disease by cardiopulmonary exercise and recovery indices

Recovery indices of CPET are important tools for assessing the exercise capacity of patients with CHF, which differ significantly from healthy subjects, as shown in our former study (Klainman et al., 2004). The kinetics of post-exercise VO_2 is shown to be delayed in relationship to the severity of the disease and closely related to exercise capacity (Cerretelli et al., 1996; Hayashida et al., 1993; Sietsema et al., 1994). The ability to estimate quantitatively the severity of CAD by a non-invasive test, such as the CPET, might be of great value for directing further management of these patients. In this study we measured three recovery O_2 kinetic indices as detailed below, in order to compare patients with varying degrees of CAD.

6.1 Methods

62 ambulatory patients were selected in this study on the basis of the following criteria:

- All patients were men to avoid gender physiological discrepances.
- All patients have performed a coronary angiogram within two months prior or post a CPET (which has been done in all patients as well).
- All the CPETs were well qualified for collecting relevant data for the purpose of the study.
- No patients with a history of pulmonary, valvular or peripheral vascular diseases, CHF, left ventricular dysfunction, or chronic atrial fibrillation were selected.
- All patients stopped all relevant medications: beta-blockers, calcium channel antagonists and nitrates at least 24 hours prior to the CPET.

17 patients who demonstrated a normal coronary angiogram were defined as the control group (group A). The other 45 patients had documented CAD based on stenosis of 60% and above, in at least one major coronary artery, excluding the left main or proximal LAD stenosis. On the basis of the coronary angiogram results, patients were divided into three additional groups: B, 26 patients with mono-artery disease (1VD); C, 11 patients with two-vessel disease (2VD), and D, 8 patients with three-vessel disease (3VD).

6.1.1 CPET protocol

The exercise protocol was carried out as described in paragraph 2.1.1. Data were recorded during exercise and recovery periods until the respiratory exchange ratio (RER) of 1 or less was reached. Three recovery indices were defined as follows: 1) half-time recovery of VO_2 (1/2tRec- VO_2), which is the time, in seconds, of peak- VO_2 reaching half of its value. 2) half-time recovery of oxygen pulse (1/2tRec- O_2-P), which is the time, in seconds, of peak- O_2-P reaching half of its value, and 3) total-time recovery of VO_2 (TtRec- VO_2), which is the time, in minutes, from peak exercise end-point till obtaining an RER value of 1 or less.

6.1.2 Statistical analysis

Data were analyzed by the SAS system, using the Duncan's Multiple Range Test to compare the variables of each group. Values were calculated as mean +/- 1 standard deviation (SD). P values <0.05 were considered statistically significant. P values of 0.06-0.1 were considered as borderline. Values of > 0.1 were not significant.

6.2 Results

The mean age of all patients (n=62) was 65.75+/-9.85 years, and when divided into the four groups: A) 62.8+/-10.9 y (n=17); B) 67.5+/-9.5 y (n=26); C) 66.9+/-9.3 y (n=11), and D) 65+/-6.5 y (n=8). No statistical differences of age were found among the groups. Table 10 summarizes the group data of the CPET as mean +/-1 SD and shows the comparison of the exercise and recovery indices among the four groups. This table shows no significant differences of peak HR, % pred. HR, Ex. time and peak O_2-P among the four groups (lines 2, 3, 4 and 7 respectively). A significant difference of peak-VO_2 was observed only between groups A and D, while borderline differences were shown between groups A vs. B; A vs. C; D vs. B; and D vs. C (line 5). Similar differences among the groups were observed in peak O_2-P (% of predicted value) variable (line 8). Significant differences of peak VO_2 (% of predicted value) were observed between group D vs. A, B and C, but not among A, B and C themselves (line 6). Similar differences were shown in VAT variables (lines 9 and 10). Lines 2-10 summarize the exercise parameters, while lines 11-13 demonstrate the recovery indices. Significant differences of 1/2tRec-VO_2 were observed between the following groups: A vs. C; A vs. D; and B vs. D, while borderline differences were shown between groups: A vs. B; B vs. C; and C vs. D (line 11). Similar differences of the indices 1/2tRec- O_2-P and TtRec-VO_2 were demonstrated among the groups (lines 12 and 13): Significant differences were apparent between A or B vs. C or D, but not between A vs. B or C vs. D.

1	Group	A (N=17)	B (N=26)	C (N=11)	D (N=8)
2	Peak HR	146+/-17*	127+/-20*	131+/-15*	117+/-18*
3	% pred. HR	92+/-5*	84+/-13*	86+/-11*	76+/-12*
4	Ex. Time (min)	8.3+/-1.9*	7.8+/-1.9*	7.8+/-1.7*	6.8+/-1.9*
5	Peak-VO_2 (ml/kg/min)	25+/-6.4*	22.5+/-6.6¶	22+/-6.2¶	18.4+/-6.2†
6	Peak-VO_2 (% pred.)	109+/-13*	110+/-24*	99+/-18*	78+/-22†
7	Peak-O_2-P (ml/beat)	15.2+/-2.6*	16+/-5*	14.4+/-4.4*	12.5+/-3.2*
8	Peak-O_2-P (% pred.)	121+/-14*	132+/-32¶	115+/-26*	104+/-25†
9	VAT (ml of VO_2)	1170+/-182*	1161+/-234*	1027+/-172*	814+/-245†
10	VAT (% of VO_2-max)	56%+/-5*	62%+/-11*	55%+/-8*	44%+/-8†
11	1/2tRec-VO_2 (sec.)	84+/-20*	100+/-35‡	123+/-36§	134+/-18†
12	1/2tRec-O_2-P (sec.)	101+/-30*	123+/-34*	162+/-37†	174+/-40†
13	TtRec-VO_2 (min.)	7.6+/-1.3*	7.9+/-1.4*	9.1+/-1.9†	9.2+/-1.7†

Pred.=predicted; Ex.=Exercise; 1/2tRec=1/2 time recovery; TtRec=Total time recovery.
P values: Significance: * vs § or †; ‡ vs †.
Borderline: * vs ‡ or ¶; ‡ vs §; § vs †; and † vs ¶.
Not Significant: * vs *; † vs †; and ¶ vs ¶.

Table 10. Group comparison of CPET indices during exercise and recovery.

6.3 Post-exercise recovery period

Few data are available in regard to VO_2 kinetics in recovery among patients with CAD. Traditionally, the rate of VO_2 recovery from exercise indicates the oxidative capacity in healthy subjects, and its decrease has been related to the oxygen debt following exercise (Barstow, 1987; Di Prampero, 1970). This oxygen debt has been considered to involve a first, fast alactatic phase and a second, slow lactatic component (Margaria et al., 1933). More recently, the term excess post-exercise oxygen consumption has been used to express more complex mechanisms which mediate the post-exercise VO_2 recovery, and absolve this entity from a total dependence on anaerobic metabolism (Gaesser, 1984). A relatively fast recovery time of oxygen consumption has been demonstrated in athletes (McCully et al., 1992), while a delay of oxygen kinetics is shown in heart failure patients. The later may involve a delay of several factors, such as circulatory transport of oxygen to and from metabolizing tissue (Koike et al., 1989), pulmonary gas exchange (Sullivan et al., 1988b), or oxygen consumption of the exercising/recovering muscles themselves. One important factor, which contributes to the delayed recovery of VO_2, is the prolonged recovery of the muscle phosphate/phosphocreatine ratio, which is determined by the blood flow as well as by the oxidative capacity of the exercising muscles (Chati et al., 1994; Sapega et al., 1987; Wiener et al., 1986). Other central factors, which may explain the slower VO_2 recovery in patients with heart failure, are higher cardiac output and increased SV during the early recovery period (Koike et al., 1990), which are directly related to VO_2 and O_2-P respectively, according to the Fick formula, as discussed previously. The arterio-venous oxygen difference, which appears in the formula, shows a rapid decline after exercise, thus supporting the direct relationship between the central factors to VO_2 and O_2-P (Sumimoto et al., 1991, 1993). Both healthy subjects and patients with CAD demonstrated elevated cardiac output and ejection fraction during early recovery (Plotnick et al., 1986), and the CAD patient levels were even higher. It is suggested that an existence of a transient mismatch between cardiac contractility and after-load reduction during recovery, even from mild-intensity exercise, in healthy subjects as well as in CAD patients, might be the mechanism of overshoot in cardiac function observed in the early-recovery phase (Kano et al., 1999). According to the above, we hypothesized that patients with CAD may also demonstrate similar changes in recovery indices since ischemic reaction during exercise might be considered as temporary LV dysfunction in correlation to the severity of the ischemic reaction. In our study, there are significant differences in the recovery VO_2 indices between the healthy group and the CAD groups, with a clear tendency of delayed recovery in parallel to the severity of the CAD. Our results demonstrate such differences, which are emphasized more in group D (3VD), where the sub-maximal exercise was mostly limited for the severity of the CAD. This supports other studies in which even mild-intensity or sub-maximal exercise was enough for showing slower recovery kinetics of VO_2 in CAD (Kano et al., 1999) and CHF patients (Cohen-Solal et al., 1995) compared to healthy subjects. Our findings do not concur with Pavia et al. which do not show significant differences between CAD and healthy subjects. In some patients the kinetics of VO_2 recovery may be complex and incorrectly described by a single exponential curve (Henry, 1951) as opposed to another later report (Hayashida et al., 1993). Thus, Cohen-Solal et al. characterized recovery kinetics by measuring the half-time of VO_2 recovery, while also measuring the time for RER to reach level 1 or less (Lim et al., 1998). In this study, the three recovery indices, mentioned above (paragraph 6.1.1) were measured. All three indices differ significantly among the four groups studied. The 1/2tRec- VO_2

shows a significant systematic progression of increased time from group A (control group) to group D, while the two other indices show only a tendency for such a progression. Moreover, these last two indices differ significantly between groups A or B vs. C or D. Group B appears closer to A while C appears closer to D, inferring that mono-artery disease should be considered for further conservative treatment rather than invasive procedures. Such significant differences were not demonstrated in most of the exercise indices (Table 1, lines 2-10). These findings validate the recovery indices as even more important than those in quantitative functional evaluation of varying degrees of CAD.

6.4 Conclusions

We have concluded that recovery cardiopulmonary indices of VO_2 kinetics are important in evaluating patients with CAD and may differ functionally according to the degree of disease. Thus, additional recovery measurement indices are recommended for the standard CPET in order to obtain a more comprehensive and quantitative assessment of the functional degree of CAD, which seems to correlate with the anatomical findings of the coronary angiogram. Additional studies are recommended to further establish these findings.

6.5 Clinical applications

The present study provides a simple, non-invasive physiological tool for evaluating the severity of ischemia in patients with CAD, following and in addition to the anatomical results of the coronary angiogram. Furthermore, this tool may be used for identifying patients with varying degrees of ischemia, prior to coronary angiogram and accordingly, indicate them for further treatment - conservative or invasive.

7. Summary

In the five studies reported in this chapter, we emphasize the important contribution of cardiopulmonary indices, during both exercise and recovery, for quantitative functional assessment of patients with CAD. The most important indices for measuring ischemic exercise responses were: Peak-VO_2; peak-O_2-P; VAT; O_2-P curve characteristics, all measured during exercise; and three relatively new indices, measured during the recovery period: total-time and half-time recovery kinetics of VO_2, and half-time recovery of O_2-P. Using these indices it was shown that it is possible to quantitatively assess the functional results following invasive procedures like PTCA in chronic CAD patients as well as exercise training results in similar patients. The results from these two groups support the assertion that benefits of regular exercise training are not inferior to the invasive procedure, at least in patients with one- or two-vessel CAD. Also illustrated here is a possible mechanism for better understanding the training effect in those patients. It is suggested that the increase in the O_2-P, which reflects an increase in SV following exercise training program, causes a gradual decrease in exercise HR, while maintaining the same or an even higher VO_2 level during exercising. As a consequence, there is a decrease in myocardial oxygen demand. This metabolic-physiologic advantage to the myocardium is expressed by significant improvement of ischemia as demonstrated by MIBI-SPECT imaging at peak-HR in trained patients compared to untrained ones. Finally, it has been shown how the recovery O_2 kinetic indices may contribute, in addition to the exercise indices, to quantitative comparison among varying degrees of CAD, as expressed during CPET. All indices mentioned above, further validate the CPET as an effective, non-invasive, and essential tool for quantitative functional assessment of CAD patients and, accordingly, may even provide an indication of further treatment required - conservative or invasive, in chronic and stable patients.

8. References

American College of Sports Medicine: Position Stand. (1990). The Recommended Quantity and Quality of Exercise for Developing and Maintaining Cardiorespiratory and Muscular Fitness in Healthy Adults. *Medical Science & Sports Exercise,* Vol.22, pp. 265-274

Barstow, TJ.; Mole, PA. (1987). Stimulation of Pulmonary O_2 Uptake during Exercise Transients in Human. *Journal of Applied Physiology,* Vol.63, pp. 2253-2261

Beaver, WL.; Wasserman, K. & Whipp, B. (1986). A New Method for Detecting Anaerobic Threshold by Gas Exchange. *Journal of Applied Physiology,* Vol.60, pp. 2020-2027

Belardinelli, R.; Georgiou, D.; Ginzton, L.; Cianci, G. & Purcaro, A. (1998). Effects of Moderate Exercise Training on Thallium Uptake and Contractile Response to Low-Dose Dobutamine of Dysfunctional Myocardium in Patients with Ischemic Cardiomyopathy. *Circulation,* Vol.97, pp. 553-561

Bengston, JR.; Mark, D.; Honan, M.; Rendall, D.; Hinhohara, T.; Stack, R.; Hjatky, M.; Califf, R.; Lee, K. & Pryor, D. (1990). Detection of Restenosis after Elective Percutaneous Transluminal Coronary Angioplasty Using the Exercise Treadmill Test. *American Journal of Cardiology,* Vol.65, pp.28-34

Blair, SN.; Kohl, HW. & Barlow, CE. (1993). Physical Activity, Physical Fitness and all Cause Mortality in Women: do Women need to be Active? *Journal of American College Nutrition,* Vol.12, pp. 368-371

Cerretelli, P.; Sikand, R. & Farhi, LE. (1996). Readjustment of Cardiac Output and Gas Exchange during Onset of Exercise and Recovery. *Journal of Applied Physiology,* Vol.21, pp. 1355-1360

Chati, Z.; Zannad, F.; Robin-Lherbier, B.; Jeandel, C.; Escanye, JM.; Robert, J. & Aliot, E. (1994). Contribution of Specific Skeletal Metabolic Abnormalities to Limitation of Exercise Capacity in Patients with Chronic Heart Failure: A 31P Nuclear Magnetic Resonance Study. *American Heart Journal,* Vol.128, pp. 781-792

Church, TS.; Barlow, CE.; Earnest, CP.; Kampert, JB.; Priest, EL. & Blair SN. (2002). Associations between Cardiorespiratory Fitness and C-reactive Protein in Men. *Arteriosclerosis, Thrombosis &Vascular Biology,* Vol.22. pp. 1869-1876

Clausen, JP. & Trap-Jensen, J. (1970). Effects of Training on the Distribution of Cardiac Output in Patients with Coronary Artery Disease. *Circulation,* Vol.42, pp. 611-624

Cohen-Solal, A.; Laperche, T.; Morvan, D.; Geneves, M.; Caviezel, B. & Gourgon R. (1995). Prolonged Kinetics of Recovery of Oxygen Consumption after Maximal Graded Exercise in Patients with Chronic Heart Failure. *Circulation,* Vol.91, pp. 2924-2932

De Groote, P.; Millaire, A.; Decoulx, E.; Nugue, O.; Guimier, P. & Ducloux, P. (1999). Kinetics of Oxygen Consumption during and after Exercise in Patients with Dilated Cardiomyopathy. *Journal of American College Cardiology,* Vol.28, pp. 168-175

Di Prampero, P.; Davies, CT.; Cerretelli, P. & Marqaria, R. (1970). An Analysis of the Oxygen Debt Contracted in Submaximal Exercise. *Journal of Applied Physiology, Vol.*29, pp. 547-551

Fioretti, PM.; Pozzoli, MMA.; Ilmer, B.; Salustri, A.; Cornel, J-H.; Reijs, AEM.; Krening, EP.; Reiber, JHC.; De-Feyter, PJ. & Roelandt, JRTC. (1992). Exercise Echocardiography versus Thallium-201 SPECT for Assessing patients before and after PTCA. *European Heart Journal,* Vol.13, pp. 213-219

Froelicher, VF.; Brammell, HR.; Davis, G.; Noguera, I.; Stewart, A. & Lancaster, MC. (1974). A Comparison of the Reproducibility and Physiological Response to Three Maximal Treadmill Exercise Protocols. *Chest,* Vol.65, pp. 512-517

Froelicher, V.; Jensen, D.; Genter, F.; Sullivan, M.; Dan-McKirnan, M.; Witztum, K.; Schart, J.; Strong, ML. & Ashburn, W. (1984). A Randomized Trial of Exercise Training in Patients with Coronary Heart Disease. *JAMA,* Vol.252, pp. 1291-1297

Gaesser, GA. & Brooks GA. (1984). Metabolic Bases of Excess Post-exercise Oxygen Consumption: A Review. *Medical Science of Sports Exercise,* Vol.16, pp. 29-43

Goldhammer, E.; Tanchilevitch, A.; Maor, I.; Beniamini, Y.; Rosenschein, U. & Sagiv M. Exercise Training Modulates Cytokines Activity in Coronary Heart Disease Patients. *International Journal of Cardiology,* Vol.100, pp. 93-99

Gordon, NF. & Scott, CB. (1995). Exercise Intensity Prescription in Cardiovascular Disease: Theoretical Basis for Anaerobic Threshold Determination. *Journal of Cardiopulmonary Rehabilitation,* Vol.15, pp. 193-196

Grodzinski, E.; Jette, M.; Blumchen, G. & Borer, J. (1987). Effect of a Four-Week Training Program on Left Ventricular Function as Assessed by Radionuclide Ventriculography. *Journal of Cardiopulmonary Rehabilitation,* Vol.7, pp. 517-524

Hambrecht, R.; Fiehn, E.; Weigl, C.; Gielen, S.; Hamann, C.; Kaiser,R.; Yu,J.; Adams,V.; Niebauer,J. & Schuler,G. (1998). Regular Physical Exercise Corrects Endothelial Dysfunction and Improves Exercise Capacity in Patients with ChronicHeart Failure. *Circulation*, Vol.98, pp. 2709-2715

Hambrecht, R.; Wolf, A.; Gielen, S.; Linke, A.; Hofer, J.; Erbs, S.; Schoene, N. & Schuler G. (2000). Effect of Exercise on Coronary Endothelial Function in Patients with Coronary Artery Disease. *The New England Journal of Medicine,* Vol. 342, pp. 454-460

Hambrecht, R.; Walther, C.; Mobius-Winkler, S.; Gielen, S.; Linke, A.; Conradi, K.; Erbs, S.; Kluge, R.; Kendziorra, K.; Sabri, O.; Sick, P. & Schuler, G. (2004). Percutaneous Cronary Agioplasty Cmpared with Eercise Taining in Patients with Stable Coronary Artery Disease: A Randomized Trial. *Circulation*, Vol.109, pp. 1371-1378

Hayashida, W.; Kumada, T. & Kohno, F. (1993). Post Exercise Oxygen Uptake Kinetics in Patients with Left Ventricular Dysfunction. *International Journal of Cardiology,* Vol. 38, pp. 63-72

Henry, FM. (1951). Aerobic Oxygen Consumption and Alactic Debt in Muscular Work. *Journal of Applied Physiology,* Vol.3, pp. 427-438

Kano, H.; Koike, A.; Yajima, T.; Koyama, Y.; Marumo, F. & Hiroe M. (1999). Mechanism of Overshoot in Cardiac Function during Recovery from Submaximal Exercise in Man. *Chest,* Vol.116, pp. 868-873

Kent, KM.; Bonow, R.; Rosing, D.; Ewels, C.; Lipson, L.; McIntosh, C.; Bacharach, S.; Green, M. & Epstein, S. (1982). Improved Myocardial Function during Exercise after Successful Percutaneous Transluminal Coronary Angioplasty. *New England Journal of Medicine,* Vol.306, pp. 441-446

Klainman, E.; Lebzelter, J.; Fink, G. & Kramer, MR. (2004). Significance of Post Exercise Oxygen Consumption Kinetics in the Evaluation of Patients with Congestive Heart Failure. *Journal of Heart Disease*; Vol.2, p. 123 (Suppl.).

Kohl, HW.; Powell, KE.; Gordon, NF.; Blair, SN. & Paffenbarger, RS. (1992). Physical Activity, Physical Fitness and Sudden Cardiac Death. *Epidemiology Review,* Vol.14, pp. 37-58

Koike, A.; Itoh, H.; Taniguchi, K. & Hiroe, M. (1989). Detecting Abnormalities in Left Ventricular Function during Exercise by Respiratory Measurements. *Circulation,* Vol.80, pp. 1737-1746

Koike, A.; Itoh, H.; Doi, M.; Taniguchi, K.; Marumo, F.; Umehara, I. & Hiroe M. (1990). Beat-to-beat Evaluation of Cardiac Function during Recovery from Upright Bicycle Exercise in Patients with Coronary Artery Disease. *American Heart Journal,* Vol.120, pp. 316-323

Koike, A.; Hiroe, M. & Marumo, F. (1998). Delayed Kinetics of Oxygen Uptake during Recovery after Exercise in Cardiac Patients. *Medical Science Sports Exercise,* Vol.30, pp. 185-189

Lim, H.; Lee, CW.; Park, SW.; Kim, JJ.; Song, JK.; Hong, MK.; Jin, YS. & Park, SJ. (1998). Effect of Percutaneos Balloon Mitral Valvuloplasty and Exercise Training on the Kinetics of Recovery Oxygen Consumption after Exercise in Patients with Mitral Stenosis. *European Heart Journal,* Vol.19, pp. 1865-1871

Margaria, R.; Edwards, HT. & Dill, DB. (1993). The Possible Mechanisms of Contracting and Paying the Oxygen Debt and the Role of Lactic Acid in Muscular Contraction. *American Journal of Physiology,* Vol.106, pp. 689-715

McCully, KK.; Vandenborne, K.; DeMeirleir, K.; Posner, JD. & Leigh, JS. Jr. (1992). Muscle Metabolism in Track Athletes Using 31P Magnetic Resonance Spectroscopy. *Acta Radiologica,* Vol.70, pp. 1353-1359

Milani, RV.; Lavie, CJ. & Sapiva, H. (1995). Limitations of Estimating Metabolic Equivalents in Exercise Assessment in Patients with Coronary Artery Disease. *American Journal of Cardiology,* Vol.75, pp. 940-942

Milani, RV.; Lavie, CJ.; Mehra, MR. & Ventura, HO. (2006). Understanding the Basis ofCardiopulmonary Exercise Testing. *Journal of Myoclinic Process,* Vol.81, No.12, pp. 1603-1615

Nigam, A. & Tardif, JC. (2008). The Place of Exercise in the Patient with Chronic StableAngina. *Heart and Metabolism,* Vol.38, pp. 34-37

O'Callaghan, W.; Teo, K.; O'Riordan, J.; Webb, H.; Dolphin, T. & Horgan, J. (1984). Comparative Responses of Male and Female Patients with Coronary Artery Disease to Exercise Rehabilitation. *European Heart Journal,* Vol.5, pp. 649-651

Pavia, L.; Myers, J. & Cesari, R. (1999). Recovery Kinetics of Oxygen Uptake and HR in Patients with Coronary Artery Disease and Heart Failure. *Chest,* Vol.116, pp. 808-813

Plotnick, GD.; Becker, LC. & Fisher, ML. (1986). Changes in Left Ventricular Function during Recovery from Upright Bicycle Exercise in Normal Persons and in Patients with Coronary Artery Disease. *American Journal of Cardiology,* Vol.58, pp. 247-251

Redwood, DR.; Rosing, DR. & Epstein, SE. (1972). Circulatory and Symptomatic Effects of Physical Training in Patients with Coronary Artery Disease and Angina Pectoris. *New England Journal of Medicine,* Vol.286, pp. 959-965

Sapega, AA.; Sokolow, DP.; Graham, TJ. & Chance, B. (1987). Phosphorous Nuclear Magnetic Resonance: A Noninvasive Technique for the Study of Muscle Bioenergetics during Exercise. *Medical Science* of *Sports Exercise,* Vol.19, pp 410-420

Sesso, HD.; Paffenbarger, RS. & Lee I-M. (2000). Physical Activity and Coronary Heart Disease in Men: The Harvard Alumni Health Study. *Circulation,* Vol.102, pp. 975-980

Sietsema, KE.; Ben-Dov, I.; Zhang, YY.; Sullivan, C. & Wasserman K. (1994). Dynamics of Oxygen Uptake for Submaximal Exercise and Recovery in Patients with Chronic Heart Failure. *Chest*, Vol.105, pp. 1693-1700

Sullivan, MJ.; Higginbotham, MB. & Cobb, FR. (1988a). Exercise Training in Patients with Severe Left Ventricular Dysfunction: Hemodynamic and Metabolic Effects. *Circulation,* Vol.78, pp. 506-515

Sullivan, MJ.; Higginbotham, MB. & Cobb, FR. (1988b). Increased Exercise Ventilation in Patients with Chronic Heart Failure: Intact Ventilatory Control Despite Hemodynamic and Pulmonary Abnormalities. *Circulation*, Vol.77, pp. 552-559

Sumimoto, T.; Sugiura, T.; Takeuchi, M.; Yuasa, F.; Hasegawa, T.; Nakamura, S.; Iwasaka, T.& Inada M. (1991). Oxygen Utilization, Carbon Dioxide Elimination and Ventilation during Recovery from Supine Bicycle Exercise 6 to 8 Weeks after Acute Myocardial Infarction. *American Journal of Cardiology,* Vol.67, pp. 1170-1174

Sumimoto, T.; Sugiura, T.; Takeuchi, M.; Yuasa, F.; Iwasaka, T. & Inada M. (1993). Overshoot in Mixed Venous Oxygen Saturation during Recovery from Supine Bicycle Exercise in Patients with Recent Myocardial Infarction. *Chest*, Vol.103, pp. 514-220

Tailefer, R. (1990). Technetium -99m Sestamibi Myocardial Imaging: Same Day Rest-Stress Studies and Dipyridamole. *American Journal of Cardiology,* Vol.66, pp. 80E-84E

Vivekananthan, K.; Lavie CJ. & Milani RV. (2000). Stress Testing. In: Lavie, CJ. Lubin, MF. Eds. *Clinical Atlas of Office Procedures – Cardiovascular Disease,* pp. 377-391, Philadelphia, Pa: WB Saunders Co.

Walther, C.; Gielen, S. & Hambrecht, R. (2004). The Effect of Exercise Training on Endothelial Function in Cardiovascular Disease in Humans. *Exercise and Sport Sciences Reviews*, Vol.32, pp. 129-134

Wasserman, K.; Hansen, JE.; Sue, DY. & Whipp, BJ. (1987). Principals of Exercise Testing and Interpretation. *Lea & Febiger, Philadelphia, PA,* pp. 1-57

Wiener, DH.; Fink, LI.; Maris, J.; Jones, RA.; Chance, B. & Wilson JR. (1986). Abnormal Skeletal Muscle Bioenergetics during Exercise in Patients with Heart Failure: Role of Reduced Muscle Blood Flow. *Circulation,* Vol.73, pp. 1127-1136

5

LBBB: The ECG Patterns and Cardiac Function in Patients With and Without Coronary Artery Disease

Marwan Badri, William Kornberg, James F. Burke,
Peter R. Kowey and Li Zhang
Lankenau Medical Center,
Lankenau Institute for Medical Research
USA

1. Introduction

Left bundle branch block (LBBB) is a common conduction abnormality. Its prevalence increases from 0.4% at age 50 to 6.5% at age 80. (Eriksson, Hansson et al. 1998) LBBB is seen in many diseases such as coronary artery disease (CAD), hypertension, valvular heart disease, non-ischemic cardiomyopathies and conduction tissue defects/degenerations. (Nisse 1929; Jain and Mehta 2003) Identifying CAD in patients with LBBB has been the subject of many studies and remains a clinical challenge.

The conduction abnormality caused by LBBB alters the ventricular activation sequence, resulting in distortion of the QRS complex, and secondary changes in the ST segment and T-wave on the surface ECG. Presence of LBBB is known to mask the ECG features of CAD. Since approximately 50% of LBBB patients have underlying CAD, identifying the ECG differences between CAD and non-CAD patients with LBBB would have considerable clinical impact in risk stratifying LBBB and in the detection of underlying CAD.

Hayat et al reported that myocardial blood velocity was markedly reduced in LBBB patients with CAD compared with those without. (Hayat, Dwivedi et al. 2008) Whether CAD can modify the QRS-ST-T patterns over time in the presence of LBBB is unclear. The first part of this study, therefore, was designed to compare QRS morphology and ST-T changes between CAD and non-CAD patients to determine if there were any subtle ECG pattern differences between the two groups.

The consequence of LBBB is the delay of left ventricular (LV) contraction, altered septal motion, and reduced diastolic filling time.(Strauss, Selvester et al.; Grines, Bashore et al. 1989) These effects impair the pump function and stimulate negative LV remodeling. (Sweeney, van Bommel et al.) An inverse relationship between the QRS duration and left ventricular ejection fraction has been observed in LBBB patients in the presence of mechanical asynchrony. (Roshan, Pati et al. 2008) This finding provides the basis for cardiac resynchronization therapy (CRT) in heart failure patients. (Strauss, Selvester et al.) It is unclear, however, if such a relationship is more pronounced when underlying CAD exists.

The second part of this study, therefore, was to examine the correlation between QRSd and LV ejection fraction (EF) in patients with LBBB, and to determine if this relationship is altered by CAD.

2. Methods

2.1 Materials and methods

A retrospective study in accordance with compliance guidelines was conducted after obtaining the approval of the Institutional Review Board of the Lankenau Medical Center. Patients' identifiable information was removed for the data analysis.

The LBBB diagnosis was first made by the automated interpretation of the ECG system. Then it was over-read by a cardiologist to confirm the diagnosis. LBBB ECGs were retrieved from the ECG library and from patients who underwent cardiac catheterization between January 1st 2005 and June 30th 2010. Electronic medical records were reviewed to extract demographic and clinical information. A cardiac catheterization database containing patients who had undergone diagnostic coronary angiography, percutaneous coronary intervention (PCI) and/or coronary artery bypass grafting (CABG) was interrogated. Patients were classified as having CAD if they had history of PCI, CABG or if they had ≥50% luminal diameter stenosis of a major coronary artery on angiography.

2.2 ECG evaluation

To determine whether LBBB ECG morphology is different between CAD and non-CAD groups, the resting supine 12-lead ECG (AC filter 60Hz, 25 mm/sec, 10 mm/mV) was evaluated for six aspects: 1) Pathologic Q waves. 2) QRS duration (QRSd), amplitude and axis. 3) Among patients with leftward QRS axis ≥ -45 degrees, QRS morphology was further evaluated for the presence of left anterior fascicular block (LAFB) pattern (Figure 1)

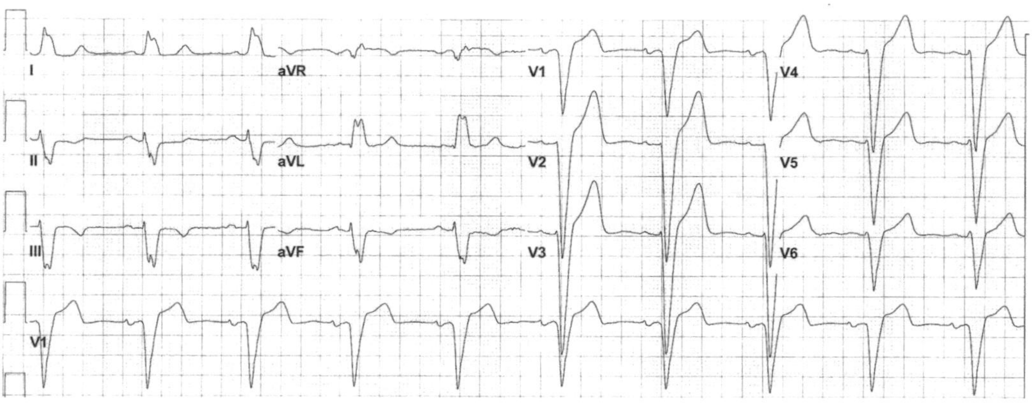

ECG from a 69-year-old man with CAD and EF 31% demonstrating QRS-ST-T pattern typical to divisional LBBB: QRSd = 188 ms. The LAFB pattern is shown as QRS axis > -45 degree, rS in II, III and aVF with deflection of $S_{III} > S_{II}$; and broad and notched R wave in I and qR in aVL with $R_{aVL} > R_{I}$; Poor R progression with rS in V6 and T wave opposite to the direction of QRS complex in precordial leads.

Fig. 1. Poor R progression V1-6 in a CAD patient with LBBB

4) Low QRS voltage in the limb leads was considered if QRS amplitude was ≤ 0.5 mV in six limb leads. 5) Poor R wave progression was diagnosed if the S wave was the dominant deflection in the QRS complex, i.e. in rS waveform, from right to left precordial leads and if the ratio of R/S was < 1 in V1-V4 or beyond. 6) Presence of ischemic ST-T changes such as ST elevation accompanying T wave inversion, or ST depression with upright T wave in the same lead. For patients with injury or ischemic ST-T changes, short term follow-up ECGs were evaluated to determine whether these ST-T changes were resolved.

2.3 QRSd-EF relationship

Cardiac output was estimated by one of two methods: 1) 2-D echocardiography using modified Simpson's biplane method, or 2) post-stress, nuclear perfusion imaging the single photon emission computed tomography (gated SPECT). The QRSd was obtained from automated interpretation of each ECG tracing and QRSd-EF curve was plotted.

2.4 Statistical analysis

Comparisons of CAD and non-CAD groups were performed using NCSS 2007 biomedical statistical software (Kaysville, UT). A two-sample t test was applied for descriptive analysis in quantitative measures showing normal distribution of data points. Nonparametric tests Mann-Whitney U or Wilcoxon Rank Tests were used for difference in medians if the normality was rejected. A chi square (X2) statistic was used to compare categorical variables. For the ECG changes that were more prevalent in one group than the other, sensitivity, specificity, positive and negative predictive values were calculated for the assessment of predictive accuracy. Univariate linear regression analysis was performed when appropriate. A p value <0.05 was considered statistically significant.

3. Results

LBBB was found in 3.7% (134/3582) of all patients screened. Among LBBB patients, 72% (96/134) had evidence of CAD. Patients with CAD were older (76 ± 9 vs. 65 ± 13 years, $p <0.001$) and more commonly of male gender (53% vs. 43%, $p < 0.05$).

3.1 ECG patterns

Table 1 demonstrates that in patients with LBBB, leftward QRS axis, QS wave in V1, poor R wave progression, and broad/notched/slurred R wave in V6 are prevalent in both CAD and non-CAD groups. RS morphologies (rS, rs or Rs) in V6 was the second most common waveform (Figure 1) next to broad/notched/slurred R wave in this lead, seen in 40% of CAD and 26% of non-CAD patients. Though it is less frequent, low QRS voltage is more common in CAD patients. Ischemic ST-T changes were infrequently seen in the CAD group. Among all ECG variables assessed, none reached statistical significance except T wave inversion in V4, present in 13.5% in CAD and in none of the non-CAD patients ($p < 0.05$). Clinical assessment of those with T wave inversion in V4 revealed that those patients were indeed having acute coronary events at the time the ECGs were taken. Since acute ischemic ST-T changes were infrequently seen in the CAD group, the sensitivity and negative predictive value (NPV) were low though the specificity and positive predictive value (PPV) were relatively high (Table 2).

QRS-ST-T Morphology	CAD	Non-CAD	p Value
QRSd; ms	148 [142;154]*	140 [136; 150]	NS
Left axis deviation (-30° to -60°)	54%	42%	NS
QS in V1	62.5%	68%	NS
Low QRS voltage	11%	5%	NS
Poor R progression	86%	87%	NS
Broad/notched/slurred R wave in V6	60%	74%	NS
T wave inversion in V2-3	5%	0	NS
QRS in LAFB pattern	21%	24%	NS
T wave inversion in V4	13.5%	0	<0.05
ST elevation with inverted T wave	5%	0	NS
ST depression with upright T wave	16%	8%	NS

*Median [95% LCL; UCL]

Table 1. QRS-ST-T morphology in LBBB patients with and without CAD

ECG changes	Sensitivity	Specificity	PPV	NPV
T wave inversion in V2-3	30%	100%	100%	5.2%
T wave inversion in V4	32%	100%	100%	13.5%
ST elevation with inverted T wave	30%	100%	100%	5.2%
ST depression with upright T wave	31%	83%	93%	15.6%

PPV: positive predictive value; NPV: negative predictive value

Table 2. The predictive accuracy of CAD by presence of ischemic ST-T changes

3.2 QRSd-EF relationship

The median QRSd values (Table 1) in our study cohort were well above 120 ms, indicating all patients had complete LBBB. The EF values (0.35±0.15 vs 0.39±0.17, p=NS) were similar between CAD and non-CAD groups. Figures 2 A-B demonstrate that an increased QRSd was inversely related to EF in both the CAD (Slope=-0.36, R^2 = 0.1, correlation = -0.319, p<0.005) and the non-CAD groups (Slope = -0.52, R2 = 0.37, correlation = -0.61, p<0.001).

4. Discussion

CAD is one of the most common findings in patients with LBBB. Recognizing CAD-associated ECG changes is of clinical importance. Among all the criteria proposed, (Havelda, Sohi et al. 1982; Fesmire 1995; Sgarbossa, Pinski et al. 1996) the Sgarbossa criteria (Sgarbossa, Pinski et al. 1996) seem very promising with good predictive values reported by the investigators. Since it is mainly targeted at ST-T changes at an acute or sub-acute phase of myocardial infarction, when applied to identify both acute and chronic ischemia, a low sensitivity was reported (Shlipak, Lyons et al. 1999; Gunnarsson, Eriksson et al. 2001).

Our study examined ECG changes associated with acute coronary syndromes (ACS) as well as in patients with stable CAD. Consistent with previous studies, there were no QRS-ST-T pattern differences between the patients with and without CAD.

Regardless of etiology poor R wave progression is highly prevalent in our study cohort (Table 1, Figure 1).

This ECG wave pattern reflects the right ventricle to septum and to left ventricle activation sequence in LBBB. Reversal of this pattern has been used in evaluating the effectiveness of CRT.(Sweeney, van Bommel et al.) Although broad/notched/slurred R waves are predominant in V6, we found that RS morphology (rS, rs or Rs) is the second most common waveform in V6, seen in 40% of CAD patients and 26% of non-CAD patients with LBBB. rS in V6, is part of poor R progression and can be well explained by the right to left activation sequence. (Sweeney, van Bommel et al.)

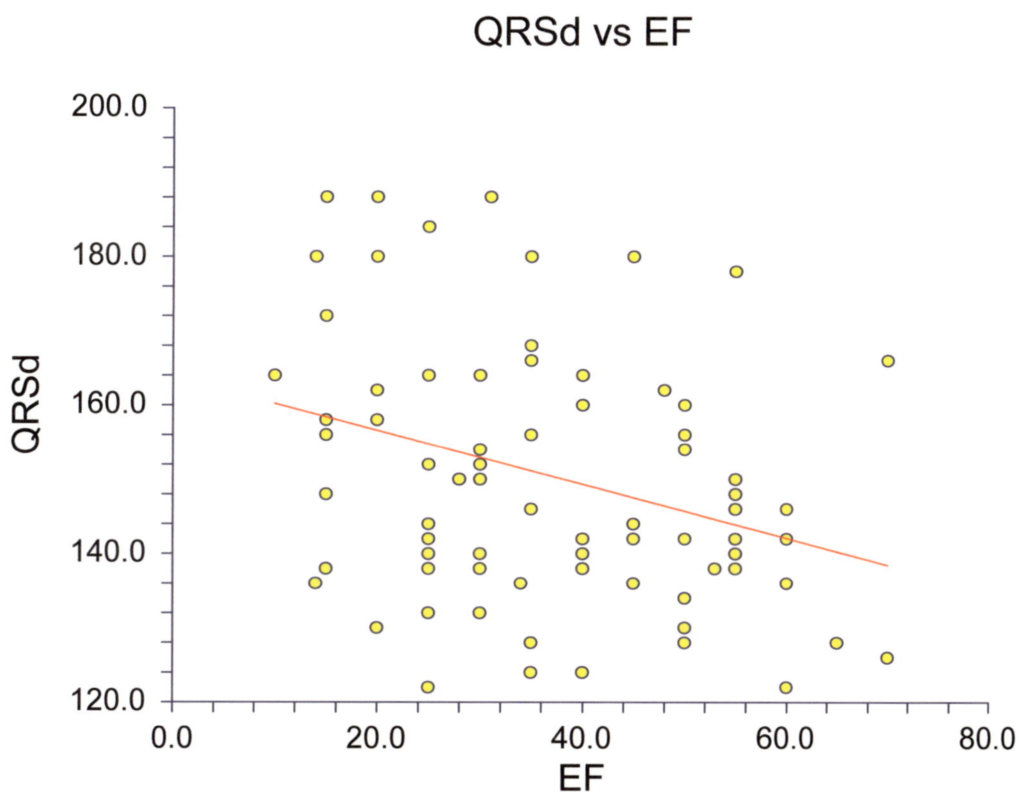

A. LBBB with CAD: QRSd = (164) + (-0.36) EF; the correlation between QRSd and EF is -0.32; the estimated slope is -0.36 [95% CI: -0.60 lower limit; -0.12 upper limit]; the estimated intercept is 164 [95% CI: 154 lower limit; 173 upper limit].

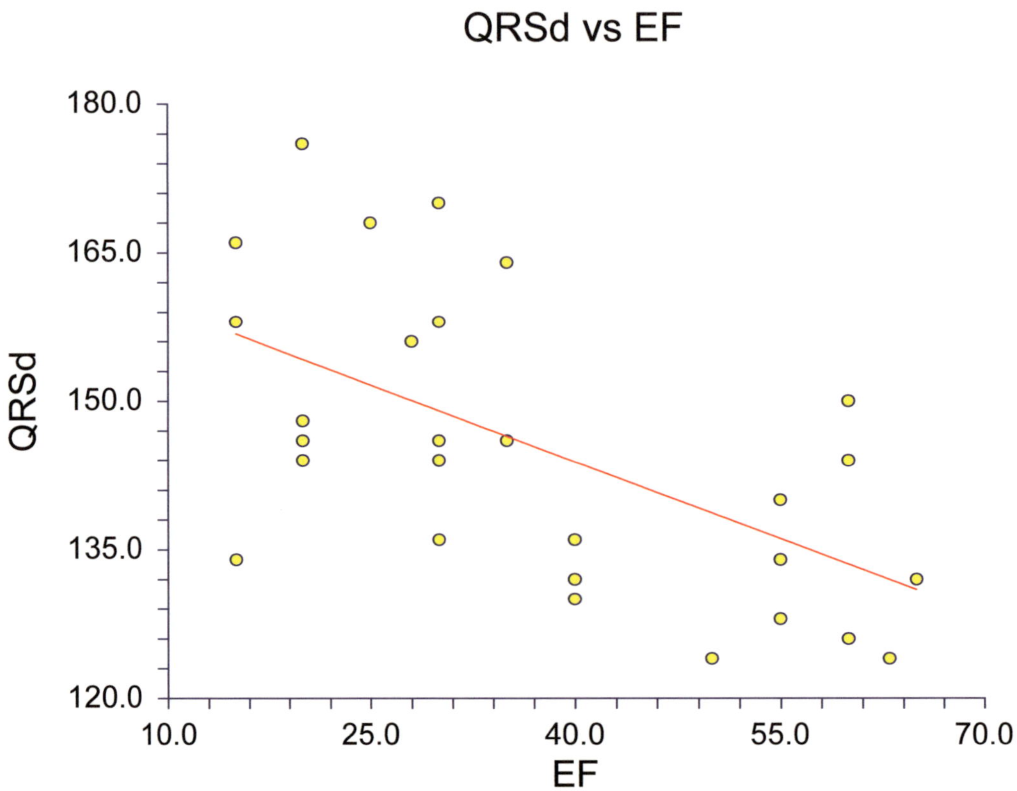

B. LBBB without CAD: QRSd = (164) + (-0.51) EF; the correlation between QRSd and EF is -0.31; the estimated slope is -0.51 [95% CI: -0.77 lower limit; -0.36 upper limit]; the estimated intercept is 164 [95% CI: 154 lower limit; 175 upper limit].

Fig. 2. QRSd-EF relationship in LBBB patients with and without CAD.

Depending on the blocking sites LBBB can be divided into pre-divisional, divisional and intramural subtypes.(Runge, Dorner et al. 1973; Jazayeri, Caceres et al. 1989; Childers, Lupovich et al. 2000) Pre-divisional block is at the level of left bundle trunk, divisional is at fascicular level and intramural at the intramyocardial Purkinje network. The lower level block is often associated with myocardial involvement and worse prognosis. In our study cohort, 21% of CAD and 24% non-CAD patients had LAFB ECG pattern, indicating the presence of divisional LBBB with complete blockage at LAF and partial blockage at left posterior fascicular branch level. Together they account for 42.6% of LBBB patients with leftward QRS axis.

Ischemic ST-T changes were only seen in patients with ACS. Since the majority of CAD patients do not have ACS at the time ECGs are taken, the sensitivity and negative predictive value (NPV) are low though the specificity and positive predictive value (PPV) are high (Table 2).

The second part of this study examined the correlation between QRS duration and LVEF in LBBB patients with and without CAD. LBBB patients are more predisposed to having LV systolic dysfunction.(Littmann and Symanski 2000; Talreja, Gruver et al. 2000) LBBB patients also have a higher mortality(Huvelle, Fay et al.) when compared to patients who also have LV systolic dysfunction without LBBB.(Abdel-Qadir, Tu et al.) This in part can be attributed to the higher than normal incidence of CAD, hypertension, cardiomyopathy and valvular heart disease in patients with LBBB.(Abdel-Qadir, Tu et al.) These co-morbidities may be responsible for the LBBB itself. However, LBBB results in alteration of both the systolic and diastolic properties of the LV. The alterations in the diastolic filling time and septal wall motion cause both systolic and diastolic dysfunction (Grines, Bashore et al. 1989), therefore reduce the global cardiac performance. This effect, as shown in this study, is possibly exaggerated by and is positively proportional to the QRS duration. Moreover, we demonstrated that the negative correlation between QRS duration and LVEF is present in both patients with and without CAD, further proof of the negative outcome independently caused by LBBB.

5. Conclusions

Other than acute ischemic ST-T changes seen in patients with ACS, the overall LBBB morphology is not different in patients with and without CAD. Increased QRS duration in LBBB has a significant negative correlation with LVEF in both CAD and non-CAD patients.

6. Acknowledgement

Dr. Li Zhang is supported by William Wikoff Smith Charitable Trust and AHA 0735474N.

7. References

Abdel-Qadir, H. M., J. V. Tu, et al. "Bundle branch block patterns and long-term outcomes in heart failure." Int J Cardiol 146(2): 213-8.

Childers, R., S. Lupovich, et al. (2000). "Left bundle branch block and right axis deviation: a report of 36 cases." J Electrocardiol 33 Suppl: 93-102.

Eriksson, P., P. O. Hansson, et al. (1998). "Bundle-branch block in a general male population: the study of men born 1913." Circulation 98(22): 2494-500.

Fesmire, F. M. (1995). "ECG diagnosis of acute myocardial infarction in the presence of left bundle-branch block in patients undergoing continuous ECG monitoring." Ann Emerg Med 26(1): 69-82.

Grines, C. L., T. M. Bashore, et al. (1989). "Functional abnormalities in isolated left bundle branch block. The effect of interventricular asynchrony." Circulation 79(4): 845-53.

Gunnarsson, G., P. Eriksson, et al. (2001). "ECG criteria in diagnosis of acute myocardial infarction in the presence of left bundle branch block." Int J Cardiol 78(2): 167-74.

Havelda, C. J., G. S. Sohi, et al. (1982). "The pathologic correlates of the electrocardiogram: complete left bundle branch block." Circulation 65(3): 445-51.

Hayat, S. A., G. Dwivedi, et al. (2008). "Effects of left bundle-branch block on cardiac structure, function, perfusion, and perfusion reserve: implications for myocardial contrast echocardiography versus radionuclide perfusion imaging for the detection of coronary artery disease." Circulation 117(14): 1832-41.

Huvelle, E., R. Fay, et al. "Left bundle branch block and mortality in patients with acute heart failure syndrome: a substudy of the EFICA cohort." Eur J Heart Fail 12(2): 156-63.

Jain, A. C. and M. C. Mehta (2003). "Etiologies of left bundle branch block and correlations with hemodynamic and angiographic findings." Am J Cardiol 91(11): 1375-8.

Jazayeri, M. R., J. Caceres, et al. (1989). "Electrophysiologic characteristics of sudden QRS axis deviation during orthodromic tachycardia. Role of functional fascicular block in localization of accessory pathway." J Clin Invest 83(3): 952-9.

Littmann, L. and J. D. Symanski (2000). "Hemodynamic implications of left bundle branch block." J Electrocardiol 33 Suppl: 115-21.

Nisse, B. S. (1929). "Congenital Heart Disease associated with Arborization Block of the Left Branch Bundle." Proc R Soc Med 22(4): 405-6.

Roshan, J., P. K. Pati, et al. (2008). "Echocardiographic evaluation of ventricular dyssynchrony in patients with left bundle branch block." Indian Heart J 60(6): 567-73.

Runge, M., V. Dorner, et al. (1973). "[Predivisional left bundle-branch block with left anterior hemiblock]." Z Kardiol 62(11): 1004-12.

Sgarbossa, E. B., S. L. Pinski, et al. (1996). "Electrocardiographic diagnosis of evolving acute myocardial infarction in the presence of left bundle-branch block. GUSTO-1 (Global Utilization of Streptokinase and Tissue Plasminogen Activator for Occluded Coronary Arteries) Investigators." N Engl J Med 334(8): 481-7.

Shlipak, M. G., W. L. Lyons, et al. (1999). "Should the electrocardiogram be used to guide therapy for patients with left bundle-branch block and suspected myocardial infarction?" JAMA 281(8): 714-9.

Strauss, D. G., R. H. Selvester, et al. "Defining left bundle branch block in the era of cardiac resynchronization therapy." Am J Cardiol 107(6): 927-34.

Sweeney, M. O., R. J. van Bommel, et al. "Analysis of ventricular activation using surface electrocardiography to predict left ventricular reverse volumetric remodeling during cardiac resynchronization therapy." Circulation 121(5): 626-34.

Talreja, D., C. Gruver, et al. (2000). "Efficient utilization of echocardiography for the assessment of left ventricular systolic function." Am Heart J 139(3): 394-8.

6

Characterization of Repolarization Alternans in the Coronary Artery Disease

Laura Burattini and Roberto Burattini
Department of Information Engineering, Polytechnic University of Marche, Ancona, Italy

1. Introduction

Repolarization alternans (RA), an electrophysiologic phenomenon consisting on every-other-beat changes of the repolarization morphology (amplitude, shape, and, sometimes, polarity) unaccompanied by gross changes in the heart-cycle length, is generally recognized as a promising electrocardiographic (ECG) predictor of sudden cardiac arrest (SCA; Bloomfield et al., 2006, Chow et al. 2006, Ikeda et al., 2006, Klingenheben et al., 2000, Leino et al., 2009, Maeda et al., 2009, Narayan, 2006, Rosenbaum et al., 1994, Sakaki et al., 2009, Salerno-Uriarte et al., 2007, Stein et al., 2008), that is one of the leading causes of death in developed countries (over 300,000 lives per year in the U.S.; Montagnana at al., 2008, Zheng et al., 2001). On the ECG tracing, RA consists of an alternation of either the ST-segment (Nearing et al., 1991, Rosenbaum et al., 1994), or the T-wave, or even the U-wave (Habbab & el-Sherif, 1992). Macroscopic and, thus, visible RA (like that reported in Fig. 1) is quite rare. After being first reported by Hering in the early 1900s (Hering, 1909), RA has later on been occasionally observed in patients affected by various diseases, among which ischemia (Kleinfeld & Rozanski, 1977), long QT syndrome (Schwartz & Malliani, 1975, Zareba et al., 1994) and ventricular arrhythmias (Verrier et al., 2003). Recent investigations on RA rely on automatic detection of microvolt RA from the digital ECG signal by means of specifically designed techniques, among which the spectral method (implemented in the commercial ECG machine CH2000 and Heartwave, Cambridge Heart Inc., Bedford, MA; Smith et al., 1988, Rosenbaum et al., 1994, Rosenbaum et al., 1996), the complex demodulation method (Nearing et al., 1991, Nearing & Verrier, 1993), the modified moving average method (implemented in the commercial ECG machine CASE-8000, GE Medical Systems, Milwaukee, WI; Nearing & Verrier, 2002), the Laplacian likelihood ratio method (Martínez & Olmos, 2005, Martínez et al., 2006), our adaptive match filter method (Burattini et al., 2008, Burattini et al., 2009b) and others (Burattini et al., 1999, Martínez & Olmos, 2005). Microvolt RA has been found to be much more common than visible RA (Adachi et al., 1999, Chow et al., 2007, Ikeda et al., 2006, Klingenheben et al., 2000, Narayan et al., 2006, Narayan et al., 2007, Reddy et al., 1984) and linked to inducible (Narayan and Smith, 2000, Rosenbaum et al., 1994, Smith et al., 1988) as well as spontaneous (Bloomfield et al., 2006, Klingenheben et al., 2000, Maeda et al., 2009, Narayan, 2006, Verrier et al., 2003) ventricular arrhythmias.

The pathophysiology underlying microvolt RA in humans has not been delineated yet. Several experimental settings have shown that RA may reflect spatial (Banville & Gray, 2002, Chinushi et al., 1998, Narayan, 2006) or temporal (Narayan, 2006, Pastore et al., 1999) dispersion of repolarization, both preceding ventricular fibrillation (Weiss et al., 1999, Smith & Cohen, 1984). Indeed, spatial variations in repolarization (action potential duration, APD) or conduction velocity may prevent depolarization in myocytes that are still repolarizing from their last cycle, causing the typical 2:1 behavior (Banville & Gray, 2002, Chinushi et al., 1998). RA may also results from an alternation of the APD (temporal dispersion of repolarization), which can occur when the relationship of the APD to its preceding diastolic interval (i.e. the APD restitution curve) has a slope greater than one. Under these conditions, mainly occurring in the presence of fast heart rates, small changes of the diastolic interval may cause large APD fluctuations that facilitate alternans (Pastore et al., 1999).

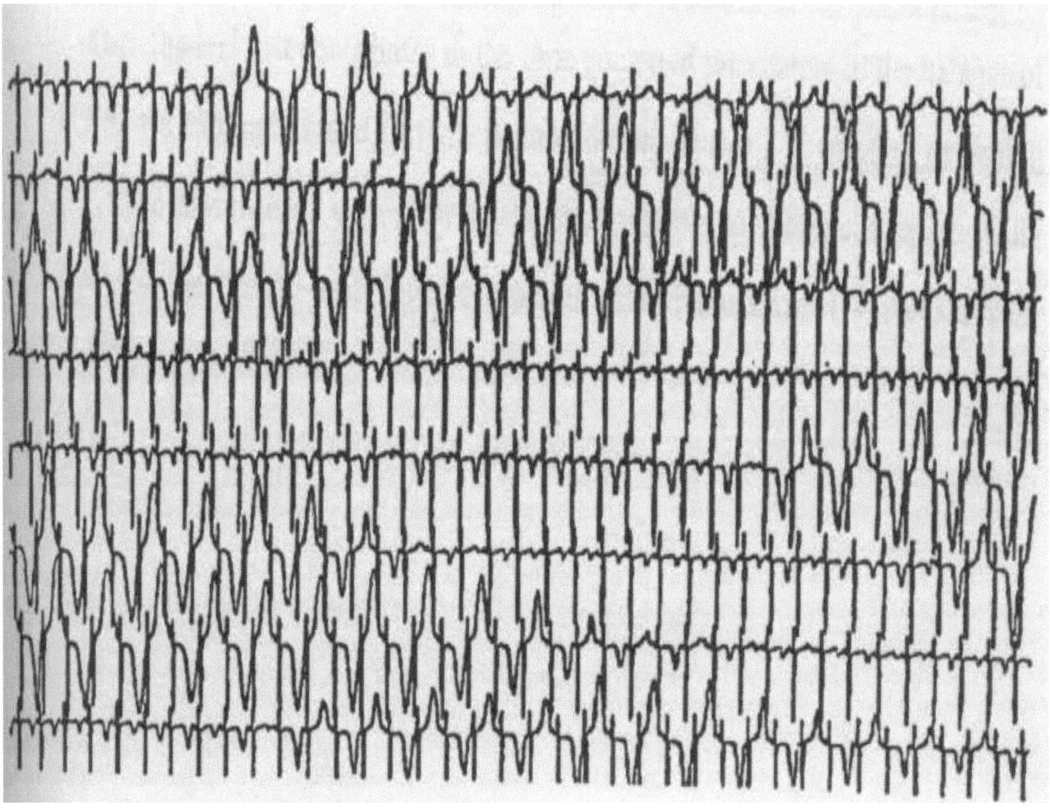

Fig. 1. ECG tracing affected by macroscopic RA.

Alternans derived from the cardiac spatial and temporal dispersion of repolarization projects onto body-surface ECG RA, which shows (Selvaraj et al., 2007) an heterogeneous temporal location along the JT segment, constituted by the ST-segment and T-wave complex. Characterization of this heterogeneity is a matter of major interest, since controversial results have been reported after attempting to identify an association of RA to different diseases. According to Narayan & Smith (Narayan & Smith, 1999) RA has been found to be more specific for inducible ventricular tachycardia when distributed late, rather than elsewhere, throughout the JT segment. In other studies (Martínez et al., 2006, Nearing et al., 1994) RA has been found to be located within the ST segment and the first half of the T wave in patients undergoing left anterior descending artery occlusion (LAD) and left circumflex artery occlusion (LCX), and to occur a little further on along the JT segment in patients undergoing right coronary artery occlusion (RCA). Eventually, RA heterogeneity along the entire JT segment has been observed in patients with cardiomyopathy (Selvaraj et al., 2007). To the best of our knowledge, quantitative investigations on RA location along the repolarization segment in the coronary artery disease have not been reported yet. Such an investigation was the aim of the present study.

Considering that our adaptive match filter (AMF) based method has been successfully used in previous clinical (Burattini et al., 2008, Burattini et al., 2009a, Burattini et al., 2010) and simulation (Burattini et al., 2006, Burattini et al., 2009b, Burattini et al., 2011) studies for characterization of T-wave alternans (which can be considered a special case of RA limited to the T-wave), this method was applied in the present study to Holter ECGs recordings from coronary artery disease (CAD) patients and control healthy (CH) subjects in order to: A) automatically identify and quantitatively characterize RA in terms of both amplitude and location with respect to the T-wave apex; and B) define a physiological RA region which allows discrimination of abnormal (RA+) from normal RA cases.

2. Methods

2.1 Study populations and clinical data

Our clinical data belong to the Intercity Digital Electrocardiology Alliance (IDEAL) Study databases, available at the Telemetric and Holter ECG Warehouse database (http://thew-project.org). The IDEAL protocol was approved by the Research Subject Review Board of the University of Rochester (Rochester, NY) and the study was conducted following required rules for human subjects' research principles, according to the Declaration of Helsinki, as well as to Title 45, U.S. Code of Federal Regulations, Part 46, Protection of Human Subjects, Revised November 13, 2001, effective December 13, 2001.

Two populations were considered, which consist of 201 coronary artery disease (CAD; 166 men) patients and 167 control-healthy (CH; 86 men) subjects, respectively. Namely, a patient was classified as belonging to the CAD-group if:

1. having positive angiogram (at least one vessel with critical narrowing >75%) with either exercise induced ischemia on ECG or evidence of previous myocardial infarction;
2. being in stable phase of the ischemic heart disease with digital ECG recordings performed on an outpatients basis. Stable post-MI patients should be enrolled at least 2 month after the index event;
3. not having evidence of congenital heart failure. Patients with clinical or echocardiographic evidence for congestive heart failure (LVD >60 mm, EF <40%) were excluded;
4. being in sinus rhythm (no atrial flutter/fibrillation, no pacemaker rhythm, no atrioventricular block, no sick sinus syndrome);
5. not having dilated cardiomyopathy (left ventricular diameter >60 mm and ejection fraction <40%);
6. not having coronary instability (unstable angina requiring hospitalization with evolving ischemic changes in standard ECG);

7. not having congestive heart failure (left ventricular diameter >60 mm and ejection fraction <40%);
8. not having had coronary artery bypass surgery (CABG) in the past. Patients with a history of non-CABG coronary revascularization (percutaneous transluminal coronary angioplasty, stent, atherectomy) were eligible to be enrolled;
9. not having major comorbidity such as malignancy, severe haptic, renal or cerebral disease.

Instead, a subject was classified as belonging to the CH-group when fulfilling the following criteria:

1. not having overt cardiovascular disease or history of cardiovascular disorders (including stroke, transient ischemic attack, and peripheral vascular disease);
2. no having history of high blood pressure (>150/90 mmHg);
3. not taking medication;
4. not being affected by other chronic illness (e.g. diabetes, asthma, chronic obstructive pulmonary disease, etc.);
5. being diagnosed as being healthy if evaluated by a physician for cardiovascular-related syndrome (chest pain, palpitation, syncope);
6. having normal physical examination;
7. having sinus rhythm in 12-lead ECG without any suspicious abnormalities (e.g. signs of ventricular hypertrophy, inverted T-wave, intraventricular conduction disturbances);
8. having normal echo and normal ECG exercise testing in presence of suspicious ECG changes;
9. not being pregnant.

Clinical parameters such as age, body max index (BMI), systolic (SAP) and diastolic (DAP) arterial pressure were measured in each subject, whereas the ventricular ejection fraction (LVEF, in %) was determined only for the CAD patients. Therapeutic treatments were also reported. In addition, a 20-minute, 3-lead (pseudo-orthogonal configuration, with bipolar leads X, Y, Z corresponding to limb lead I, augmented limb lead aVF, and precordial lead V3, respectively) digital Holter ECG recording was obtained from each individual in supine and resting conditions, making use of Burdick recorders (Burdick Inc., Milton, WI; sampling frequency: 200 Hz, resolution: 10 μV). ECG tracings were used to determine the heart rate (mRR; computed as the mean time interval RR between two consecutive sinus beats in a 5-min window) and heart-rate variability (sdRR; determined as the standard deviation of the RR intervals in a 5-min window) as well as RA parameters (see below).

2.2 RA identification and characterization

Repolarization alternans (RA) was identified in the first 5 minutes of each ECG recording. More specifically, ECG segments consisting of 16 consecutive heart beats were recursively (every 2 s) submitted to a preprocessing stage performing noise removal, R-peak detection, baseline removal and identification, and replacement of ectopic or noisy beats (Burattini et al., 2006, Martínez. & Olmos, 2005), before being processed by our heart-rate adaptive match filter for RA identification (see below). Only 16-beat ECG strings characterized by a stable heart rate (RR-interval standard deviation less than 10% mean RR interval) and by the presence of a low level of noise or ectopic beats (no more than 1 replaced beats in each ECG string) were considered eligible for the subsequent RA analysis.

In the presence of a fixed heart rate (and, thus, of a constant time-interval RR between two consecutive sinus beats) RA is, by definition, characterized by a specific frequency of half heart rate: f_{RA}=0.5 cycles per beat, or f_{RA}= 1/(2×RR) Hz. In clinical cases in which heart rate may be considered stable but presenting some physiological variation, the RA phenomenon is assumed to be characterized by a narrow frequency band, 2×df_{RA} wide, centered around f_{RA}= 1/(2×meanRR) (Fig. 2; Burattini et al., 2006, Burattini et al., 2008, Burattini et al., 2009a, Burattini et al., 2010). On this basis, our AMF is designed as a pass-band filter with its passing band centered in f_{RA} (Burattini et al., 2006, Burattini et al., 2008).

Technically, the AMF is implemented as a 6th order bidirectional Butterworth band-pass filter having the passing band 0.12 Hz wide (i.e. df_{RA}=0.06 Hz) and centered at a frequency that adapts to mean RR interval. More specifically, our AMF is a cascade of a low-pass filter (LPF) with cut-off frequency f_{LPF}= f_{RA}+ df_{RA}, and a high-pass filter (HPF) with a cut-off frequency f_{HPF}= f_{RA}-df_{RA}. The squared module of the AMF transfer function is expressed by the following equation:

$$|H_{AMF}(f)|^2 = |H_{LPF}(f)|^2 \cdot |H_{HPF}(f)|^2 == \frac{1}{1+\left(\frac{f}{f_{LPF}}\right)^6} \cdot \frac{\left(\frac{f}{f_{HPF}}\right)^6}{1+\left(\frac{f}{f_{HPF}}\right)^6} \qquad (1)$$

Being the AMF applied in a bidirectional fashion, no group delay occurs. Thus, the AMF is expected to detect RA by filtering out noise as well as every other ECG component but the RA typical one.

The input signal of the AMF is the 16-beat ECG tracing over which f_{RA} has been computed. In the absence of RA, the output of the AMF, called RA signal (Fig. 2), is a zero constant signal. Instead, in the presence of RA, the RA signal is a sinusoidal signal, possibly amplitude-modulated, characterized by the same length of the ECG and by a frequency equal to f_{RA}.

The time occurrences of the sinusoid maxima or minima, which are expected to fall inside the JT intervals when pertaining to RA, provide the center of mass of the alternations in each beat, and, thus, a localization of the alternans inside the repolarization (Fig. 3). After having identified a reference point (T_{ref}), inside the repolarization segment, as the T-wave apex for monophasic T waves, or as the amplitude-weighted mean point between T apexes for biphasic T waves, an RA delay (RAD, in ms) parameter was computed, for each beat, as the difference between the instant at which T_{ref} occurs and the instant at which the sinusoidal RA signal maximum or minimum occurs. Thus, a negative RAD value indicates the presence of early repolarization, which mostly involves the ST segment or the first half of the T wave. Instead, an RAD value close to zero indicates the presence of central RA, which mostly occurs over the T-wave apex. Eventually, a positive RAD value indicates the presence of late RA, characterized by the alternation of the final portion of the T wave. Within the same beat, the amplitude value of the sinusoidal RA signal provides an estimate of the RA amplitude (RAA, in μV).

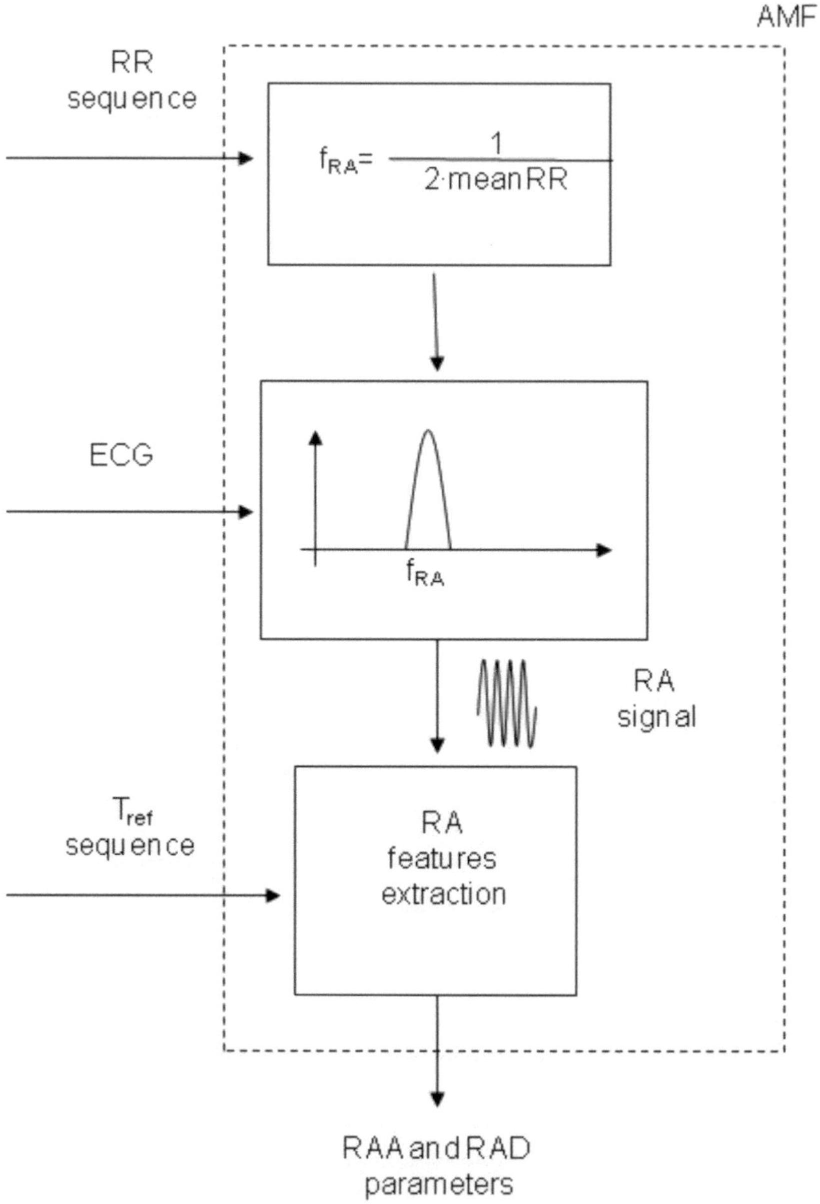

Fig. 2. Block diagram describing the AMF-based procedure for characterization of RA in terms of RAA and RAD parameters.

In the present study, RA analysis was initially performed in each ECG lead as follows. RAD and RAA values were first averaged over the 16 beats of each single-lead ECG segment (M16b_RAD_X and M16b_RAA_X, M16b_RAD_Y and M16b_RAA_Y, and M16b_RAD_Z and M16b_RAA_Z for leads X, Y, and Z, respectively); the resulting values were then averaged over the entire 5 minutes of each single-lead recording (M5m_RAD_X and

M5m_RAA_X, M5m_RAD_Y and M5m_RAA_Y, and M5m_RAD_Z and M5m_RAA_Z for leads X, Y, and Z, respectively). Eventually, the latter values were averaged over the three leads (M5m_RAD and M5m_RAA) for a comprehensive RA characterization relative to a single patient.

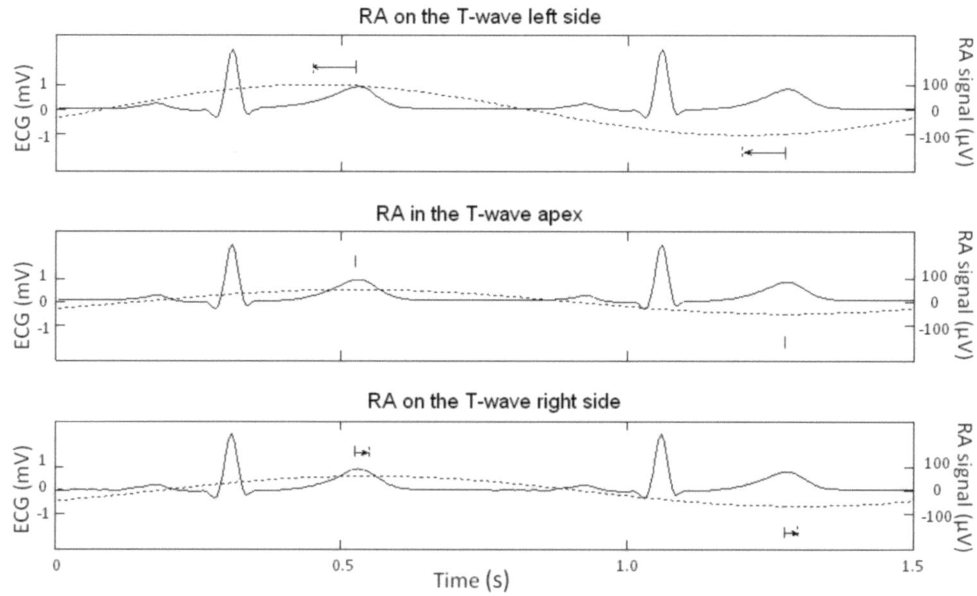

Fig. 3. Simulated ECG tracing (solid lines) and relative RA signal (dotted lines) at the output of the heart-rate adaptive match filter (AMF) in the presence of early (panel A), central (panel B), and late (panel C) repolarization alternans.

2.3 Definition of an RA normality region

The M5m_RAD and M5m_RAA distributions over the CH population were used to identify an RA normality region delimited by three thresholds. Two of them (THR_RADmin and THR_RADmax) were defined for the M5m_RAD parameter as the 0.5th and the 99.5th percentiles of the M5m_RAD distribution, respectively. The third one (THR_RAA) was defined for the non-negative M5m_RAA parameter as the 99.5th percentile of the M5m_RAA distribution. A subject, independently of the belonging population, was classified as characterized by normal RA levels if the following conditions were simultaneously satisfied:

$$\begin{cases} M5m\_RAD \geq THR\_RAD\min \\ M5m\_RAD \leq THR\_RAD\max \\ M5m\_RAA \leq THR\_RAA \end{cases} \quad (2)$$

These conditions define a physiologic RA region in the M5m_RAD vs. M5m_RAA plane (Fig. 4). Thus, no satisfaction of at least one condition denotes an abnormal RA case (RA+).

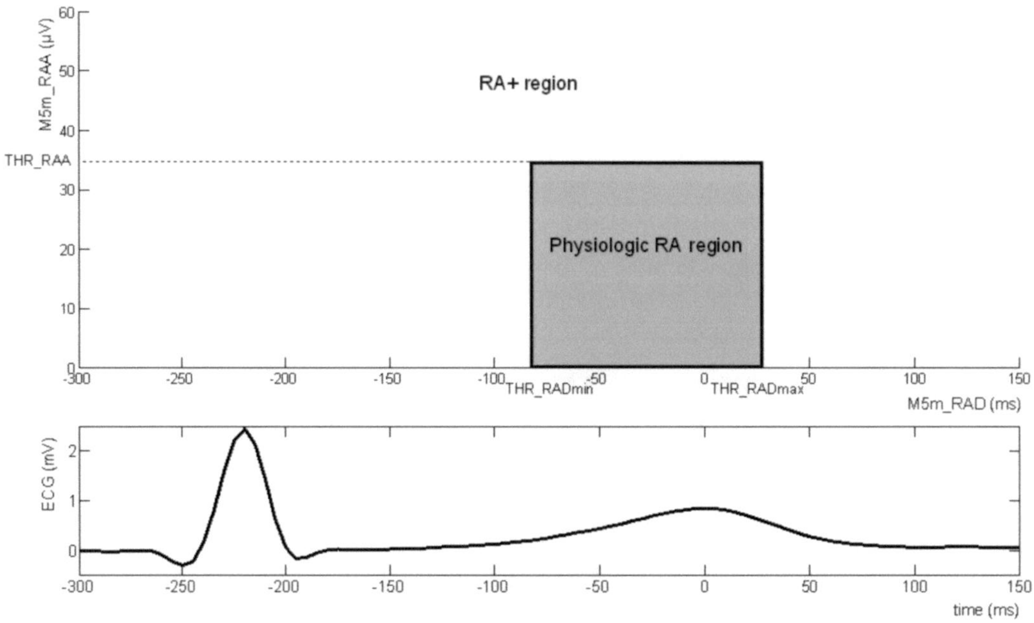

Fig. 4. Definition of a physiologic RA region in the M5m_RAD vs. M5m_RAA plane (shaded area in the upper panel). RA cases falling outside the physiologic RA region are considered abnormal RA cases (RA+). The ECG beat in the lower panel shows RA location along the JT interval.

2.4 Statistics

To be independent of normal distributions, non-parametric tests were used to perform comparisons among quantities. In the specific, comparisons between the distributions of the clinical and ECG parameters over the two populations (CAD vs. CH) were performed using the Wilcoxon rank sum test for equal medians. The Kruskal-Wallis test was used to perform the one-way ANOVA test to evaluate if, in a population, the RA parameters distributions over the three ECG leads were characterized by the same median value. Information about which pairs of leads had different median values was obtained using the multiple comparison procedure. The χ^2 test was used to compare number of treated subjects between the two populations. Eventually, the existence of a possible relationship of the RA parameters with the clinical or the other ECG parameters was evaluated computing the correlation coefficient ρ. Statistical significance level was set at 5%.

3. Results

A summary of the clinical and ECG parameter values characterizing the CAD and the CH populations are reported in Table 1, where pharmaceutical treatments are also specified. Compared to the CH subjects, the CAD patients were significantly older and characterized by significantly higher BMI, SAP, and DAP, and by significantly lower heart rate (longer mRR) and heart-rate variability (lower sdRR).

	CAD patients (201)	CH subjects (167)	P value
Clinical parameters:			
Age (years)	58±11	38±15	$<10^{-32}$
BMI (kg/m²)	27±4	24±5	$<10^{-13}$
SAP (mmHg)	129±18	118±12	$<10^{-11}$
DAP (mmHg)	79±10	75±8	$<10^{-3}$
LVEF	58±11	NA	-
Treatments:			
Beta blocker	150	0	<0.005
Digoxin	0	0	NS
Diuretic	11	0	<0.01
ACE inhibitor	57	0	<0.005
Antiarrhythmic	6	0	NS
ECG parameters:			
mRR (ms)	960±155	904±140	$<10^{-3}$
sdRR (ms)	37±40	43±24	$<10^{-6}$
M5m_RAD_X (ms)	-29±52	-25±29	NS
M5m_RAA_X (μV)	17±10	15±5	NS
M5m_RAD_Y (ms)	-34±51	-24±30	NS
M5m_RAA_Y (μV)	21±12	20±8	NS
M5m_RAD_Z (ms)	-38±44	-32±31	NS
M5m_RAA_Z (μV)	18±9	15±5	$<10^{-3}$
M5m_RAD(ms)	-33±37	-27±23	NS
M5m_RAA (μV)	19±9	17±15	<0.05

Table 1. Clinical parameters, therapeutic treatments and ECG parameters relative to the CAD patients and the CH subjects. NA: not available; - : not applicable; NS: not significant.

Some levels of RA were detected in all 201 CAD patients and 167 CH subjects. In both populations, RA amplitude values were significantly greater in lead Y (CAD: M5m_RAA_Y=21±12 μV; CH: M5m_RAA_Y=20±8 μV) than in leads X and Z (CAD: M5m_RAA_X=17±10 μV, M5m_RAA_Z=18±9 μV, $P<10^{-5}$; CH: M5m_RAA_X=15±5 μV, M5m_RAA_Z=15±5 μV, $P<10^{-9}$). Instead, comparable values of RA delay were measured over the leads in the CAD patients (M5m_RAD_X=-29±52 ms, M5m_RAD_Y=-34±51 ms, M5m_RAD_Z=-38±44 ms), while the CH subjects were characterized by a significantly lower RA delay value in lead Z (M5m_RAD_Z=-32±31 ms) compared to both lead X and Y (M5m_RAD_X=-25±29 ms, M5m_RAD_Y=-24±30 ms, P<0.01). Although RA amplitude appears systematically higher for the CAD patients than for the CH subjects in all leads, statistically significant differences were observed only in correspondence of lead Z (M5m_RAA_Z). No significant differences were found between the two populations in terms of RAD parameters, independently of the lead.

A comprehensive description of the RA phenomenon in the two populations was provided by M5m_RAA and M5m_RAD parameters. In the specific, the CAD population showed RA episodes characterized by higher amplitude (CAD M5m_RAA: 19±9 μV, CH M5m_RAA: 17±5 μV, $P<0.05$; Table 1) and comparable delay (CAD M5m_RAD: -33±37 μV, CH M5m_RAD: -27±23 μV; Table 1). Still, M5m_RAD and M5m_RAA standard deviation values (Table 1) as well as the their distribution histograms (Fig. 5) indicate a greater M5m_RAD and M5m_RAA variability among the CAD patients than the CH subjects. According to these results, RA is localized over the first half of the T wave in most cases of the CH population, and only occasionally overcomes the T-wave apex. Instead, among the CAD patients, RA is distributed along the entire repolarization segment (ST/T wave), with several cases occurring over the ST segment or over the T-wave right-hand side.

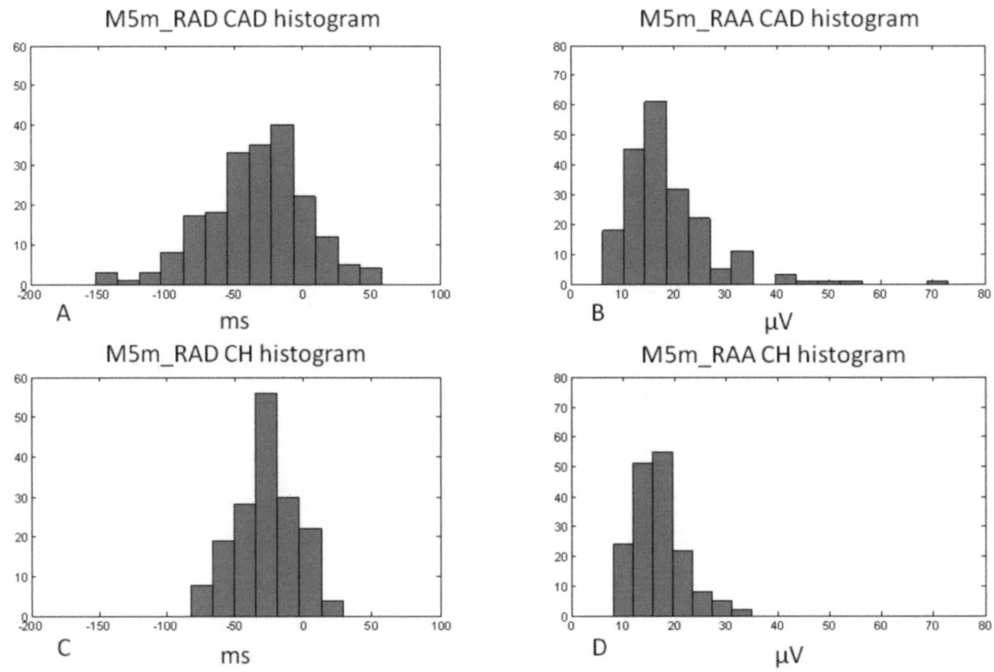

Fig. 5. Histograms of M5m_RAD and M5m_RAA distributions for the CAD (panels A and B) and CH (panels C and D) populations showing a greater M5m_RAD and M5m_RAA variability among the CAD patients than the CH subjects.

The definition of an RA normality region (Fig. 6) delimited by THR_RADmin=-82 ms, THR_RADmax=28 ms, and THR_RAA=35 μV (as defined in Methods) allowed the identification of 29 (14.4%) RA+ CAD patients with abnormal M5m_RAD. Specifically, 22 (10.9%) had abnormally low M5m_RAD (M5m_RAD <THR_RADmin) while the remaining 7 (3.5%) had abnormally high M5m_RAD (M5m_RAD >THR_RADmax). RA+ CAD patients characterized by abnormally high M5m_RAA (M5m_RAA >THR_RAA) were 11 (5.5%). Among these, 4 were also characterized by abnormally low M5m_RAD. Thus, altogether, 36 (17.9%) RA+ cases were identified among the CAD patients. By contrast, only 3 (1.8%) cases at the verge of abnormal condition were identified among the CH subjects (Fig. 6).

Correlative analysis showed that, in both CAD and CH populations, RA parameters distributions were not significantly linked to the other clinical and ECG ($|\rho|\leq 0.44$; Table 2) parameters distributions. Moreover, CAD patients under pharmaceutical treatments showed RA levels comparable to those characterizing not-treated patients (Table 3).

	CAD patients (201)		CH subjects (167)	
	M5m_RAD (ms)	M5m_RAA (μV)	M5m_RAD (ms)	M5m_RAA (μV)
Clinical parameters:				
Age (years)	0.11	-0.01	0.20*	-0.28*
BMI (kg/m²)	0.19*	-0.10	-0.09	-0.30*
SAP (mmHg)	0.11	-0.08	-0.06	-0.11
DAP (mmHg)	0.16*	-0.07	-0.11	-0.16*
LVEF	-0.17*	0.01	-	-
ECG parameters:				
mRR (ms)	-0.44*	0.29*	-0.42*	0.20*
sdRR (ms)	0.00	0.10	-0.35*	0.39*

Table 2. Correlation coefficient values linking RA parameters with the other clinical and ECG parameters. - : not applicable; *: statistically significant (P<0.05).

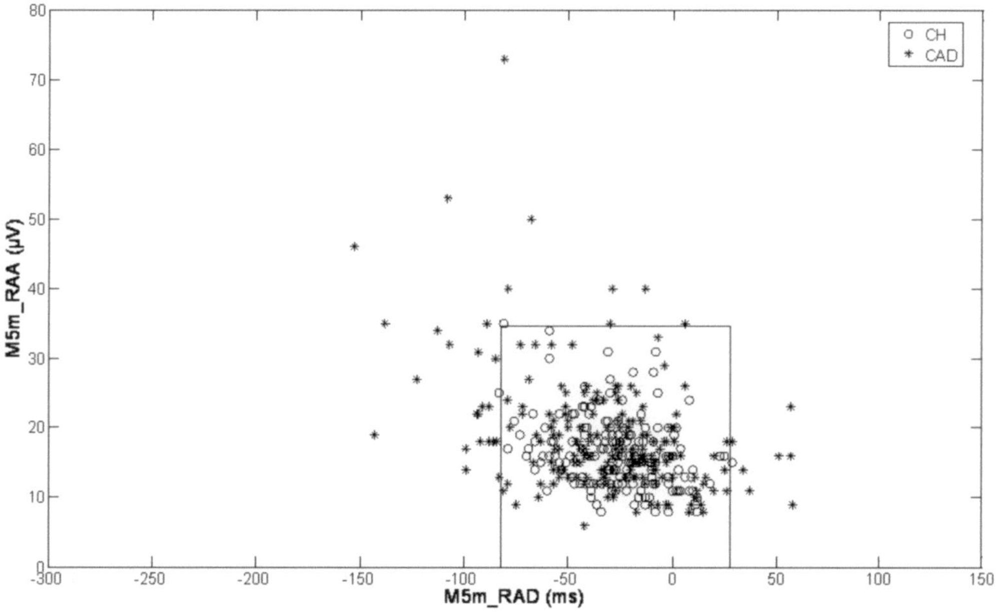

Fig. 6. Representation of the RA cases for CH subjects (o) and the CAD patients (*) in relation to the RA normality region (internal solid-line square) in the M5m_RAD vs. M5m_RAA plane.

	Beta blocker		Diuretic		ACE inhibitor		Anti-arrhythmic	
	Treated (N=150)	Not Treated (N=51)	Treated (N=11)	Not Treated (N=190)	Treated (N=57)	Not Treated (N=144)	Treated (N=6)	Not Treated (N=195)
Clinical parameters:								
Age (years)	58±10	59±12	65±11	58±11	59±10	58±11	54±13	58±11
BMI (kg/m^2)	27±4	27±4	28±5	27±3	27±3	27±4	29±3	27±4
SAP (mmHg)	130±18	127±16	130±14	129±18	134±21	127±16	133±14	129±18
DAP (mmHg)	80±10	76±10	76±9	79±10	81±12	78±9	82±12	79±10
LVEF	58±11	58±10	49±12*	59±10	58±12	58±10	51±11	58±10
ECG parameters:								
mRR (ms)	979±156*	903±137	924±158	962±155	943±143	967±159	865±122	963±155
sdRR (ms)	37±41	35±35	71±72	35±36	42±39	35±40	30±31	37±40
M5m_RAD (ms)	-34±39	-33±32	-19±41	-34±37	-30±31	-35±39	-13±23	-34±37
M5m_RAA (µV)	19±7	19±11	20±7	19±9	19±9	19±8	21±8	19±9

Table 3. Comparison of clinical and ECG parameteres between CAD patients under vs. not under pharmaceutical treatment. *: statistical signisficance (P<0.05) when comparing treated vs. not treated CAD patients groups.

4. Discussion

Our study represents the first attempt to quantify RA heterogeneity in the coronary artery disease (CAD) in terms of the traditional RA amplitude as it combines with a temporal parameter that allows RA localization along the JT segment as a delay from the T-wave apex. This characterization was accomplished by analyzing RA in 5-minute resting ECG recordings by means of our AMF-based technique, previously tested for T-wave alternans detection and quantification in both simulated and clinical settings (Burattini et al., 2006, Burattini et al., 2008, Burattini et al., 2009a, Burattini et al., 2009b, Burattini et al., 2010, Burattini et al., 2011).

Previous studies reported by others identified temporal RA localization in cases other than CAD, either by computing the time-interval from the R peak to the RA instant of occurrence (Martínez et al., 2006, Nearing et al., 1994, Selvaraj et al., 2007) or by identifying three windows of half JT duration (localized at the beginning, at the middle and at the end of repolarization, respectively) and, subsequently, determining which of these was more affected by RA (Narayan & Smith, 1999). The former approach has the major limitation of not taking into account the physiological variability of the RR interval and the JT duration, so that the same time interval localizing RA can be associated to different alternating portions of the JT segment. The latter approach tries to overcome this limitation by use of three windows half-overlapped. However, because of the large variability characterizing the ST segment in clinical cases, the middle window does not necessarily include the T-wave apex, as it is expected to do. Our AMF-based approach resolves these limitations by measuring the "delay" (RAD) of the alternans with respect to the T-wave apex, so that large negative values of RAD are necessarily due to RA occurring along the ST segment and the T-wave left-hand side. Instead, RAD values close to zero indicate the presence of RA mainly localized over the T wave, while positive values of RAD indicate alternation of the T-wave right-hand side. Since each portion of the JT segment pertains to a specific phase of the ventricular repolarization, our AMF-based method is expected to provide a more accurate identification of the ventricular repolarization phase involved in the alternation.

Besides RA heterogeneity characterization, our AMF-based method has the further peculiarity of relying on the RA continuity hypothesis. Other techniques, such as the spectral method, the RA identification technique most commonly used in clinics (Smith et al., 1988, Rosenbaum et al., 1994, Rosenbaum et al., 1996), and the Laplacian likelihood ratio method (Martínez & Olmos, 2005, Martínez et al., 2006) ascribe to noise the low-TWA levels, not associated with cardiac instability, which are even detected under physiological conditions. This methodological approach aroused from the early hypothesis that RA could be an on-off phenomenon, usually not present in health (Bloomfield et al., 2002). After the recent experimental study by Pruvot et al.(Pruvot et al., 2004) who demonstrated the possibility of inducing various levels of RA, some of which not necessarily associated to cardiac instability, the hypothesis that RA is a phenomenon characterized by a continuously changing amplitude and/or location from physiological to pathological condition has gained increasing consideration. This assumption requires the set up of methods, like our AMF-based one, that allow identification of an RA normality region to improve reliability in the discrimination of non-physiological or abnormal RA (RA+) levels potentially at risk of cardiac instability. In the present study the RA normality region was delimited by three thresholds (THR_RADmin, THR_RADmax, THR_RAA, respectively), computed from the

RA parameters distribution over the CH population (Burattini et al., 2008, Burattini et al., 2009a). More specifically, THR_RADmin and THR_RADmax were defined as the 0.5th and 99.5th percentiles of the M5m_RAD distribution, whereas one other threshold was defined as the 99.5th percentile over the THR_RAA distribution, being it a non-negative parameter. Use of percentiles, rather than mean and SD, makes the procedure independent of the assumption of normal distribution for parameter estimates. These threshold definitions strongly optimize specificity rather than sensitivity. The rationale for our choice is that, as mentioned above, RA was initially supposed not be present in healthy conditions (Bloomfield, 2002), so that the number of positive detections among healthy subjects was forced to be negligible (Burattini et al., 2008). Due to our recent studies highlighting the hypothesis that RA is a phenomenon characterized by an amplitude continuously changing from physiological to abnormal conditions (Burattini et al., 2009a, Burattini et al., 2010), identification of thresholds levels at 0.5th and 99.5th percentile may be too restrictive and, thus, not appropriate for an optimal identification of abnormal RA cases. Optimization of thresholds for RA+ identification in relation to risk stratification, however, is beyond the scope of this work, which is mainly focused on RA characterization in the coronary artery disease.

With this aim, our AMF-based technique was applied to ECG tracings from CAD patients, who, compared to CH subjects, are known to show increased levels of T-wave alternans (Bigger & Bloomfield, 2007, Bloomfield et al., 2006, Burattini et al., 2009a, Burattini et al., 2010, Ikeda et al., 2006, Zacks et al., 2007) and to be prone to experience major cardiac events related to it (Narayan et al., 2006). Our results indicate that, in agreement with what previously found (Burattini et al., 2008, Burattini et al., 2009a, Burattini et al., 2010), RA affects all subjects, either diseased or healthy, with different characteristics though. First of all, the CAD patients were, on average, characterized by higher RA amplitude than the CH subjects (CAD: 19±9 μV, CH: 17±15 μV; $P<0.05$). The most interesting results, however, concern the RA localization, which was distributed all over the entire JT segment (ST segment, or T-wave left-hand side, or T-wave right-hand side) in the CAD patients, whereas it occurred mainly over the T-wave left-hand side, and occasionally in correspondence of the T-wave apex, among the CH subjects. Similarly to our CAD patients, RA was found to be distributed all along the JT segment also in the cardiomyopathy (Selvaraj et al., 2007). In spite of the fact that our choice of the threshold values delimiting the RA normality region tends to minimize the number of RA+ cases, the greater RA heterogeneity observed in our CAD patients compared with CH subjects allowed discrimination of a relevant percentage (17.9%) of RA+ cases in the coronary artery disease (Fig. 6). In these abnormal cases RA was characterized by high amplitude (5.5%), as previously reported in other studies on the CAD (Narayan et al., 2006), or occurred either early (11.0%), as in other diseased states (Martínez et al., 2006, Nearing et al., 1994), or late (3.5%) along the JT segment. According to Narayan & Smith (1999), RA occurring late is mainly associated to ventricular tachycardia. Thus, the characterization of RA in terms of both RA amplitude (generally used to discriminate RA+ cases in most studies using other techniques) and RA delay (a parameters which instead is a peculiarity of our AMF-based method) allowed a significant increment in the identification of RA+ cases among the CAD patients, which raised from 11 (identified when using only the RA amplitude parameter) to 36.

According to our results, increased RA heterogeneity observed in the CAD population was not associated to other clinical factors (age, BMI, SAP, DAP and LVEF) or pharmaceutical treatments (beta blocker, digoxin, diuretic, and ACE inhibitor), with the only exception of heart rate. Indeed, a significant, though low ($-0.44 \leq \rho \leq -0.42$; $P<0.05$), correlation was found between M5m_RAD and RR in both populations, indicating that early RA tends to characterize patients with prolonged RR. Instead, a negligible correlation ($0.20 \leq \rho \leq 0.29$, $P<0.05$) was found between M5m_RAA and RR distributions. This result is complementary and not in contradiction with the findings from several other studies, which have previously related RA amplitude to hart rate (Bloomfield et al., 2002, Narayan & Smith, 1999, Narayan & Smith, 2000, Smith et al., 1988). Such studies have indeed demonstrated that, within a subject, RA increases when heart rate is forced to increase (by pacing, exercise or drug) over 90 beats/min (Bloomfield et al., 2002). Identification of RA at rest, as in the present study, was often neglected because it requires sophisticated RA identification methods, such as our AMF-based one (Burattini et al., 2011), suitable to detect low levels of RA even in the presence of physiological levels of heart-rate variability (heart-rate variability is indeed strongly reduced at high heart rates).

5. Conclusion

Our quantitative investigation of RA heterogeneity in CAD patients yields the conclusion that, compared to the CH subjects, the former population shows higher RA amplitude and greater variability of RA localization along the JT segment. Especially, in the coronary artery disease, the RA occurs not only over the left-hand side of the T wave, as it is generally observed in health, but also along the ST segment (early repolarization) or along the T-wave right-hand side (late repolarization). Identification of patients characterized by RA occurring in early or late repolarization is relevant since in the literature these kinds of RA phenomena are associated to an increased risk of ventricular arrhythmias. Thus, our AMF-based method appears as a useful tool to identify RA characteristics that help enhancing pathophysiological interpretation and, with it, the ability to discriminate patients at increased risk of sudden cardiac death, who might be appropriately treated before they experience a major cardiac event.

6. References

Adachi, K., Ohnishi, Y., Shima, T., Yamashiro, K., Takei, A., Tamura, N. & Yokoyama, M. (1999). Determinant of microvolt-level T-wave alternans in patients with dilated cardiomyopathy. *Journal of the American College of Cardiology,* Vol.34, No.2, (August 1999), pp. 374-380, ISSN 0735-1097.

Banville, I. & Gray, R.A. (2002). Effect of action potential duration and conduction velocity restitution and their spatial dispersion on alternans and the stability of arrhythmias. *Journal of Cardiovascular Electrophysiology,* Vol. 13, No.11, (November 2002), pp. 1141-1149, ISSN 1045-3873.

Bigger, J.T. & Bloomfield D.M. (2007). Microvolt T-wave alternans: An effective approach to risk stratification in ischemic cardiomyopathy? *Nature Clinical Practice Cardiovascular Medicine,* Vol. 4, No.6, (June 2007), pp. 300-301, ISSN 1743-4297.

Bloomfield, D.M., Hohnloser, S.H. & Cohen, R.J. (2002). Interpretation and classification of microvolt T wave alternans tests. *Journal of Cardiovascular Electrophysiology*, Vol.13, No.5 (May 2002), pp.502-512, ISSN 1045-3873.

Bloomfield, D.M., Bigger, J.T., Steinman, R.C., Namerow, P.B., Parides, M.K., Curtis, A.B., Kaufman, E.S., Davidenko, J.M., Shinn, T.S. & Fontaine, J.M. (2006). Microvolt T-wave alternans and the risk of death or sustained ventricular arrhythmias in patients with left ventricular dysfunction. *Journal of the American College of Cardiology*, Vol.47, No.2, (January 2006), pp. 456-463, ISSN 0735-1097.

Burattini, L., Zareba, W. & Moss, A.J. (1999). Correlation method for detection of transient T-wave alternans in digital Holter ECG recordings. *Annals of Noninvasive Electrocardiology*, Vol. 4, No.4, (October, 1999), pp. 416-424, ISSN 1082-720X.

Burattini, L., Zareba, W. & Burattini, R. (2006). Automatic detection of microvolt T-wave alternans in Holter recordings: Effect of baseline wandering. *Biomedical Signal Processing and Control*, Vol.1, (2006), pp.162-168, ISSN 1746-8094.

Burattini, L., Zareba, W. & Burattini, R. (2008). Adaptive match filter based method for time vs. amplitude characterization of microvolt ECG T-wave alternans. *Annals of Biomedical Engineering*, Vol.36, No.9, (September 2008), pp. 1558-1564, ISSB 0090-6964.

Burattini, L., Zareba, W. & Burattini, R. (2009a). Assessment of physiological amplitude, duration and magnitude of ECG T-wave alternans. *Annals of Noninvasive Electrocardiology*, Vol.14, No.4, (October 2009), pp. 366-374, ISSN 1082-720X.

Burattini, L., Bini, S. & Burattini, R. (2009b). Comparative analysis of methods for automatic detection and quantification of microvolt T-wave alternans. *Medical Engineering & Physics*, Vol. 31, No.10, (December 2009), pp. 1290-1298, ISSN 1350-4533.

Burattini, L., Zareba, W. & Burattini, R. (2010). Identification of gender-related normality regions for T-wave alternans. *Annals of Noninvasive Electrocardiology*, Vol.15, No.4, (October 2010), pp. 328-336, ISSN 1082-720X.

Burattini, L., Bini, S. & Burattini, R. (2011). Automatic microvolt T-wave alternans identification in relation to ECG interferences surviving preprocessing. *Medical Engineering & Physics*, Vol.33, No.1, (January 2011), pp. 17-30, ISSN 1350-4533.

Chinushi, M., Restivo, M., Caref, E.B. & El-Sherif, N. (1998). Electrophysiological basis of arrhythmogenicity of QT/T alternans in the long-QT syndrome: tridimensional analysis of the kinetics of cardiac repolarization. *Circulation Research*, Vol.83, No.6, (September 1998), pp. 614-628, ISSN 0009-7330.

Chow, T., Kereiakes, D.J., Bartone, C., Booth, T., Schloss, E.J., Waller, T., Chung, E.S., Menon, S., Nallamothu, B.K. & Chan, P.S. (2006). Prognostic utility of microvolt T-wave alternans in risk stratification of patients with ischemic cardiomyopathy. *Journal of the American College of Cardiology*, Vol.47, No.9, (May 2006), pp. 1820-1827, ISSN 0735-1097.

Chow, T., Kereiakes, D.J., Bartone, C., Booth, T., Schloss, E.J., Waller, T., Chung, E., Menon, S., Nallamothu, B.K. & Chan, P.S. (2007). Microvolt T-wave alternans identifies patients with ischemic cardiomyopathy who benefit from implantable cardioverter-defibrillator therapy. *Journal of the American College of Cardiology*, Vol.49, No.1, (January 2007), pp.50-58, ISSN 0735-1097.

Habbab, M.A. & El-Sherif N. (1992). TU alternans, long QTU, and torsade de pointes: clinical and experimental observations. *Pacing and Clinical Electrophysiology,* Vol.15, No.6, (June 1992), pp. 916-931, ISSN 0147-8389.

Hering H. (1909). Experimentelle studien an saugentieren uber das electrocardiogram. *Zchr Exper Path Therapie,* Vol. 7. p. 363.

Ikeda, T., Yoshino, H., Sugi, K., Tanno, K., Shimizu, H., Watanabe, J., Kasamaki, Y., Yoshida, A. & Kato, T. (2006). Predictive value of microvolt T-wave alternans for sudden cardiac death in patients with preserved cardiac function after acute myocardial infarction: results of a collaborative cohort study. *Journal of the American College of Cardiology,* Vol.48, No.11, (December 2006), pp. 2268-2274, ISSN 0735-1097.

Kleinfeld, M.J. & Rozanski J.J. (1977). Alternans of the ST segment in Prinzmetal's angina. *Circulation,* Vol.55, No.4, (April 1977), pp. 574-577, ISSN 0009-7322.

Klingenheben, T., Zabel, M., D'Agostino, R.B., Cohen, R.J. & Hohnloser, S.H. (2000). Predictive value of T-wave alternans for arrhythmic events in patients with congestive heart failure. *Lancet,* Vol.356, No. 9230, (August 2000), pp. 651-652, ISSN 0140-6736.

Leino, J., Minkkinen, M., Nieminen, T., Lehtimäki, T., Viik, J., Lehtinen, R., Nikus, K., Kööbi, T., Turjanmaa, V., Verrier, R.L. & Kähönen, M. (2009). Combined assessment of heart rate recovery and T-wave alternans during routine exercise testing improves prediction of total and cardiovascular mortality: the Finnish Cardiovascular Study. *Heart Rhythm,* Vol.6, No.12, (December 2009), pp.1765-1771, ISSN 1547-5271.

Maeda, S., Nishizaki, M., Yamawake, N., Ashikaga, T., Shimada, H., Asano, M., Ihara, K., Murai, T., Suzuki, H., Fujii, H., Sakurada, H., Hiraoka, M. & Isobe, M. (2009). Ambulatory ECG-based T-wave alternans and heart rate turbulence predict high risk of arrhythmic events in patients with old myocardial infarction. *Circulation Journal,* Vol.73, No.3, (December 2009), pp. 2223-2228, ISSN 1346-9843.

Martínez, J.P. & Olmos, S. (2005). Methodological principles of T wave alternans analysis: a unified framework. *IEEE Transactions on Bio-Medical Engineering,* Vol.52, No.4, (April 2005), pp.599-613, ISSN 0018-9294.

Martínez, J.P., Olmos, S., Wagner, G. & Laguna, P. (2006). Characterization of repolarization alternans during ischemia: time-course and spatial analysis. *IIEEE Transactions on Bio-Medical Engineering,* Vol.53, No.4, (April 2006), pp. 701-711, ISSN 0018-9294.

Montagnana, M., Lippi, G,. Franchini, M., Targher, G. & Cesare Guidi, G. (2008). Sudden cardiac death: prevalence, pathogenesis, and prevention. *Annals of Medicine,* Vol.40, No.5, (2008), pp. 360-375, ISSN 0785-3890.

Narayan, S.M. & Smith, J.M. (1999). Differing rate dependence and temporal distribution of repolarization alternans in patients with and without ventricular tachycardia. *Journal of Cardiovascular Electrophysiology,* Vol.10, No.1, (January 1999), pp.61-71, ISSN 1045-3873.

Narayan, S.M. & Smith, J.M. (2000). Exploiting rate-related hysteresis in repolarization alternans to improve risk stratification for ventricular tachycardia. *Journal of the American College of Cardiology,* Vol.35, No.6, (May 2000), pp. 1485-1492, ISSN 0735-1097.

Narayan, S.M. (2006). T-wave alternans and the susceptibility to ventricular arrhythmias. *Journal of the American College of Cardiology,* Vol.47, No.2, (2006), pp. 269-281, ISSN 0735-1097.

Narayan, S.M., Smith, J.M., Lindsay, B.D., Cain, M.E. & Dávila-Román, V.G. (2006). Relation of T-wave alternans to regional left ventricular dysfunction and eccentric hypertrophy secondary to coronary heart disease. *The American Journal of Cardiology*, Vol.97, No.6, (March 2006), pp. 775-780, ISSN 0002-9149.

Narayan, S.M., Franz, M.R., Lalani, G., Kim, J. & Sastry, A. (2007). T-wave alternans, restitution of human action potential duration, and outcome. *Journal of the American College of Cardiology,* Vol.50, No.25, (December 2007), pp. 2385-2392, ISSN 0735-1097.

Nearing, B.D., Huang, A.H. & Verrier, R.L. (1991). Dynamic tracking of cardiac vulnerability by complex demodulation of the T wave. *Science,* Vol.252, No.5004, (April 1991), pp.437-440, ISSN 0036-8075.

Nearing, B.D. & Verrier, R.L. (1993). Personal computer system for tracking cardiac vulnerability by complex demodulation of the T wave. *Journal of Applied Physiology,* Vol.74, No.5, (May,1993), pp. 2606-2612, ISSN 8750-7587.

Nearing, B.D., Oesterle, S.N. & Verrier, R.L. (1994). Quantification of ischaemia induced vulnerability by precordial T wave alternans analysis in dog and human. *Cardiovascular Research,* Vol.28, No.9, (September 1994), pp. 1440-1449, ISSN 0008-6363.

Nearing, B.D. & Verrier, R.L. (2002). Modified moving average analysis of T-wave alternans to predict ventricular fibrillation with high accuracy. *Journal of Applied Physiology,* Vol.92, No.2, (February 2002), pp.541-549, ISSN 8750-7587.

Pastore, J.M., Girouard, S.D., Laurita, K.R., Akar, F.G. & Rosenbaum, D.S. (1999). Mechanism linking T-wave alternans to the genesis of cardiac fibrillation. *Circulation,* Vol.99, No.10, (March 1999), pp.1385-94, ISSN 0009-7322.

Pruvot, E.J., Katra, R.P., Rosenbaum, D.S. & Laurita, K.R. (2004). Role of calcium cycling versus restitution in the mechanism of repolarization alternans. *Circulation Research,* Vol.94, No. 8, (April 2004), pp. 1083–1090, ISSN 0009-7330.

Reddy, C.V., Kiok, J.P., Khan, R.G. & El-Sherif, N. (1984). Repolarization alternans associated with alcoholism and hypomagnesemia. *The American Journal of Cardiology,* Vol.53, No.2, (January 1984), pp. 390-391, ISSN 0002-9149.

Rosenbaum, D.S., Jackson, L.E., Smith, J.M., Garan, H., Ruskin, J.N. & Cohen, R.J. (1994). Electrical alternans and vulnerability to ventricular arrhythmias. *The New England Journal of Medicine*, Vol.330, No. 4, (January 1994), pp. 235-241, ISSN 0028-4793.

Rosenbaum, D.S., Albrecht, P. & Cohen, R.J. (1996). Predicting sudden cardiac death from T wave alternans of the surface electrocardiogram: promises and pitfalls, *Journal of Cardiovascular Electrophysiology,* Vol.7, No.11, (November 1996), pp. 1095-1111, ISSN 1045-3873.

Sakaki, K., Ikeda, T., Miwa, Y., Miyakoshi, M., Abe, A., Tsukada, T., Ishiguro, H., Mera, H., Yusu, S. & Yoshino, H. (2009). Time-domain T-wave alternans measured from Holter electrocardiograms predicts cardiac mortality in patients with left ventricular dysfunction: a prospective study. *Heart Rhythm,* Vol.6, No.3, (March 2009), pp. 332-337, ISSN 1547-5271.

Salerno-Uriarte, J.A., De Ferrari, G.M., Klersy, C., Pedretti, R.F., Tritto, M., Sallusti, L., Libero, L., Pettinati, G., Molon, G., Curnis, A., Occhetta, E., Morandi, F., Ferrero, P., Accardi, F. & ALPHA Study Group Investigators (2007). Prognostic value of T-wave alternans in patients with heart failure due to nonischemic cardiomyopathy: results of the ALPHA Study. *Journal of the American College of Cardiology,* Vol.50, No. 19, (November 2007), pp. 1896-1904, ISSN 0735-1097.

Schwartz, P.J. & Malliani, A. (1975). Electrical alternation of the T-wave: clinical and experimental evidence of its relationship with the sympathetic nervous system and with the long Q-T syndrome. *American Heart Journal,* Vol.89, No.1, (January 1975), pp.45-50, ISSN 0002-8703.

Selvaraj, R.J., Picton, P., Nanthakumar, K., Mak, S. & Chauhan, V.S. (2007). Endocardial and epicardial repolarization alternans in human cardiomyopathy: evidence for spatiotemporal heterogeneity and correlation with body surface T-wave alternans. *Journal of the American College of Cardiology,* Vol.43, No.3 (January 2007), pp. 338-346, ISSN 0735-1097.

Smith, J.M. & Cohen, R.J. (1984). Simple finite-element model accounts for wide range of cardiac dysrhythmias. *Proceedings of the National Academy of Sciences of the United States of America,* Vol. 81, No.1, (January 1984), pp. 233-237.

Smith, J.M., Clancy, E.A., Valeri, C.R., Ruskin, J.N. & Cohen, R.J. (1988). Electrical alternans and cardiac electrical instability. *Circulation.* Vol.77, No.1,(January 1988), pp. 110-121, ISSN 0009-7322.

Stein, P.K., Sanghavi, D., Domitrovich, P.P., Mackey, R.A. & Deedwania, P. (2008). Ambulatory ECG-based T-wave alternans predicts sudden cardiac death in high-risk post-MI patients with left ventricular dysfunction in the EPHESUS study. *Journal of Cardiovascular Electrophysiology,* Vol.19, No.10, (October 2008), pp. 1037-1042, ISSN 1045-3873.

Verrier, R.L., Nearing, B.D., La Rovere, M.T., Pinna, G.D., Mittleman, M.A., Bigger, J.T. Jr, Schwartz, P.J. & ATRAMI Investigators. (2003). Ambulatory electrocardiogram-based tracking of T wave alternans in postmyocardial infarction patients to assess risk of cardiac arrest or arrhythmic death. *Journal of Cardiovascular Electrophysiology,* Vol.14, No.7, (July 2003), pp. 705-711, ISSN 1045-3873.

Weiss, J.N., Garfinkel, A., Karagueuzian, H.S., Qu, Z. & Chen, P.S. (1999). Chaos and the transition to ventricular fibrillation: a new approach to antiarrhythmic drug evaluation. *Circulation,* Vol.99, No.21, (June 1999), pp. 2819-2826, ISSN 0009 -7322.

Zacks, E.S., Morin, D.P., Ageno, S. Janik, M., Mauer, A.C., Markowitz, S.M., Mittal, S., Iwai, S., Shah, B.K., Lerman, B.B. & Stein, K.M. (2007). Effect of oral betablocker therapy on microvolt T-wave alternans and electrophysiology testing in patients with ischemic cardiomyopathy. *American Heart Journal,* Vol.153, No.3, (March 2007), pp. 392-397, ISSN 0002-8703.

Zareba, W., Moss, A.J., le Cessie, S. & Hall, W.J. (1994). T wave alternans in idiopathic long QT syndrome. *Journal of the American College of Cardiology,* Vol.23, No.7,(June 1994), pp. 1541-1546, ISSN 0735-1097.

Zheng, Z.J., Croft, J.B., Giles, W.H. & Mensah, G.A. (2001). Sudden cardiac death in the United States, 1989 to 1998. *Circulation*, Vol.104, No.18, (October 2001), pp. 2158-2163, ISSN 0009-7322.

7

Relatioship Between Serum 7-Ketocholesterol Concentrations and Coronary Artery Disease

Takashi Hitsumoto and Kohji Shirai
The Department of Internal Medicine, Sakura Medical Center, School of Medicine, Toho University, Chiba, Japan

1. Introduction

Coronary artery disease is a major health problem and a major cause of death in most industrialized and developing countries. On the other hand, recent basic and clinical studies have illustrated that oxidative stress plays an important role in the progression of coronary atherosclerosis (Kunsch C & Medford RM., 1999; Azumi H et al., 2002). Oxidative stress leads to oxidation of products in vivo and numerous oxidation products have been investigated and their significance examined in atherosclerotic disease (Steinberg D et al., 1997; Ehara S et al., 2001). 7-Ketocholesterol is known to be a major component of the cholesterol oxidation product, oxysterols, and is found in high concentrations in atherosclerotic plaques which contribute to the development of atherosclerosis (Brown AJ & Jessup W., 1998; Smith LL et al., 1996). Thus, 7-ketocholesterol is considered to be an important target factor in the prevention of coronary events and reflects the pathogenesis of coronary artery disease, and therefore has clinical applications. However, the clinical significance of blood 7-ketocholesterol concentrations (7KCHO) are not fully understood, because it is difficult to analyze these concentrations accurately. In the present study, we established a measuring system for serum 7-ketocholesterol concentrations (s-7KCHO) using gas chromatography mass spectrometry technique and attempted to clarify the clinical significance of s-7KCHO in the progression of coronary atherosclerosis using coronary angiography and intra-vascular ultrasound (IVUS).

2. Measurement of s-7KCHO

7KCHO was purchased from Sigma Chemicals Co. (St. Louis, MO, USA). 24,25,25,25,26,26,26,-d7-7-Ketocholesterol (d7-7KCHO) was prepared by Isotec (Miamisburg, OH, USA), and used as an internal standard. Dried pyridine was purchased from Merck (Darmstadt, Germany). Serum blood samples were stored immediately at −80°C , and were used as samples for the s-7KCHO assay within 1 week. A 500 µl aliquot of serum was mixed with 50 µl internal standard stock solution (10 µg/ml of d7-7KCHO dissolved in 1 ml toluene/ethyl acetate = 1:1, v/v), and 3 ml of diethyl ether/hexane (2:3, v/v) containing 0.01% BHT. The mixture was flushed with nitrogen gas and mixed in a rotary shaker for 30 min at room temperature. After centrifugation at 2000 × *g* for 15 min, the organic phase was collected and dried under nitrogen gas. The residue was dissolved in 1 ml of toluene/ethyl acetate (1:1, v/v), and applied to 3 ml "Diol" extraction columns (Bakerbond Spe, J.T. Baker Inc., Phillipsburg, NJ) that had been conditioned with the same solvent. After collection of the first eluted fraction under mild vacuum, the columns were eluted with another 2 ml of the same solvent. Three ml the of eluent was dried under nitrogen gas, and the residues were dissolved in 2 ml of diethyl ether, following which 500 μl of 20% potassium hydroxide dissolved in methanol was added. After mixing in a rotary shaker for 3 h, the mixture was neutralized by 20% acetic acid. To separate the organic phase from the aqueous phase, 1 ml of water was added and centrifuged. The organic phase was s eparated, added again to 1 ml of water, and centrifuged. The pooled organic fractions were dried under nitrogen gas. Dried samples were derivatized with 200 μl of *o*-methylhydroxylamine/hydrochloride dissolved in dried pyridine at 70°C for 2 h, and 100 μl of *N,O*-bis(trimethyl-silyl)trifluoroacetamide (BSTFA) at 70°C for 2 h. Then 1 μl aliquots were injected into a Varian GC/MS system consisting of a gas chromatography (CP-3800), an ion trap mass spectrometry (Saturn-2000), and an auto-sampler (CP-8400). The whole instrument set was controlled by a computer. The column used was a commercial product "WCOT Fused Silica (30 m × 0.25 mm i.d.) Coating CP-SIL 8 CB Low Bleed/MS" (Varian Inc., Palo Alto, CA, USA). Helium was used as carrier gas at a flow rate of 0.8 ml/min. The injection temperature was set at 270 °C (split ratio 1:4) and the initial column temperature at 60 °C. The analysis was run by holding the initial temperature for 1 min, and then increasing it at a rate of 20°C/min up to 280°C and 10°C/min up to 300°C. Thereafter the temperature was held at 300 °C for 10 min and was then increased again at a rate of 15 °C/min until 330 °C. The total running time was 31 min. The transfer line was maintained at 250 °C and the ion source at 220 °C. The electron ionization was performed by 70 eV ionized energy. The number of monitoring ions used was 471 for 7KCHO and 478 for internal standard (d7-7KCHO). In this assay system, recovery test was 95%, intra-assay coefficients of variation were <5%, and the detection limit of the assay was 6.2ng/ml.

3. Angiographic study

3.1 Study population

One hundred and thirty-nine subjects with coronary artery disease (CAD; subjects with stable angina pectoris or acute myocardial infarction) and 43 subjects with normal coronary arteries were enrolled. We examined relation of s-7-KCHO and findings of coronary angiography or coronary risk factors.

3.2 Methods of coronary angiography

Coronary angiography was performed by transfemoral or transbrachial approaches using a standard technique. Two experienced angiographers who were single blinded to the study reviewed all coronary angiograms. The severity of coronary stenosis was assessed with a worst-view projection. The percentage of luminal narrowing was recorded according to the American Heart Associations reporting system. Significant stenotic lesion was defined as ≥75% diameter stenosis, and the extent of coronary atherosclerosis was classified by the number of vessels with significant stenotic lesions. Lesions in the left main trunk were not observed in the present study. Of the study population, 68 subjects suffered from acute myocardial infarction (AMI). All AMI subjects had confirmed culprit lesion, which was a total or subtotal occlusion by coronary angiography. Diagnosis of AMI was based on: (1) a clinical history of central chest pressure pain, or tightness for 30 min or more, (2) ST-segment elevation greater than 0.1 mV in at least one standard or precordial lead, and (3) a rise in the serum creatine kinase concentration to more than twice the normal laboratory value. All subjects with normal coronary artery (NCA) were performed coronary angiography for evaluation of chest pain and/or abnormality of electrocardiograph and NCA was defined as the absence of significant stenosis and spastic reaction which was provoked by intracoronary administration of acetylcholine.

3.3 Results

Patient characteristics are shown in Table 1. Age, proportion of male subjects, diabetes mellitus and smoking were significantly higher in subjects with CAD than in those with NCA. Considering the serum lipid concentrations, there were significantly higher TC, LDL-C and triglyceride concentrations in subjects with NCA than in those with CAD; however, the serum lipid data were similar in subjects without antihyperlipidemic treatment (data not shown). HDL-C concentrations were significantly lower in subjects with CAD than in those with NCA. hs-CRP concentrations were significantly higher in subjects with CAD than in those with NCA.

	NCA (n=43)	CAD (n=139)
Age (yrs)	62±9	66±10*
Sex (male/female)	21/22	105/33**
Hypertension	16 (37)	70 (51)
Diabetes mellitus	5 (12)	45 (33)**
Obesity (BMI ≧25)	12 (28)	44 (32)
Smoking	12 (28)	68 (49)*
Family history of CAD	6 (14)	18 (13)
Total cholesterol (mg/dl)	217±38	189±34**
LDL-cholesterol (mg/dl)	127±36	114±30*
Triglyceride (mg/dl)	142±103	114±53*
HDL-cholesterol (mg/dl)	55±13	45±13*
Antihyperlipidemic treatment	8 (19)	73 (53)**
Statin use	5 (11)	63 (45)**
High sensitive CRP (mg/L)	0.9±0.7	1.8±1.7*

Data are expressed mean ± SD( ): %
*p<0.05 vs NCA, **p<0.01 vs NCA
NCA: Normal coronary artery
CAD: Coronary artery disease
BMI: body mass index
LDL: low-density lipoprotein
HDL: high-density lipoprotein

Table 1. Baseline clinical characteristics

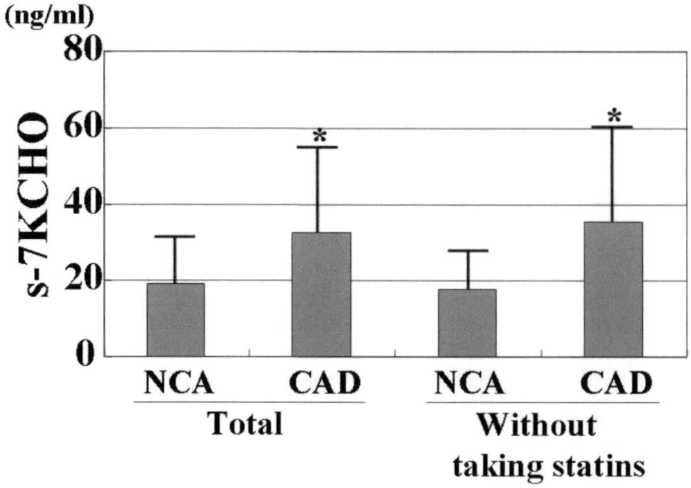

Data are expressed mean ± SD *p<0.01 vs NCA

Fig. 1. Comparisons of 7-ketocholesterol concentrations between subjects with normal coronary artery and coronary artery disease

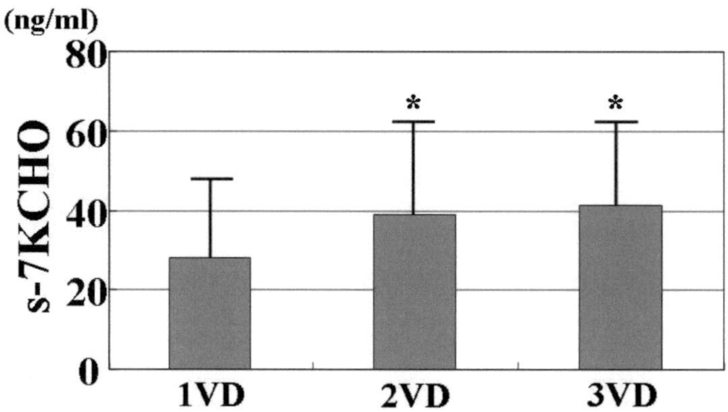

Data are expressed mean ± SD
*p<0.05 vs 1VD
1VD (n=85): 1-vessel disease
2VD (n=36): 2-vessel disease
3VD (n=18): 3-vessel disease

Fig. 2. Relation of 7-ketocholesterol concentrations and number of affected vessels.

Comparisons of s-7KCHO between NCA and CAD subjects are shown in Fig. 1. s-7KCHO were significantly higher in subjects with CAD than in those with NCA ($p < 0.01$) (NCA: 19.0 ± 11.3 ng/ml, CAD: 32.4 ± 23.1 ng/ml). We also examined s-7KCHO in subjects without taking statins. s-7KCHO were significantly higher in subjects with CAD than in those with NCA ($p < 0.01$) (NCA: 17.7 ± 9.6 ng/ml, CAD: 35.4 ± 25.4 ng/ml). The relationship between s-7KCHO and the number of affected vessels is shown in Fig. 2. s-7KCHO were significantly higher in subjects with 2 or 3 vessel disease than those with single vessel disease ($p < 0.05$, p

< 0.05, respectively) (1-vessel disease: 28.0 ± 21.1 ng/ml, 2-vessel disease: 39.0 ± 25.6 ng/ml, 3-vessel disease: 41.3 ± 23.2 ng/ml). Comparisons of s-7KCHO between subjects with stable angina pectoris and those with AMI are shown in Fig. 3. s-7KCHO were significantly higher in subjects with AMI than in those with stable angina pectoris even though the number of affected vessels were similar in the two groups ($p < 0.01$) (Stable angina pectoris: 26.1 ± 15.2 ng/ml, AMI: 39.1 ± 27.7 ng/ml).

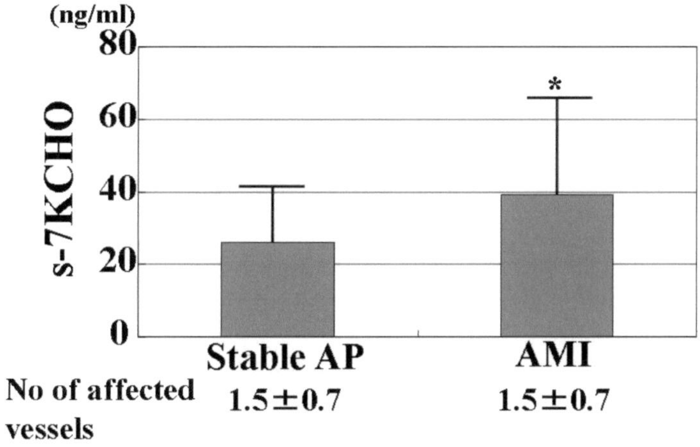

Data are expressed mean ± SD
*p<0.01 vs stable AP
Stable AP (n=69): stable angina pectoris
AMI (n=68): acute myocardial infarction

Fig. 3. Comparisons of 7-ketocholesterol concentrations between subjects with stable angina pectoris and acute myocardial infarction.

	r	p value
Total cholesterol	-0.03	NS
LDL-cholesterol	-0.04	NS
Log-Triglyceride	0.01	NS
HDL-cholesterol	-0.23	<0.01
Log-hs-CRP	0.24	<0.01

Table 2. Correlation between 7-keto cholesterol concentration and serum parameters.

Correlation between serum parameters and s-7KCHO in CAD subjects were shown in Table 2. There were no significant correlations between TC or LDL cholesterol concentrations and s-7KCHO. Conversely, s-7KCHO had significant correlations with HDL-cholesterol and hs-CRP concentrations. Other coronary risk factors such as age, sex, hypertension, diabetes mellitus, obesity, smoking, and family history of CAD were not related to s-7KCHO (data not shown). We also examined relationship between statin use and s-7KCHO. Subjects with statin use showed higher s-7KCHO than those without statin use, although the difference was not significant (p=0.09) (without statin use: 28.9 ± 19.9 ng/ml, statin use: 35.4 ± 25.7 ng/ml).

Multivariate analysis revealed that s-7KCHO were selected as an independent variable for CAD ($p < 0.01$, Table 3). In CAD subjects, the presence of acute myocardial infarction, number of affected vessels, and high sensitive C-reactive protein concentrations strongly correlated with s-7KCHO ($p < 0.01$, < 0.05, < 0.05, respectively, Table 4).

	OR (95%CI)	p value
s-7KCHO	1.06 (1.02-1.09)	<0.01
Age	1.08 (1.03-1.13)	<0.01
Sex (male)	5.04 (1.81-13.98)	<0.01
Diabetes mellitus	2.29 (0.85-6.13)	NS
HDL-cholesterol	0.97 (0.94-1.01)	NS
Smoking	1.66 (0.62-4.42)	NS
hs-CRP	1.10 (0.36-3.41)	NS

OR: odds ratio, CI: confidence interval, (n=182)

Table 3. Results of multivariate logistic regression analysis for coronary artery disease.

	Standard regression coefficent	t value	p value
Explanatory factor			
AMI	0.32	3.9	<0.01
No of affected vessels	0.25	3.0	<0.05
hs-CRP	0.24	2.9	<0.05
Subordinate factor			
s-7KCHO (actual value)			

R2=0.27, F value=3.8, p<0.0001, (n=139)

Table 4. Results of multiple regression analysis for 7-ketocholesterol concentrations in subjects with coronary artery disease.

Our angiographic study indicated that high s-7KCHO were closely associated with acute myocardial infarction. On the other hand, recent clinical studies using IVUS have clarified that coronary artery plaque already exists in subjects with normal coronary artery, which is diagnosed by coronary angiography. Furthermore, it has been reported that almost 70% of culprit lesion on acute myocardial infarction, now called acute coronary syndrome, which is highly correlated with mortality, occurs in less than 50% of angiographic stenosis (Falk E et al., 1995). Therefore, it is difficult to predict the occurrence of acute coronary syndrome and it is important that we consider the presence of coronary atherosclerosis; especially presence of vulnerable plaque, before angiographic stenosis. IVUS studies have clarified the future of plaque on acute coronary syndrome; plaque volume is large and shows abnormal plaque quality (Yamagishi M et al., 2000; Namiki N et al., 1999; Kotani J et al., 2003) such as eccentricity, lipid pool and mild calcified lesions. Therefore, next, we examined relation of s-7KCHO and coronary plaque in angiographic normal stage using IVUS.

4. IVUS study

4.1 Study population

66 subjects with normal coronary artery diagnosed by coronary angiography were enrolled. Proxymal range of left anterior descending coronary artery was observed by intravascular ultrasound using auto-pullback methods and examined relation of s-7KCHO and coronary plaque.

4.2 Methods of IVUS study

Coronary angiography was performed the transfemoral approach using a standard technique. Two experienced angiographers reviewed all coronary angiograms and confirmed that there were no stenotic lesion, and consequently performed IVUS study. To avoid spasm, 1 to 2 mg of nitroglycerin was administrated before insertion of the 0.014-inch coronary guidewire and IVUS catheter through a coronary guiding catheter. After the IVUS catheter was inserted more than 20 mm beyond proximal of left descending coronary artery (LAD), a motorized auto pullback was performed at 1 mm/second velocity and the percent plaque volume was calculated for 20 mm length of LAD proximal side as plaque quantity. We also evaluated plaque quality, such as eccentricity, calcification and lipid pool into plaque. Eccentricity was identified when the minimum dimension of plaque thickness/dimension of the other side plaque thickness at max plaque area was less than 0.5. Calcification was defined when a high echo area with back reflection was detected and lipid pool was defined as when echo lucent zone was detected during the observation period.

4.3 Results

There were significantly positive correlation between s-7-KCHO and %Plaque volume ($r=0.37$, $p<0.001$, Fig. 4.); furthermore, multiple regression analysis showed that high s-7-KCHO were selected as independent variables for %Plaque volume ($p<0.05$). On the other hand, subjects with high s-7-KCHO (≧20ng/ml, n=33) were detected high incidence of abnormal plaque quality such as eccentric plaque (76%), mild calcified lesion (64%) and lipid pool (30%) (Table 5). Fig. 5. shows the relationship of high s-7-KCHO and degree of calcification. Subjects with high s-7-KCHO had mild degree and plural number of calcification into plaque.

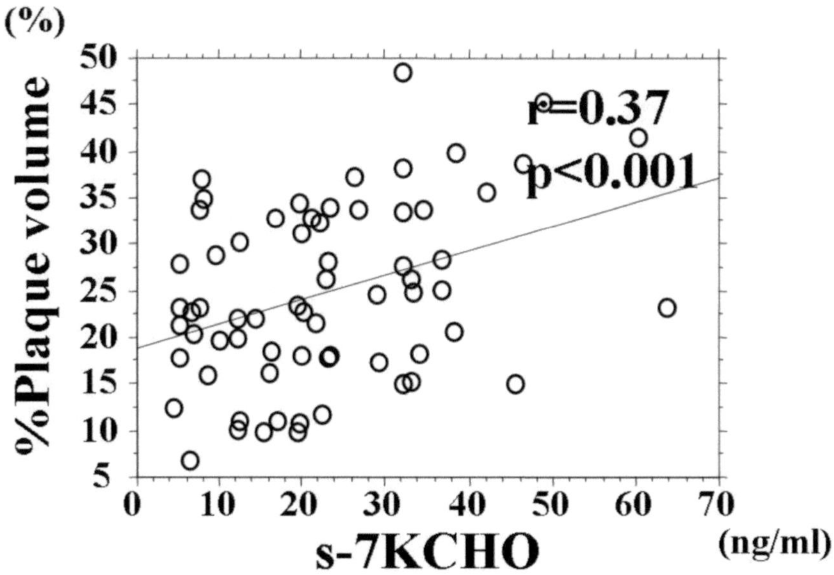

Fig. 4. Correlation between 7-keto cholesterol concentration and %Plaque volume.

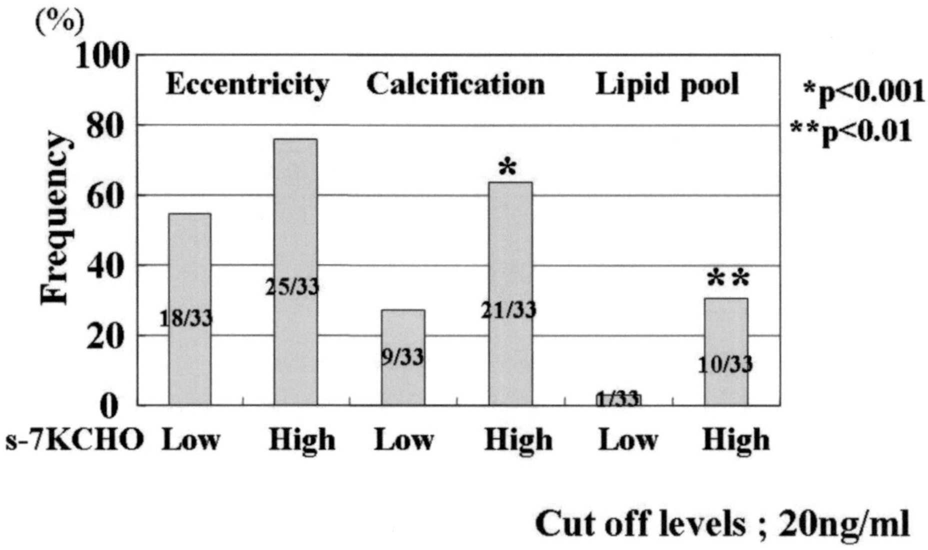

Table 5. 7-ketocholesterol concentrations and abnormality of plaque quality.

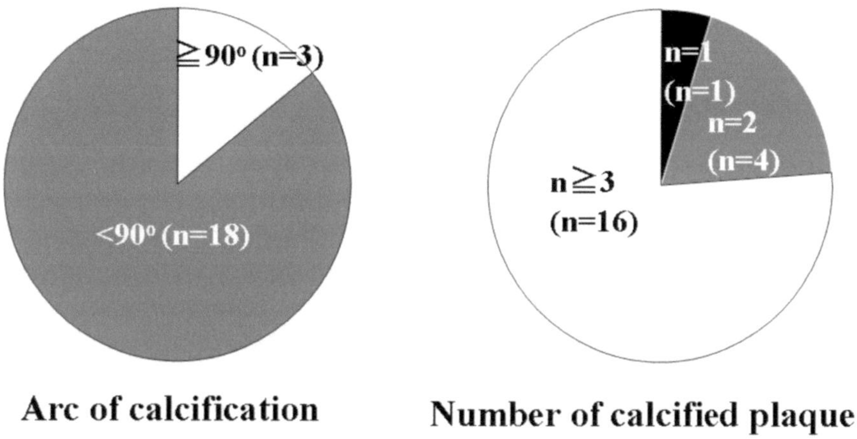

Fig. 5. Feature of calcification in subjects with high 7-ketocholesterol concentrations.

5. Discussion

In angiographic study, s-7KCHO were significantly higher in subjects with CAD than in those with NCA; furthermore, multiple regression analysis revealed that s-7KCHO were selected as independent variable for the presence of CAD as a subordinate factor. The presence of AMI, number of affected vessels, and hs-CRP concentrations strongly correlated with s-7KCHO in CAD subjects. Furthermore, IVUS study indicated that s-7KCHO reflected vulnerable coronary plaque which is not detectable by coronary angiography.

7KCHO is excessive in advanced atherosclerotic plaques (Brown AJ & Jessup W., 1998), and contributes to the development of atherosclerosis (Smith LL et al., 1996). Furthermore, 7KCHO causes apoptosis (Miyashita Y et al., 1997) and inhibits migration of smooth muscle cells (Oyama T et a.l, 2001). These findings suggest that accumulation of 7KCHO in atherosclerotic lesions may decrease the amount of cells and render atherosclerotic plaques unstable. Thus, 7KCHO is important not only in the progression of coronary atherosclerosis but is also the cause of plaque rupture which is a major factor of AMI. In the present study, s-7KCHO reflected the severity of coronary atherosclerosis, estimated by coronary angiography; furthermore, s-7KCHO strongly correlated with presence of AMI and vulnerable coronary plaque. Therefore, s-7KCHO may reflect 7KCHO in the coronary artery plaque and is expected to be a predictor of AMI occurrence which is strongly associated with mortality.

Hypercholesterolemia is established as one of the most important coronary risk factors; however, the average serum TC or LDL-C concentration in subjects with CAD often appears to be within the normal range. The present study also indicated that serum TC or LDL-C concentrations were not higher in CAD subjects than in NCA subjects. Furthermore, there is no relationship between serum TC or LDL-C concentrations and s-7KCHO. Another study also indicated that blood 7KCHO had no relationship with blood cholesterol concentrations in CAD subjects (Tomasik A et al., 2000). Therefore, these results suggest that s-7KCHO is a different marker from blood cholesterol concentrations even though 7KCHO were oxidation products of cholesterol. This allows us to predict coronary events which are not detectable by serum TC or LDL-C concentrations if we can measure s-7KCHO in the clinic. In a basic study, degenerative LDL such as small sized LDL or glycated LDL was shown to be easily oxidized (de Graaf J et al., 1991; Lyons TJ., 1992), consequently, promoting atherosclerotic lesion. Some clinical studies emphasized an increase in degenerative LDL in CAD (Austin MA & Krauss RM., 1984; Krauss RM., 1994). 7KCHO may relate to oxidation products of degenerative LDL, however, the relationship is not fully understood. Therefore, further studies are required to investigate the significance of s-7KCHO from the perspective of precise lipid profiles.

Among the serum lipid concentrations, only HDL-C had significant relationship with s-7KCHO. A number of studies reported that low HDL-C concentrations were inversely related to the risk of cardiovascular disease (Castelli WP et al., 1986; Rhoads GG et al., 1976) and the present study may indicate that HDL retards the progression of coronary atherosclerosis by decreasing 7KCHO in the coronary vessel wall or blood flow. The relationship between HDL-C concentrations and s-7KCHO in coronary atherosclerosis is not fully understood. Recently, however, Terasaka reported that HDL exerted a protective effect against apoptosis induced by 7KCHO using ATP-binding cassette transporter ABCG1+/+ mice (Terasaka N et al., 2007). The ATP-binding cassette transporter ABCG1 was recently shown to promote efflux of cholesterol from macrophage to HDL and reverse the relationship between HDL-C concentrations and s-7KCHO. This may be partly explained by the role of ATP-binding cassette transporter ABCG1.

In the present study, there was a significant correlation between s-7KCHO and hs-CRP concentrations in CAD subjects. Furthermore, these two factors had a significant association with each other after adjustment of related factors. Thus, this result suggests that s-7KCHO are closely associated with inflammation in coronary atherosclerosis. Recent clinical investigations showed that inflammation plays an important role in the progression of atherosclerosis (Ross R., 1999; Libby P et al., 2002) and epidemiological studies clarified the link between high levels of CRP concentration and cardiovascular events (Ridker PM et al., 2002; Matsumoto K et al., 2003). Paul et al. showed that CRP is present in the human arterial intima of the atherosclerotic lesion by histological examination (Paul A et al., 2004); furthermore, Kobayashi et al. reported that, by using a sample of directional coronary atherectomy, expression of CRP was colocalized with p22phox and CRP directly induced p22phox expression generating reactive oxygen species in cultured smooth muscle cells (Kobayashi S et al., 2003). Therefore, CRP may promote the production of 7-KCHO in coronary artery plaques; consequently, increasing s-7KCHO. However, some reports indicate that oxysterol influences proinflammatory properties (Wang N et al., 1996; Liu Y et al., 1997). Joffre et al. reported that 7KCHO enhanced interleukin-8 gene expression using porcine retinal pigment epithelial cells (Joffre C et al., 2007). Interleukin-8 is a proinflammatory and chemotactic cytokine which might play a crucial role in the recruitment of monocytes and T lymphocytes into the arterial subendothelial space, consequently, promoting atherosclerotic lesion (Terkeltaub R et al., 1998). Furthermore, interleukin-8 could have a potential atherogenic role by inhibiting the local tissue inhibitor of metalloproteinase-1 expression, thereby leading to an imbalance between matrix metalloproteinases and metalloproteinase-1 at focal sites of atherosclerotic plaque, and to local extracellular degradation, causing the rupture of atheromatous plaques (Moreau M et al., 1999). Thus, 7KCHO and inflammation in coronary atherosclerosis are closely associated with each other and may promote vulnerable plaque formation.

In IVUS study, calcification was frequently detected in subjects with high s-7KCHO compared with low s-7KCHO.

Calcification into plaque is vulnerable and has been controversial. However, some clinical studies have shown that coronary calcification, which is detected by computed tomography is a powerful predictor for cardiac events (Kondos GT et al., 2003; Greenland P et al., 2004). Raggi et al (Raggi P et al., 2003) reported that coronary calcification identified by electron-beam computed tomography was highly prevalent in patients with acute myocardial infarction; thus, coronary calcification might be indicated in the presence of vulnerable plaque. Furthermore, a recent IVUS study (Ehara S et al., 2004) reported that culprit lesion on acute coronary syndrome had significantly high incidence of mild calcification than those with stable angina pectoris. Therefore, our results can be interpreted as follows: from the viewpoint of calcification, subjects with high s-7KCHO already have vulnerable plaque in early stage coronary atherosclerosis.

6. Conclusion

Our data which is accurately measured s-7KCHO indicate that high s-7KCHO are closely associated with not only progression of coronary atherosclerosis but also formation of vulnerable plaque. To achieve the clinical usefulness, simple and reliable methods to measure blood 7KCHO concentrations are needed and examination of many clinical studies investigating the significance of s-7KCHO in diagnosis and treatment are required.

7. References

Azumi H, Inoue N, Ohashi Y, Terashima M, Mori T, Fujita H, Awano K, Kobayashi K, Maeda K, Hata K, Shinke T, Kobayashi S, Hirata K, Kawashima S, Itabe H, Hayashi Y, Imajoh-Ohmi S, Itoh H, &Yokoyama M (2002). Superoxide generation in directional coronary atherectomy specimens of patients with angina pectoris: important role of NAD(P)H oxidase. *Arterioscler Thromb Vasc Biol,* 22:1838-1844

Austin MA & Krauss RM (1986). Genetic control of low density lipoprotein subclasses. *Lancet,* 2: 592-595

Brown AJ & Jessup W (1998). Oxysterols and atherosclerosis. *Atherosclerosis,* 142: 1–28

Castelli WP, Garrison RJ, Wilson PW, Abbott RD, Kalousdian S, & Kannel WB (1986). Incidence of coronary heart disease and lipoprotein cholesterol levels. The Framingham Study. *J Am Med Assoc,* 256: 2835–2838

de Graaf J, Hak-Lemmers HL, Hectors MP, Demacker PN, Hendriks JC, & Stalenhoef AF (1991). Enhanced susceptibility to in vitro oxidation of the dense low density lipoprotein subfraction in healthy subjects. *Arterioscler Thromb,* 11: 298-306

Ehara S, Ueda M, Naruko T, Haze K, Itoh A, Otsuka M, Komatsu R, Matsuo T, Itabe H, Takano T, Tsukamoto Y, Yoshiyama M, Takeuchi K, Yoshikawa J, & Becker AE (2001). Elevated levels of oxidized low density lipoprotein show a positive relationship with the severity of acute coronary syndromes. *Circulation,* 103: 1955-1960

Ehara S, Kobayashi Y, Yoshiyama M, Shimada K, Shimada Y, Fukuda D, Nakamura Y, Yamashita H, Yamagishi H, Takeuchi K, Naruko T, Haze K, Becker AE, Yoshikawa J, & Ueda M (1995). Spotty calcification typifies the culprit plaque in patients with acute myocardial infarction: an intravascular ultrasound study. *Circulation,* 110: 3424-3429

Falk E, Shah PK, & Fuster V (1995). Coronary plaque disruption. *Circulation,* 92: 657-671

Greenland P, LaBree L, Azen SP, Doherty TM, & Detrano RC (2004). Coronary artery calcium score combined with Framingham score for risk prediction in asymptomatic individuals. *JAMA,* 291: 210-215

Joffre C, Leclère L, Buteau B, Martine L, Cabaret S, Malvitte L, Acar N, Lizard G, Bron A, Creuzot-Garcher C,& Bretillon L (2007). Oxysterols induced inflammation and oxidation in primary porcine retinal pigment epithelial cells. *Curr Eye Res,* 32: 271-280

Kunsch C & Medford RM (1999). Oxidative stress as a regulator of gene expression in the vasculature. *Circ Res,* 85: 753-766

Kobayashi S, Inoue N, Ohashi Y, Terashima M, Matsui K, Mori T, Fujita H, Awano K, Kobayashi K, Azumi H, Ejiri J, Hirata K, Kawashima S, Hayashi Y, Yokozaki H, Itoh H,& Yokoyama M (2003). Interaction of oxidative stress and inflammatory response in coronary plaque instability: important role of C-reactive protein. *Arterioscler Thromb Vasc Biol,* 23: 1398-1404

Krauss RM (1994). Heterogeneity of plasma low-density lipoproteins and atherosclerosis risk. *Curr Opin Lipidol,* 5: 339-349

Kondos GT, Hoff JA, Sevrukov A, Daviglus ML, Garside DB, Devries SS, Chomka EV,& Liu K (2003) Electron-beam tomography coronary artery calcium and cardiac events: a 37-month follow-up of 5635 initially asymptomatic low- to intermediate-risk adults. *Circulation,* 107: 2571-2576

Kotani J, Mintz GS, Castagna MT, Pinnow E, Berzingi CO,

Bui AB, Pichard AD, Satler LF, Suddath WO, Waksman R, Laird JR Jr, Kent KM, & Weissman NJ (2003). Intravascular ultrasound analysis of infarct-related and non-infarct-related arteries in patients who presented with an acute myocardial infarction. *Circulation,* 107: 2889-2893

Libby P, Ridker PM, & Maseri A (2002). Inflammation and atherosclerosis. Circulation, 105:1135-1143

Lyons TJ (1992). Lipoprotein glycation and its metabolic consequences. *Diabetes,* 41: 67-73

Liu Y, Hulten LM, & Wiklund O (1997). Macrophages isolated from human atherosclerotic plaques produce IL-8, and oxysterols may have a regulatory function for IL-8 production. *Arterioscler Thromb Vasc Biol,* 17: 317–323

Miyashita Y, Shirai K, Ito Y, Watanabe J, Urano Y, and Murano T & Tomioka H (1997). Cytotoxicity of some oxysterols on human vascular smooth muscle cells was mediated by apoptosis. *J Atheroscler Thromb,* 4: 73–78

Matsumoto K, Sera Y, Abe Y, Ueki Y, Tominaga T, & Miyake S (2003). Inflammation and insulin resistance are independently related to all-cause of death and cardiovascular events in Japanese patients with type 2 diabetes mellitus. *Atherosclerosis,* 169: 317-21

Moreau M, Brocheriou I, Petit L, Ninio E, Chapman MJ, &Rouis M (1999). Interleukin-8 mediates downregulation of tissue inhibitor of metalloproteinase-1 expression in cholesterol-loaded human macrophages: relevance to stability of atherosclerotic plaque. *Circulation,* 99: 420-426

Namiki N, Uchiyama T, Nagai Y, & Yamashina A (1999). Graphical comparison of coronary arterial culprit lesions in acute myocardial infarction and unstable angina pectoris. *Intern Med,* 38: 849-855

Oyama T, Miyashita Y, Kinoshita K, Watanabe H, Shirai K, & Yagima T (2001). Effect of deposited lipids in atheromatous lesions on the migration of vascular smooth muscle cells. *J Atheroscler Thromb,* 9: 109–113

Paul A, Ko KW, Li L, Yechoor V, McCrory MA, Szalai AJ, & Chan L (2004). C-reactive protein accelerates the progression of atherosclerosis in apolipoprotein E-deficient mice. *Circulation,* 109: 647-655

Rhoads GG, Gulbrandsen CL,& Kagan A (1976). Serum lipoproteins and coronary heart disease in a population study of Hawaii Japanese men. N *Engl J Med,* 294: 293–298

Ridker PM, Rifai N, Rose L, Buring JE, & Cook NR (2002). Comparison of C-reactive protein and low-density lipoprotein cholesterol levels in the prediction of first cardiovascular events. *N Engl J Med,* 347: 1557-1565

Ross R (1999). Atherosclerosis--an inflammatory disease. *N Engl J Med,* 340: 115-126

Raggi P, Cooil B, Shaw LJ, Aboulhson J, Takasu J, Budoff M, & Callister TQ (2003). Progression of coronary calcium on serial electron beam tomographic scanning is greater in patients with future myocardial infarction. *Am J Cardiol,* 92: 827-829

Steinberg D (1997). Low density lipoprotein oxidation and its pathobiological significance. *J Biol Chem,* 272: 20963-20966

Smith LL (1996). Review of progress in sterol oxidations: 1987-1995. *Lipids,* 31: 453-487

Tomasik A, Jacheć W, Skrzep-Poloczek B, Wojciechowska C, Tarnawski R, Wodniecki J, Poloński L, & Szczurek-Katański K (2000). Impact of baseline level of 7-ketocholesterol on the rate of coronary reintervention in coronary artery disease patients--results of an observational study with questionnaire-based follow up. *Med Sci Monit,* 6: 751-758

Terasaka N, Wang N, Yvan-Charvet L, & Tall AR (2007). High-density lipoprotein protects macrophages from oxidized low-density lipoprotein-induced apoptosis by promoting efflux of 7-ketocholesterol via ABCG1. *Proc Natl Acad Sci U S A,* 104: 15093-15098

Terkeltaub R, Boisvert WA, & Curtiss LK (1998). Chemokines and atherosclerosis. *Curr Opin Lipidol,* 9: 397-405

Wang N, Tabas I, Winchester R, Ravalli S, Rabbani LE,& Tall A (1996). Interleukin 8 is induced by cholesterol loading of macrophages and expressed by macrophage foam cells in human atheroma. *J Biol Chem,* 271: 8837-8842

Yamagishi M, Terashima M, Awano K, Kijima M, Nakatani S, Daikoku S, Ito K, Yasumura Y, & Miyatake K (2000). Morphology of vulnerable coronary plaque: insights from follow-up of patients examined by intravascular ultrasound before an acute coronary syndrome. *J Am Coll Cardiol,* 35: 106-111

8

Oxidized Low Density Lipoprotein, Statin Therapy and Carotid Stenosis

Elias Skopelitis, Dimitrios Levisianou,
Theodore Gialernios and Sofoklis Kougialis
General Hospital of Nikaia and Piraeus
Greece

1. Introduction

1.1 Carotid stenosis and atheromatous process

Carotid artery stenosis due to atherosclerosis is a major complication of hyperlipidemia, diabetes mellitus and hypertension. Moreover, the extent of carotid intima media thickness is a measure of atheromatosis and therefore of cardiovascular disease (CVD).

The effect of cholesterol in the process of atheromatosis is now well established. High levels of total cholesterol (TC), as well as of low-density lipoprotein (LDL), very low-density lipoprotein (VLDL), intermediate-density lipoprotein (IDL), lipoprotein a (Lp-α), and triglycerides (TG), coupled with decreased levels of high-density lipoprotein (HDL) are responsible for the creation of atheromatous plaques (Assmann & Schulte, 1992; Hokanson & Autsin, 1996; Katsouras et al., 2001). Of the above factors, LDL cholesterol, and especially the oxidized LDL (oxLDL) is considered as the most important contributor of atheromatosis (Anderson et al., 1996).

The atheromatous process is completed in the following three stages:

1. In the first stage, LDL cholesterol enters the vessel wall, binds to glucosaminoglucanes, which are part of the extracellular matrix of the intima. This binding is facilitated by apolipoprotein B-100 (ApoB–100). The accumulation of LDL in the vessel wall contributes to the formation of fatty strikes. Following adhesion to the vessel wall, LDL undergoes oxidation by free radicals produced locally, the molecule is altered and chemokines are produced by adjacent vessel wall cells, such as monocyte chemoattractant protein-1 (MCP–1), together with growth factors, which are responsible for the accumulation of monocytes and macrophages. The latter cause further oxidation of LDL, resulting in negative charge, recognition by scavenger receptors located on macrophage membrane and increased uptake of LDL inside the macrophages, as these receptors are not inhibited by increased intracellular concentration of cholesterol. The final result is an enormous accumulation of LDL in the macrophages, which are transformed to foam cells. These cells represent the first step in the atheromatous process (Durrington & Sinderman, 2002) (figure 1).
2. During the second stage, the atheromatous plaque is formed. Foam cells produce growth factors and together with oxLDL result to the attraction of smooth muscle cells.

The latter are then differentiated to fibroblasts and start producing collagen. This collagen covers foam cells, which either are destroyed or are forced to apoptosis. The final result is the formation of a pool of extracellular cholesterol trapped under a fibrous capsid (figure 2). The part which is close to the yet intact vessel wall is the active site of the plaque, where the foam cells are produced. As the plaque extents to the inner layers of the vessel wall, the point of foam cell formation becomes instable and may cause rapture of the plaque (Durrington & Sinderman, 2002) (figure 3).

3. In the third stage, that of the complicated lesion, the rapture of the fibrous capsid of the atheromatous plaque leads to massive evacuation of the cholesterol reservoir. The artery may occult due to the accumulation of platelets and subsequent clotting, leading to acute ischemia or infarction (figure 4). If not so, then the plaque will be further enlarged (Durrington & Sinderman, 2002).

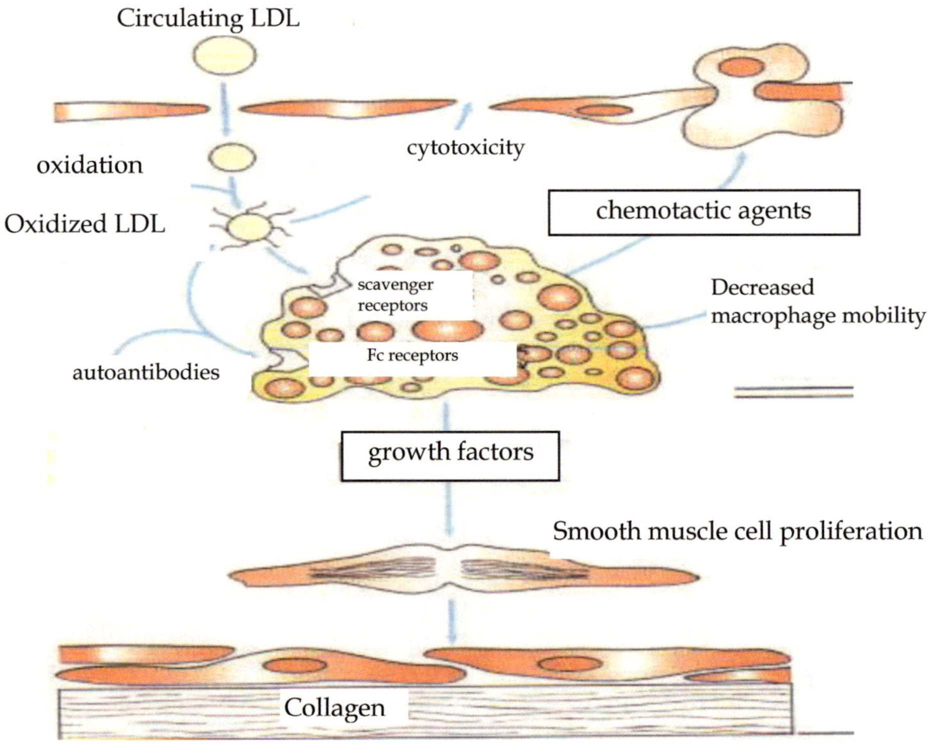

Fig. 1. Atherogenesis. Fatty strikes are characterized by macrophages containing an excess of lipids (foam cells). Foam cells are derived by blood monocytes which are attracted to vessel intima and start phagocytosing lipoproteins, such as oxLDL. The conversion of fatty strike to atheroma depends on proliferation and differentiation of smooth muscle cells to fibroblasts. The latter produce collagen resulting in intima thickening. As the lesion extents further, foam cells are destroyed releasing large amounts of cholesterol trapped in a fibrous capsid. The active site of atheroma is the point which is adjacent to normal endothelium, where foam cells are formed (adopted with persmission from Durrington & Sinderman, 2002).

Avoiding the formation and the instability of the atheromatous plaque is top priority for patients at risk for cardiovascular events. Statins may contribute towards this direction (Corti et al., 2002; Nissen et al., 2004)

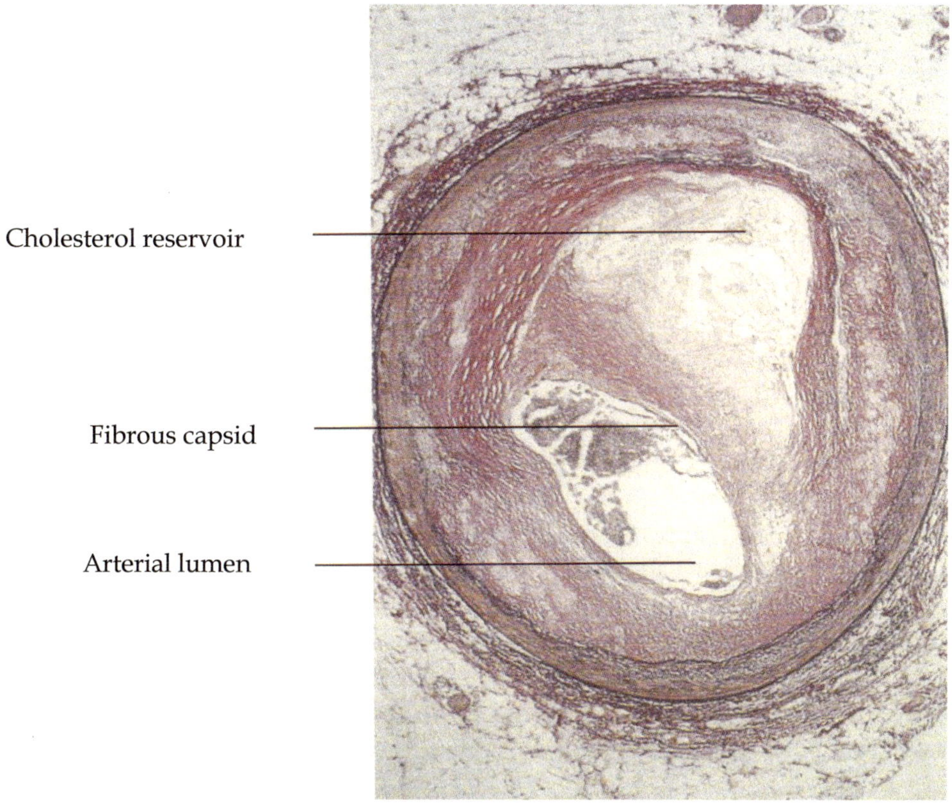

Fig. 2. Advanced atheromatous plaque causing arterial lumen occlusion of 70% (adopted from Durrington & Sinderman, 2002).

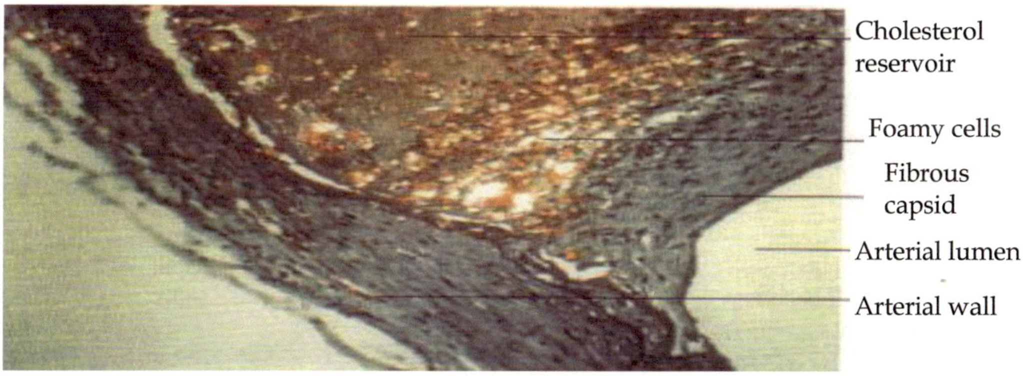

Fig. 3. The point of the atheromatous plaque, on which active enlargement occurs: formation of new foam cells and increased cholesterol uptake contribute to increased plaque instability (adopted from Durrington & Sinderman, 2002).

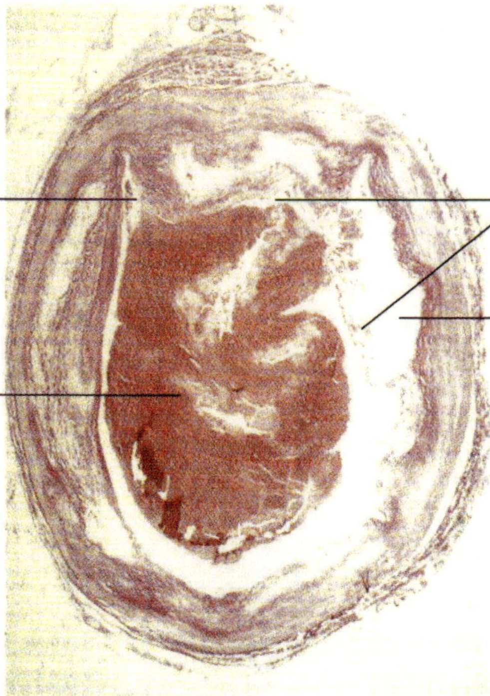

Fig. 4. A raptured ahteromatous plaque, in which the cholesterol reservoir has evacuated itself under the fibrous capsid. A clot in the endothelial surface at the site of rapture occults the lumen completely (adopted from Durrington & Sinderman, 2002).

1.2 Oxidized LDL

Oxidized LDL cholesterol in humans is found mainly in two types:

a. conjugated form, attached to the atheromatous plaque and
b. circulating form found in serum.

Oxidized LDL is produced following oxidation of LDL by free radicals and other oxidadive factors, a procedure called oxidative stress. The circulating oxLDL is the measurable fraction of oxLDL in plasma. Oxidized LDL is a key element of the pathway leading to the formation of the atheromatous plaque and has been extensively studied both as a marker of atheromatosis and as a possible target of therapeutic intervention. Circulating oxLDL is considered a risk marker for atherosclerosis (Toshima, 2000) and coronary heart disease (CHD) (Ehara et al., 2001; Holvoet et al., 2003; Toshima et al., 2000). Increased oxLDL levels in circulation and the vessel wall are associated with endothelial dysfunction (Penny et al., 2001) in such patients (Ehara et al., 2001; Holvoet et al., 1999; Nishi et al., 2002), contributing to atheromatous plaque instability (Ehara et al., 2001).

Oxidative modification of LDL leads to rapid focal accumulation in macrophages (Witztum & Steinberg, 1991), which is the first step of the atheromatous process. The increased retention time of LDL in the intima offers enhanced probability to be oxidized by free radicals produced by endothelium, smooth muscle cells or macrophages (Steinbrecher et al.,

1984). Oxidized LDL then acts chemotactic for monocytes and smooth muscle cells through binding to scavenger receptors (D. Li et al., 2002), leading to the formation of foamy cells. Oxidized LDL is also capable to elicit endothelial dysfunction by altering the secretory activity of endothelial cells (D. Li et al., 2002), inhibiting the nitric oxide-mediated vasodilatation through reduction of the expression of endothelial nitric-oxide synthase (eNOS), inducing the expression of adhesion molecules on the endothelium thus mediating the adhesion of monocytes to intima (D. Li et al., 2002), and inducing the expression of inflammatory cytokines (Steinberg, 1997). Indeed, oxLDL is a potent inducer of inflammation (Steinberg et al., 1989), contributing to the chronic inflammatory process which results to atherosclerosis (Ross, 1999).

1.3 Statins

The 3-hydroxy-3-methylglutaryl-coenzyme A reductase inhibitors, or statins, reduce serum TC, LDL cholesterol, apolipoprotein B (apoB), and, to a lesser degree, TG and Lp-a levels. Statins also have pleiotropic effects (Bellosta et al., 2000), such as the modulation of inflammatory molecules and monocyte maturation and differentiation (Bellosta et al., 2000), the suppression of smooth muscle-cells migration and proliferation (Bellosta et al., 2000), the reduction of the monocyte adhesion to the endothelium (Weber et al., 1997), the restoration of the impaired endothelium-dependent vessel wall relaxation (Jarvisalo et al., 1999), and the modification of cell-mediated LDL oxidation (Giroux et al., 1993; Aviram et al., 1998). All of the above mechanisms contribute to the reversion of atheromatosis. Undeniably, statins reduce the incidence of coronary events and are a cornerstone in the primary and secondary prevention of CHD (D.Y. Li et al., 2001). Previous studies have detected some efficacy in reducing the circulating oxLDL levels, but whether this effect is due to the reduction of LDL or is an independent, pleiotropic phenomenon remains a matter of controversy (Kwak & Mach, 2001; Robinson et al., 2005). Furthermore, little is known about the definite clinical benefit of such oxidative marker reduction.

The aim of the present study was to evaluate the efficacy of atorvastatin in reducing stenosis, to investigate the effect on oxLDL and to search for possible associations of oxLDL modification with changes of stenosis in patients managed conservatively and in pre-treated with percutaneous catheter interventional procedures patients with carotid atheromatosis. We hypothesise that atorvastatin therapy will confer remission of oxLDL levels in vivo and this will be associated with significant reduction of carotid artery stenosis.

2. Patients and methods

Between January 2005 and February 2008 a total of 100 patients were randomly selected from the lipid clinic and the carotid angioplasty clinic of a large tertiary hospital in Athens for inclusion in the study. Informed consent was obtained from each patient at recruitment according to our institutional policies. Eligible were patients with carotid artery atheromatosis from various causes (not only dyslipidemia) and with a range of predisposing factors. Exclusion criteria included: acute cardiovascular disease, severe or unstable angina pectoris, clinically evident cardiac failure, severe arrhythmias, recent surgical procedures, inflammatory diseases, active liver disease or liver impairment, excessive alcohol consumption (>4 drinks / day) or history of alcohol abuse, known allergic reaction to statins, poorly controlled diabetes mellitus as defined by a haemoglobin A1c (HbA1c) level of >7 %, uncontrolled hypertension indicated by systolic blood pressure (SBP) >140 mmHg and/or diastolic pressure >85 mmHg, history of deep vein thrombosis, bleeding tendency, serum triglycerides >350 mg/dl, evidence of thyroid dysfunction, use of systemic steroids or other anabolics, pernicious anaemia, impaired vitamin B12 or folate acid levels, abnormal serum urate at baseline, serum creatinine phosphokinase elevation of >1.5 fold at baseline, pregnancy or lactation, and end-stage renal disease or dialysis.

Patients were allocated into two groups according to the degree of carotid artery stenosis: those with arterial lumen occlusion of ≥70% in at least one common or internal carotid vessel consisted group A; those with stenosis <70% comprised group B. Patients in both groups were naive to statin therapy or if otherwise, a 6-month washout period was allowed before enrolment in the study. Group A underwent percutaneous transluminal carotid angioplasty with stenting by the same interventional cardiologist, prior to the initiation of statin therapy. Those patients were additionally administered clopidrogrel and salicylate. Both groups had to follow an American Heart Association step II diet and were encouraged to exercise.

According to the study protocol, all patients were placed on atorvastatin once daily at bedtime in individualised doses, tittered to achieve and maintain serum LDL cholesterol levels of <100 mg/dl (and ideally <70 mg/dl, if hypertension, renal impairment, smoking, hyperlipidemia, symptomatic peripheral arterial obstructive disease, or diabetes mellitus were present). Patients were prescribed statins even in the absence of hyperlipidemia, as the aim of the study was to investigate the effect of statin on oxLDL and carotid stenosis in a common atherogenic patient population. The most common doses used to achieve the above levels of LDL ranged between 10 to 40 mg, while seldom it was required to administer higher doses such as 60 mg (median atorvastatin dose for the total population = 20 mg, range 10 - 60 mg). The use of other drugs known to act synergistically with statins causing rhabdomyolysis was prohibited during the study. Adverse events were assessed in every visit in a non-specific manner: every newly reported symptom was documented as possible adverse reaction due to statin therapy and subsequently evaluated by an expert in clinical biochemistry. Adherence to the medication regimen was assessed indirectly by the low LDL levels compared with baseline.

Medical anamnesis, anthropometrics, smoking habits, blood pressure, and laboratory investigations comprising of complete blood count, fasting glucose, HbA1c, liver and kidney biochemistry, detailed lipid profile (TC, LDL cholesterol, HDL cholesterol, serum TG, apoB, and apolipoprotein A), urate, B12 and folate, thyroid function tests, homocysteine, Lp-a, and oxLDL were obtained at baseline and during follow-up visits, which were arranged at baseline, one, three, and six months; the final assessment was carried out in 12 months. Blood samples were collected after an at least 12-hour fast and a light, low-fat meal the night before sample collection was advised. Venous blood samples were collected in standard biochemistry vacutainer tubes. For the analysis of homocysteine and whole blood count, ethylenediaminetetraacetic acid (EDTA) vacutainer was used. Serum for biochemistry analysis was obtained by centrifugation (4000 g) at 4°C for 7 min and was immediately tested.

Lipid profiles (TC, HDL, TG) were determined using commercially available enzymatic colourimetric methods (Dade Behring, Newark, USA) with a Dade Behring analyser. LDL was calculated with the use of Friedewald's formula as all had TG <350 mg/dl (Puccetti et al., 2002). For the measurement of circulating oxLDL, a commercially available kit (Mercodia, Uppsala, Sweden), based on a double antibody (4E6 and mouse monoclonal antiapoB) (Holvoet et al., 1996) capture ELISA test, was used. This method primarily detects malondialdehyde LDL (MDA-LDL). The normative range (reference range) in our lab was 31-61 mU/l. Apolipoprotein A, B and Lp-a were measured using immuno-nephelometry with rabbit antisera (Dade Behring, Newark, USA) in a Dade Behring analyser.

The evaluation of stenosis was conducted by Triplex ultrasonography using an Apogee 800 plus scanner with a 7.5 MHz transducer (ATL Inc., Bothell WA, USA) at baseline and 12 months. The stenosis was calculated in three sections in each common and internal carotid artery, and the final measure was the mean value of the three. The value of stenosis in the most occluded vessel was used in the statistical analysis. Specifically, the internal carotid artery (ICA) and common carotid artery (CCA) bilaterally were evaluated for each patient using coloured and grey Doppler ultrasonography. An effort was made to completely visualize the vessels. Additionally, the pulse wave was estimated with Doppler phasmatometry as well as the blood flow velocity of the two vessels. Results were recorded in a validated form. Stenosis was defined as the presence of visual plaque in coloured or grey Doppler. The degree of stenosis was calculated by measuring the decrease of the lumen diameter and the maximum systolic blood flow velocity. In difficult cases, other parameters were taken into account, such as ICA/CCA max blood flow velocity ratio and the ICA end-diastolic velocity. A degree of stenosis >70% was considered as sever and angioplasty was advised. A degree of stenosis between 60 - 70% was defined as high, between 50 - 60% as moderate and <50% as mild. High, moderate and mild stenoses were treated conservatively. The intima media thickness (IMT) and plaque morphology were not studied due to specific lab requirements, not readily available in our institution.

2.1 Statistical analysis

Continuous variables were presented as mean values ± standard deviation, while qualitative variables were presented as absolute and relative frequencies. Normality tests were applied using the Kolmogorov-Smirnov criterion as well as Shapiro-Wilk test. Univariate analysis was initially applied to test the associations of oxLDL with carotid stenosis for each patient group as well as to identify first order correlations with various clinical parameters. Correlations between skewed continuous or discrete variables were evaluated using Spearman's p-coefficient, whereas correlations of normally distributed variables were evaluated by calculating the Pearson's r-coefficient. Comparisons between normally distributed, continuous variables and categorical variables were made using the Student t-test. Analysis of categorical data was carried out with the [chi]2 test or Fischer's exact test when appropriate.

The association of oxLDL with carotid stenosis was also tested through multiple Cox proportional hazard model. The results obtained were presented as Hazard Ratios (HR) and the 95% Confidence Intervals (CI). A backward elimination procedure was applied to all multivariate models (using P<5% as the threshold for removing a variable from the models). All models were adjusted for age, gender, SBP and TC. Kaplan-Meier curves concerning stenosis over the study period were plotted and Log rank test was performed. All reported P-values were based on two-sided tests and compared to a significance level of 5%. STATA 8.0 software (Stata Corporation, 2003, Texas, USA) was used for the analysis.

3. Results

3.1 Patients' characteristics

A total of 612 patients were evaluated, of which 123 fulfilled the eligibility criteria; finally, 100 had complete data to enter the analysis, 76 males and 24 females, median age 68 years (range 45-81). Diabetes mellitus was recorded in 26 of the 100 patients and hypertension in 66. Twenty patients had metabolic syndrome according to the national cholesterol education programme-adult treatment panel III (NCEP-ATP III) criteria (National Cholesterol Education Program (NCEP), 2001). Active smoking (defined as current of discontinued as far back as 5 years) was reported by 58 patients. Mean atorvastatin dose at baseline was 24.31±11.49 mg for group A and 20.62±10.39 mg for group B (p=0.1). By the end of the study period, the respective mean values were significantly increased to 30.45±16.27 mg for group A (p=0.044) and 28.75±17.57 mg for group B (p=0.007).

Each of the study group (A and B) comprised 50 patients. The two groups were comparable with regard of their baseline characteristics (table 1).

3.2 Lipid profile and oxidzed LDL

Mean serum TC, LDL-cholesterol, TG, Lp-a, homocysteine, and oxLDL were significantly reduced at 12 months compared to baseline (table 2). Specifically, mean oxLDL dropped from 62.26±22.03 to 44.49±21.75 mU/l (p<0.001). A marked decrease was noticed during the first 6 months and a plateau thereafter (figure 5).

Characteristic	Total	Group A	Group B	P value
Males / females	72 / 28	36 / 14	36 / 14	
Mean age in years ± SD	67.57±7.15	68.46±5.71	66.68±8.31	0.21
Number of pts with DM (percentage)	37 (37%)	18 (36%)	19 (38%)	0.83
Number of pts with HTN (percentage)	67 (67%)	36 (72%)	31 (62%)	0.29
Number of smokers (percentage)	54 (54%)	29 (54%)	25 (46%)	0.33
Number of pts with CAD (percentage)	51 (51%)	24 (47%)	27 (53%)	0.55
Mean ± SD TC (mg/dl)	232.23±47.8	235.24±49.2	229.22±46.7	0.53
Mean ± SD LDL cholesterol (mg/dl)	151.27±41.7	154.16±42.8	148.84±40.9	0.52
Mean ± SD HDL cholesterol (mg/dl)	51.97±12.7	52.12±12.1	51.82±13.4	0.9
Mean ± SD TG (mg/dl)	145.59±73.1	146.04±73.2	145.14±73.7	0.95
Mean ± SD oxLDL (mU/l)	64.66±24.8	65.8±25.3	63.53±24.5	0.65
Mean ± SD homocysteine (mU/l)	13.99±4.8	13.5±4.6	14.47±5.1	0.32

Pts: patients, DM: diabetes mellitus, HTN: arterial hypertension, MS: metabolic syndrome, SD: standard deviation, LDL: low density lipoprotein, HDL: high density lipoprotein, CAD: coronary artery disease, TC: total cholesterol, TG: triglycerides, oxLDL: oxidized LDL

Table 1. Study population baseline characteristics.

A significant correlation between LDL and oxLDL levels was detected (Pearson's correlation coefficient r=0.7, p<0.01) (figure 6). Similar correlation was found between oxLDL and apoB levels (r=0.65, p<0.001), while no significant correlation was shown with Lp-a.

Between smokers mean oxLDL was reduced from 60.68±24.09 at baseline to 45.84±24.89 mU/l at the end of study period (difference 14.84 mU/l, p = 0.0036). Similarly, between non-smokers it was reduced from 69.33±25.11 to 40.36±5.6 mU/l (difference 28.97 mU/l, p<0.001). Non-smokers had approximately double decline of oxLDL levels compared to smokers. Carotid artery stenosis was reduced between smokers from 29.68±25.59% at baseline to 23.06±21.71% at 12 months (p = 0.002). Non-smokers also presented significant reduction of stenosis during the study period (24.67 ± 26.22% vs 20 ± 21.45%, p = 0.004). Non-smokers and smokers had similar decline of carotid stenosis in 12 months (6.61% vs 4.67%, table 3).

Investigations	Total	Group A	Group B
TC (mg/dl) baseline	232.23 ± 47.8	235.24±49.1	229.22±46.7
TC (mg/dl) 12 months	153.36±17.2	154.24±16.9	152.48±17.7
p value	<0.0001	<0.0001	<0.0001
LDL cholesterol (mg/dl) baseline	151.5±41.7	154.16±42.8	148.84±40.9
LDL cholesterol (mg/dl) 12 months	79.75±12.7	79.54±13.2	79.96±12.3
p value	<0.0001	<0.0001	<0.0001
TG (mg/dl) baseline	145.59 ± 73.1	146.04±73.2	145.14±73.7
TG (mg/dl) 12 months	111±53.1	112.1±54.7	109.9±51.96
p value	0.0002	0.01	0.0069
OxLDL (mU/l) baseline	64.67±24.8	65.8±25.3	63.53±24.6
OxLDL (mU/l) 12 months	43.38±18.9	42.16±17.6	44.65±26.1
p value	<0.0001	<0.0001	0.0007
HDL cholesterol (mg/dl) baseline	51.97±12.7	52.12±12.1	51.82±13.4
HDL cholesterol (mg/dl) 12 months	51.32±15.5	52.22±16.3	50.42±14.8
p value	0.74	0.97	0.62
Homocysteine (mg/dl) baseline	13.99±4.8	13.5±4.6	14.48±5.1
Homocysteine (mg/dl) 12 months	11.89±3.5	11.88±3.8	11.9±3.4
p value	0.0006	0.057	0.0036
Apolipoprotein A (mg/dl) baseline	156.57±26.7	156.46±27.3	156.68±26.4
Apolipoprotein A (mg/dl) 12 months	160.35±25.3	162.02±23.7	158.68±27.1
p value	0.3	0.28	0.7
Apolipoprotein B (mg/dl) baseline	129.95±31.3	131.84±31.4	128.05±31.4
Apolipoprotein B (mg/dl) 12 months	77.1±11.8	77.58±13.1	76.62±10.47
p value	<0.0001	<0.0001	<0.0001
Lp-a (mg/dl) baseline	25.08±23.8	25.67±24.1	24.47±23.8
Lp-a (mg/dl) 12 months	27.72±29.1	29.42±29.8	26.01±28.7
p value	0.48	0.49	0.77

LDL: low density lipoprotein, HDL: high density lipoprotein, TC: total cholesterol, TG:triglycerides, oxLDL: oxidized LDL, Lp-a: lipoprotein a

Table 2. Comparison of mean ± standard deviation and respective P-values of measured laboratory investigations at baseline and 12 months, in the total population, and the two groups.

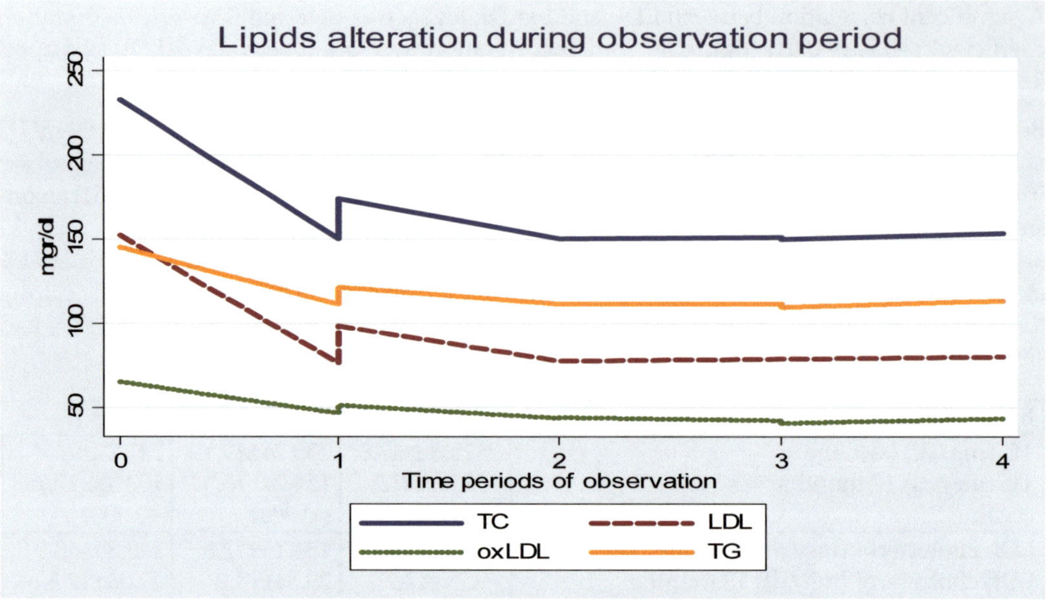

TC: total cholesterol, LDL: low density lipoprotein cholesterol, oxLDL: oxidized LDL, TG: triglycerides, 0=baseline, 1=one month, 2=three months, 3=six months, 4=twelve months.

Fig. 5. Time curve of change of total cholesterol, LDL cholesterol, triglycerides and oxidized LDL levels during the observation period.

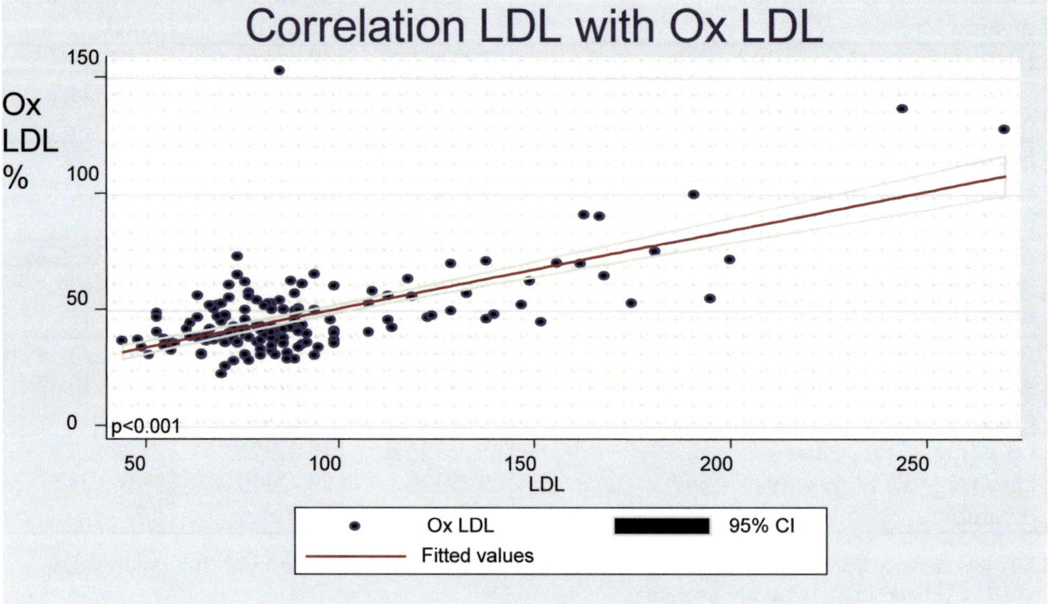

LDL: low density lipoprotein cholesterol, oxLDL: oxidized LDL, CI: confidence intervals.

Fig. 6. Correlation of low density lipoprotein with oxidized LDL levels at baseline (Pearson's correlation coefficient r=0.7, $p<0.001$).

In further analysis, the group of smokers was subdivided to mild (≤5 cigarettes/day), moderate (5 – 15 cigarettes/day) and heavy (≥15 cigarettes/day) smokers. The statistical significant reduction of oxLDL levels and degree of carotid stenosis was apparent in the subgroup of mild smokers (oxLDL at baseline 48.24±8.74 mU/l vs 41.54±9 mU/l at 12 months, $p = 0.027$ and stenosis at baseline 27.63±25.68% vs 23.42±21.74% at 12 months, $p = 0.009$), while it was not apparent in the subgroups of moderate and heavy smokers (oxLDL at baseline 86.82±37.7 mU/l vs 42.92±10.77 mU/l at 12 months, $p = 0.077$ and stenosis at baseline 34±31.9% vs 22±24.9% at 12 months, $p = 0.186$, for moderate smokers; respective values for oxLDL were 66.29±15.88 mU/l vs 34.81±5.48 mU/l, $p = 0.06$ and for stenosis 32.14±24.13% vs 22.86±22.8%, $p = 0.174$, for heavy smokers). The above described effect of smoking was taken into consideration during Cox-regression analysis.

	Smokers	P value	Non Smokers	P value
OxLDL (mU/l) baseline 12 months difference	 60.68±24.09 45.48±24.89 14.84	0.0036	 69.33±25.11 40.36±5.6 28.97	0.001
Stenosis (%) baseline 12 months difference	 29.68±25.59 23.06±21.71 6.61	0.002	 24.67±26.22 20±21.45 4.67	0.004
Correlation of oxLDL change with stenosis change in 12 months	Pearson's r = 0.412	0.021	Pearson's r = 0.198	0.03

oxLDL: oxidized LDL.

Table 3. Comparison of mean oxidized LDL values and degree of carotid stenosis change during the 1 year follow-up period, between smokers and non-smokers.

Within group B, the subgroup of patients with high degree of stenosis (>60%) had oxLDL 63.47±19.18 mU/l at baseline, while those with moderate and mild degree of stenosis (<60%) had 40.32±20.72 mU/l ($p<0.001$). Corresponding values at 12-months were 33.18±17.78 mU/l and 38.81±29.02 mU/l, representing a marked decline for patients with >60% initial stenosis and a far less decline for patients with <60% initial stenosis; yet those differences were not statistically significant (table 4).

	Stenosis >60<70%	Stenosis <60%	P value
Baseline Mean oxLDL	63.47±19.18 mU/l	40.32±20.72 mU/l	< 0.001
12 months Mean oxLDL	33.18±17.78 mU/l	38.81±29.02 mU/l	NS

LDL: low density lipoprotein cholesterol, oxLDL: oxidized LDL, NS: non significant.

Table 4. Comparison of mean oxidized LDL levels at baseline and 12 months within patients of group B (n = 50), according to degree of stenosis at enrollment.

3.3 Anthropometrics

Body mass index (BMI), weight, waist circumference and waist:hip ratio did not change significantly during the study period.

3.4 Carotid stenosis

Patients in group A had null stenosis at recruitment due to prior angioplasty with stenting. At the end of the 12-month statin therapy, no case of clinically important restenosis (>70%) was reported in this group (as restenosis was defined any increase of the carotid lumen diameter >5%). Patients in group B had mean percentage of stenosis at baseline 47.6±13.2%, which was significantly reduced following 12-month statin therapy (37.7±15.7%, p<0.001) (table 5).

	Baseline	12 months	P value
Mean (%) carotid stenosis ± standard deviation	47.6 ± 13.2	37.7 ± 15.7	0.001

Table 5. Change of the percentage of carotid artery stenosis between baseline and 12months for patients in group B.

3.5 Association of stenosis with oxidized LDL

Group B patients in the highest quartile of oxLDL values had a 12-month risk ratio for restenosis of 1.025, 95%CI=1.006-1.044, p=0.0083 (figure 7). After adjusting for gender, age, smoking, SBP, TC, and LDL levels, these patients demonstrated a HR for restenosis of 4.319 compared with those in the lowest quartile (p<0.001, figure 7). This means that an increase of oxLDL by one unit increases the degree of carotid stenosis by 2.5%, for patients in group B. A weak but significant correlation was detected between oxLDL levels and the degree of carotid artery stenosis (r=0.17, p=0.018). Similar correlation was found between LDL cholesterol levels and carotid stenosis (r=0.18, p=0.0085). The strength of Pearson's correlation of mean oxLDL change with degree of carotid stenosis change during the 12-month period was greater for smokers compared to non-smokers (table 3).

3.6 The effect of LDL levels

Patients in group B who achieved LDL levels <70 mg/dl during the observation period had a greater (28.08±28% vs 22.31±22.7%, difference 5.77%, p = 0.06) reduction of carotid stenosis compared to those with LDL levels between 70 and 100 mg/dl (26.98±25.3% vs 21.35±21.3%, difference 5.63%, p < 0.001), but this difference was not statistically significant. Thus, in conservatively treated group B, further reduction of LDL than the limit of 100 mg/dl was not associated with additional improvement of stenosis.

4. Discussion

This study demonstrates that atorvastatin administered in indivudualised doses, tittered to maintain serum LDL cholesterol levels <100 mg/dl, significantly decreased lipid profile and oxLDL, reduced carotid artery stenosis in patients managed conservatively and prevented restenosis in patients with prior angioplasty. Oxidized LDL in this study correlated positively with the degree of carotid artery stenosis; it was also shown by multivariate analysis that oxLDL represented an independent risk factor for restenosis. To our knowledge this is the first prospective study with a long observation period of 12 months to report such a clear, significant reduction of oxLDL levels following atorvastatin therapy for carotid atheromatosis of various causes and to report an association of the degree of oxLDL reduction with remission of carotid stenosis. It is also of major importance that this robust, long-standing decline of oxLDL was achieved with doses of atorvastatin used in everyday clinical practice. Interestingly, this beneficial effect was completed in the first six months, while practically no further reduction was noticed past this time point.

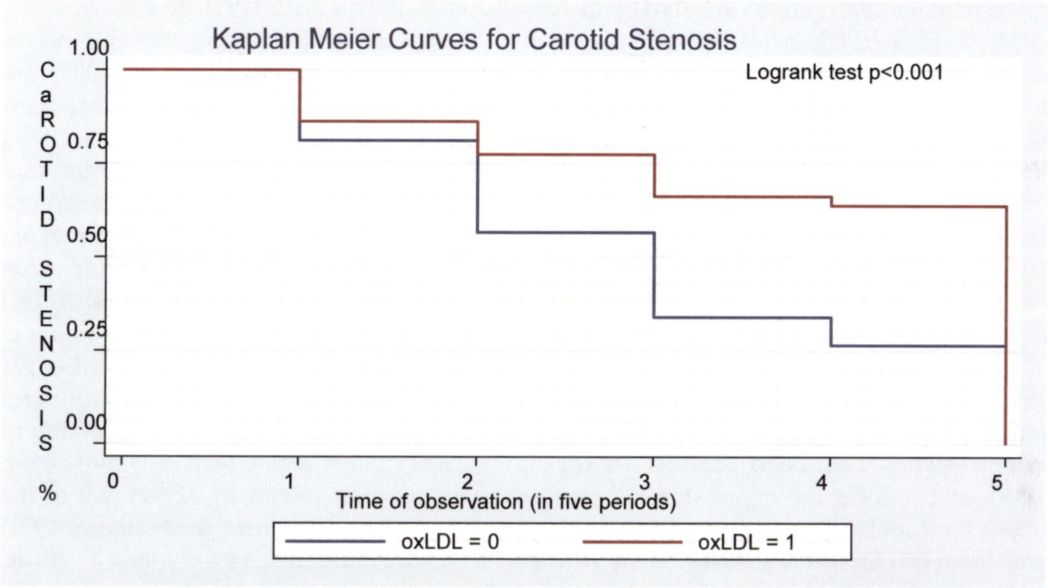

oxLDL=0: low quartile of oxLDL levels, oxLDL=1: high quartile of oxLDL levels, 0=baseline, 1=one month, 2=three months, 3=six months, 4=twelve months.

Fig. 7. Kaplan Meier survival analysis for the estimation of the risk ratio for restenosis according to the levels of oxidized LDL (oxLDL). With red line those with oxLDL levels in the highest quartile of the values. With blue line those with oxLDL levels in the lowest quartile of the measurements (risk ratio 1.025, logrank test $p<0.001$).

The mechanism by which statins modulate oxLDL levels has been controversial in the literature. Moreover, the association of oxLDL level modification with improvement of carotid atheromatosis and clinical outcome is not unequivocally established by large, double-blinded, randomised trials. Under this perspective, the present observational study provides reasonable evidence that reducing oxLDL may independently improve carotid stenosis.

Carotid IMT is a validated measure of carotid atherosclerosis. It is well established that carotid atherosclerosis, serves as an independent surrogate marker for CHD (Vasankari et al., 2001) and CVD (van Tits et al., 2006). Nevertheless, in the present study it was preferred to estimate the degree of carotid stenosis with a more direct approach, because this is more readily available in most hospital settings and because there is an obvious relation with clinical symptoms and signs. Besides, it represents a reliable method with sufficient reproducibility and it is practically the method of choice when evaluated patients candidate for endarterectomy or angioplasty. Evaluating carotid stenosis in turn, is an established method for estimating coronary risk (Vasankari et al., 2001) and cardiovascular risk (van Tits et al., 2006). Other parameters of vessel wall function, such as IMT and plaque morphology, even if clearly associated with cardiovascular risk in the literature, require well equipped laboratory and are not readily available in our hospital. Future research on the field should, ideally, comprise such measurements.

Oxidized LDL has long been recognized as a risk factor for carotid atherosclerosis in asymptomatic men (Liu et al., 2004) and has also been linked with CVD (Robbesyn et al., 2004). Oxidized LDL levels (Papathanasiou et al., 2008), autoantibodies against epitopes of oxLDL (Papathanasiou et al., 2008) and oxLDL:LDL ratio (Vasankari et al., 2001) are independently associated with increased risk for coronary atheromatosis and ischemic heart disease. Increased levels of oxLDL (Ehara et al., 2001) and MDA-LDL (Holvoet et al., 1999) in such cases are related to plaque instability. On the other hand, it has been reported that oxLDL is weakly associated with carotid IMT, but not with carotid plaque occurrence (Hulthe & Fagerberg, 2002). Oxidized LDL impairs endothelium relaxation (Harrison et al., 1987) by inhibition of the expression of eNOS and of the transport pathways of nitric oxide (NO) from the endothelial cell, reduces the responsiveness of smooth muscle cell to NO (Keaney et al., 1996), inhibits the NO-mediated vasodilation (Harrison et al., 1987; Simon et al., 1990; Steinberg, 1997), induces the expression of adhesion molecules (Frostegard et al., 1990), acts directly chemotactic to circulating monocytes (Steinberg, 1997), stimulates endothelial cells to produce MCP-1 (Cushing et al., 1990), facilitates monocyte adhesion to intima (Mehta et al., 1995), exhibits cytotoxic properties against endothelial cells (Steinberg, 1997), and induces the expression of inflammatory molecules (Steinberg, 1997). All of the above contribute directly to dysfunction of the endothelium (Witztum & Steinberg, 1991) and foam cell formation, which is the first step in the development of fatty streaks (Ross, 1999), the first visible step of atherosclerosis. These effects are mediated by preferential binding of oxLDL with type A scavenger receptors (SRA, SRA-II and CD36) on subendothelial resident macrophages and smooth muscle cells (Li et al., 1995) and lectin-like oxLDL receptor-1 (LOX-1) on endothelial cells (Sawamura et al., 1997) rather than the typical LDL receptor, resulting in an unrestricted uptake of cholesterol.

Statins reduce the incidence of cardiovascular events, an effect attributable to their hypocholesterolemic properties (Archbold & Timmis, 1999). However, the extent of clinical benefit and accumulating laboratory evidence suggest additional mechanisms of action, the so-called pleiotropic effects (Bellosta et al., 2000). The most important among such effects are the suppression of smooth muscle cell migration and proliferation (Bellosta et al., 1998), the reduction of monocyte adhesion to the vascular endothelium (Weber et al., 1997), the improvement of endothelial function (Jarvisalo et al., 1999), the inhibition of cell-mediated LDL oxidation (Aviram et al., 1998; Giroux et al., 1993), the immuno-modulation of monocyte maturation and differentiation, and the modification of production of inflammatory cytokines (Rothe et al., 1999).

Atorvastatin suppresses cellular uptake of oxLDL from differentiating monocytes by reducing the expression of LOX-1 and scavenger receptors (Fuhrman et al., 2002) and accelerates the LDL-receptor-mediated removal of the non oxidized LDL particles (Vasankari et al., 2005). Hydroxymetabolites of atorvastatin protect the LDL against oxidation (van Tits et al., 2006). The antioxidant potency of atorvastatin metabolites has been confirmed by the reduction of IgG antibodies against LDL, a marker well-associated with CHD (Aviram et al., 1998). It has even been reported that these active atorvastatin metabolites may have greater anti-atherosclerotic effects than other statin molecules (Mason et al., 2004).

In acute coronary syndromes, atorvastatin therapy was linked to modulation of short- and long-term immune response towards LDL due to inhibition of lipoprotein-associated phospholipase A2 (Lp-LPA2) enzyme (Papathanasiou et al., 2008). The apparent benefit from statin therapy after acute coronary events may also be attributed to the stabilization of the plaque and removal of oxLDL from the vessel wall (Tsimikas et al., 2004). Increased mobilization of oxidized phospholipids from the vessel wall, transient binding with apoB-100 particles and clearance from the circulation may be the possible underlying mechanism. Under this perspective the increase in oxLDL:apoB ratio detected with atorvastatin therapy might represent a marker of oxLDL efflux from the vessel wall. Removal of oxLDL contributes to improved endothelial function as oxLDL is highly immunogenic and vasoconstrictive. In our study there was no significant change in oxLDL:apoB ratio. Atorvastatin also inhibits the oxLDL-mediated LOX-1 expression by endothelial cells, the uptake of oxLDL in endothelium and the oxLDL-mediated reduction of protein kinase B (PKB) phosphorylation (Li et al., 2001). The activation of PKB is critical for the expression of eNOS, which promotes vessel relaxation. However, a meta-analysis provided no clear evidence that statin therapy have a favourable effect on oxLDL (Balk et al., 2003).

In STAT trial (Mulder et al., 2007) the antibodies against oxLDL were equally decreased with both aggressive and conventional lipid-lowering therapy. This indicates that the statin-related reduction of oxLDL is not a dose-dependent phenomenon, a finding which is in agreement with our results. It might therefore represent a pleiotropic effect, independent -at least partially- from the hypo-cholesterolemic action. A study by Orem et al. (2002) detected a significant decrease of autoantibodies against oxLDL with low doses of atorvastatin (10 mg), similar to doses used in our study. In statin exposed patients, intensification of the regimen offers no additional benefit and only those with LDL >125 mg/dl benefited from a more aggressive statin therapy (Mulder et al., 2007). Statins have a dose-related response with regard to clinical outcome, but this dose-related response has not been confirmed with regard to oxidative stress (Ky et al., 2008). This might alternatively be explained by the hypothesis that statins achieve their uttermost benefit on oxLDL within a certain time point (Mulder et al., 2007), after which further continuation of treatment serves only the purpose of maintenance. Atorvastatin has been shown to reduce small dense LDL subfractions, remnant-like particles cholesterol and oxLDL, and improve endothelial function, after just few weeks of therapy (Miyagishima et al., 2007; Sakabe et al., 2003). Such time-related effect has not been fully elucidated, but may possibly account for our finding that in the first six months there was an accelerated decline of oxLDL levels followed by a milder reduction rate thereafter.

Additional pleiotropic effects of statins have been reported in the literature and might account for the observed beneficial effects in the current study. Lysophosphatidylcholine is elevated during LDL oxidation and is responsible for some of the biological effects of oxLDL. Atorvastatin alters the ability of oxLDL to impair the endothelium relaxation, by modulating the hydrolysis of phosphatidylcholine to lysophosphatidylcholine when LDL is being oxidized (Zhu et al., 2000). Statins remove predominately "aged LDL" from plasma, which is more prone to oxidation (Orem et al., 2002), through stimulation of hepatic LDL receptor activity and inhibition of very-low density lipoprotein (VLDL) and LDL production by the liver cells (Orem et al., 2002). Statins also reduce oxygen species generation (Ky et al., 2008). Atorvastatin promotes adipocyte uptake of oxLDL in rabbits by increasing the expression of CD36 and peroxisome proliferators-activated receptor γ (PPARγ) in adipocytes (Zhao & Zhang, 2004). The increased expression of such receptors by adipocytes results to internalization of oxLDL and clearance from plasma, converting adipocytes to an oxLDL-buffering pool (Zhao & Zhang, 2004). Reduction of oxLDL in patients with CHD with atorvastatin 10 mg parallel with an increase of adiponectin, which has anti-atherogenic, anti-inflammatory and anti-diabetic properties through reduction of insulin resistance (Miyagishima et al., 2007). The CARDS study reported a significant degree of preventive activity of atorvastatin against myocardial infarction in eucholesterolemic diabetic patients, conceivably attributed to such improvement of insulin sensitivity (Miyagishima et al., 2007). Statins also diminish the expression of CD40 and CD40 ligand in vascular cells, smooth muscle cells and macrophages, which are promoted by oxLDL and are considered proatherogenic (Schonbeck et al., 2002). Other anti-inflammatory pathways include reduction of C-reactive protein (Hogue et al., 2008), chemokines, major histocompatibility complex II molecules, matrix-degrading enzymes, and procoagulant tissue factor (Schonbeck et al., 2002). Atorvastatin reverses the oxLDL-mediated inhibition of vascular endothelial growth factor-induced endothelial progenitor cell differentiation via the phosphatidylinositol 3 kinase/Akt pathway (Imanishi et al., 2003), which restores the oxLDL-related inhibition of mature endothelial cells migration (Imanishi et al., 2003). This could improve neovascularization and collateral vessel formation in response to tissue ischemia. Atorvastatin also suppresses platelet activity (Puccetti et al., 2005) by reducing the expression of CD36 and LOX-1, which are present in platelets (Puccetti et al., 2005; Sawamura et al., 1997), thus inhibiting the oxLDL-mediated platelet hyperactivity (Puccetti et al., 2005). Statins reduce the oxLDL-derived expression of adhesion molecules (E- and P-selectins, vascular cell adhesion molecule 1 [VCAM-1] and intercellular adhesion molecule 1 [ICAM-1]) in human coronary artery endothelial cells, through up-regulation of eNOS expression, which regulates the expression of adhesion molecules in endothelial cells (Li et al., 2002). Statins also diminish the oxLDL-mediated activation of nuclear factor-κB (NF-κB) (D. Li et al., 2002), which regulates the transcription of adhesion molecule genes (Robbesyn et al., 2004). In diabetic patients with dyslipidemia atorvastatin reduced CVD and markers of inflammation, adhesion and oxidation, such as C-reactive protein (CRP), soluble ICAM-1, soluble VCAM-1, E-selectin, matrix metalloproteinase 9, secretory phospholipase A2 (sPLA2), and oxLDL, the latter by 38,4% (Hogue et al., 2008). Moreover, the change of oxLDL levels correlated with the change of sICAM-1 and E-selectin levels, suggesting that statins could possibly counteract the oxLDL-associated increase of NF-κB, and therefore, the production of such cell adhesion molecules (Hogue et al., 2008). Statins also enhance scavenger receptor expression in macrophages, and increase plaque stability via reduction of metalloproteinases (Hogue et al., 2008).

The reduction of oxLDL and of carotid stenosis in our study was relevant for both smokers and non-smokers. However, subsequent subgroup analysis showed that the beneficial effect of statin use concerns mostly the subgroup of mild smokers, while no such effect was noticed for moderate and heavy smokers. How smoking may diminish the beneficial effect of statins on oxLDL and carotid stenosis is not yet clarified in the literature. A reasonable assumption might be that, since smoking increases the oxidative stress, it contributes to enhanced LDL oxidation (Van Himbergen et al., 2004). Moreover, studies in animal models, have demonstrated that smoking alters the immunologic response to oxLDL by reducing the production of antibodies against these molecules, i.e. causing a kind of immune suppression regarding the response to oxLDL. Thus, it has been shown to increase carotid IMT (Tani et al., 2004).

The Mercodia oxLDL detects the MDA-modified apoB (Holvoet et al., 1996). It has been proposed that oxLDL looses its predictive value for CVD when adjustment for apoB level is performed (Ky et al., 2008). In several studies though, a significant reduction of Mercodia oxLDL with atorvastatin 10 mg was still detected even after adjustment for apoB, (Holvoet et al., 2003; Ky et al., 2008; van Tits et al., 2006), while in other studies no adjustment for LDL or apoB levels was made (Ky et al., 2008; Sasaki et al., 2002). In our study the oxLDL:apoB ratio remained unchanged, but in the multivariate analysis the reduction of oxLDL was still significant after adjustment for apoB and LDL levels.

In patients with familial hypercholesterolemia a lack of association between oxLDL and IMT was reported at baseline, however two years therapy with atorvastatin 80 mg was associated with regression of carotid IMT (van Tits et al., 2004). The LDL subfraction profile and autoantibodies against oxLDL remained unchanged. Nevertheless, the rate of oxidation and the amount of dienes formed decreased and this was linked to lessening of atherosclerosis. In our study the reduction of carotid stenosis was associated with decreased oxLDL levels. Besides, the unchanged oxLDL autoantibodies levels do not preclude the reduction of oxLDL, as was indicated in another study involving dialysis patients, where atorvastatin therapy reduced plasma oxLDL, whereas oxLDL autoantibodies did not changed significantly (van den Akker et al., 2003).

Disadvantages of the study were the relatively small size, the lack of a control group comprising of patients with carotid stenosis not on statin therapy, which would be unethical, the fact that researchers were not blinded to the patients' status, the lack of randomization of the dose-schedules and the use of only one method to detect oxLDL.

5. Conclusion

This prospective, cross-sectional study with such a long observation period provided enough evidence to postulate a favourable effect of low-dose atorvastatin therapy on oxLDL, which was additionally associated with improvement of stenosis in patients with carotid atheromatosis. We thus, assume that oxLDL may represent a far more sensitive risk factor for carotid stenosis, than LDL itself or apoB. Further studying is required to confirm such findings and to establish a clear clinical and pathophsiologic link between oxLDL and carotid stenosis.

6. Acknowledgment

The authors wish to acknowledge Dr. Antonios Polydorou for performing the catheterizations and stenting of the carotid arteries in the group of patients that underwent intervention prior entering the study. We also thank him for allowing us access to the records of the angioplasty laboratory. Finally we are grateful for valuable advice and reviewing this manuscript before publishing.

We also wish to acknowledge Dr. Ioannis Dermitzakis for the critical contribution in evaluating the degree of stenosis of our patient population, as director of the ultrasonography laboratory in our institution. Without his help and valuable assistance this whole project would not have been completed.

The authors finally acknowledge Mrs. Anna Zervou for carrying out the biochemical laboratory measurements with diligence and accuracy, overlooking tiredness, physical and emotional strain. We thank her for her personal commitment in the success of this research.

7. References

Anderson TJ, Meredith IT, Charbonneau F, Yeung AC, Frei B, Selwyn AP, Ganz P. (1996) Endothelium - dependant coronary vasomotion relates to the susceptibility of LDL to oxidation in humans. *Circulation*, vol. 93, No. 9, (May 1996), pp. 1647-1650, ISSN 0009-7322

Archbold RA., Timmis AD. (1999) Modification of coronary artery disease progression by cholesterol-lowering therapy: the angiographic studies. *Current Opinion in Lipidology*, vol. 10, No. 6, (Dec 1999), pp 527-534, ISSN 0957-9672

Assmann G, Schulte H. (1992) Relation of high density lipoprotein cholesterol and triglycerides to incidence of atherosclerotic coronary artery disease (the PROCAM experience). Prospective cardiovascular Münster study. *The American Journal of Cardiology*, vol. 70, No. 7, (Sep 1992), pp. 733–737, ISSN 0002-9149

Aviram M., Rosenblat M., Bisgaier CL., Newton RS. (1998) Atorvastatin and gemfibrozil metabolites, but not the parent drugs, are potent antioxidants against lipoprotein oxidation. *Atherosclerosis*, vol. 138, No. 2, (Jun 1998), pp 271-280, ISSN 0021-9150

Balk EM., Lau J., Goudas LC., Jordan HS., Kupelnick B., Kim LU., Karas RH. (2003). Effects of statins on nonlipid serum markers associated with cardiovascular disease: a systematic review. *Annals of Internal Medicine*, vol. 139, No. 8, (Oct 2003), pp. 670-682, ISSN 0003-4819

Bellosta S., Bernini F., Ferri N., Quarato P., Canavesi M., Arnaboldi L., Fumagalli R., Paolleti R., Corsini A. (1998) Direct vascular effects of HMG-CoA reductase inhibitors. *Atherosclerosis, Suppl. 137, (Apr* 1998), pp. 101-119, ISSN 0021-9150

Bellosta S., Ferri N., Bernini F., Paoletti R., Corsini A. (2000) Non-lipid-related effects of statins. *Annals of Medicine*, Vol. 32, No. 3, (Apr 2000), pp. 164-176, ISSN 0785-3890

Corti R., Fuster V., Fayad ZA., Worthley SG., Helft G., Smith D., Weinberger J., Wentzel J., Mizsei G., Mercuri M., Badimon JJ. (2002) Lipid lowering by simvastatin induces regression of human atherosclerotic lesions: two years' follow-up by high-resolution noninvasive magnetic resonance imaging. *Circulation*, Vol. 106, No. 23, (Dec 2002), pp. 2884–2887, ISSN 0009-7322

Cushing SD, Berliner JA, Valente AJ, Territo MC, Navab M, Parhami F, Gerrity R, Schwartz CJ, Fogelman AM. (1990) Minimally modified low density lipoprotein induces monocyte chemotactic protein 1 in human endothelial cells and smooth muscle cells. *Proceedings of the National Academy of Sciences of the United States of America,* Vol. 87, No. 13, (Jul 1990), pp. 5134-5138, ISSN 1091-6490

Durrington P, Sniderman A. (2002) Epidemiology and pathophysiology. In: *Hyperlipidemia.* Durrington P, Sniderman A. pp. 29–31 Health Press, ISBN 1-903734-23-1, Oxford, UK

Ehara S, Ueda M, Naruko T, Haze K, Itoh A, Otsuka M, Komatsu R, Matsuo T, Itabe H, Takano T, Tsukamoto Y, Yoshiyama M, Takeuchi K, Yoshikawa J, Becker AE.(2001) Elevated levels of oxidized low density lipoprotein show a positive relationship with the severity of acute coronary syndromes. *Circulation,* vol. 103, No. 15, (Apr 2001), pp. 1955-1960, ISSN 0009-7322

Expert Panel on Detection, Evaluation, and Treatment of High Blood Cholesterol in Adults. (2001) Executive Summary of The Third Report of The National Cholesterol Education Program (NCEP) Expert Panel on Detection, Evaluation, And Treatment of High Blood Cholesterol In Adults (Adult Treatment Panel III). *JAMA,* vol. 285, No. 19, (May 2001), pp. 2486-2497, ISSN 0098-7484

Frostegard J, Nilsson J, Haegerstrand A, Hamsten A, Wigzell H, Gidlund M. (1990) Oxidized low density lipoprotein induces differentiation and adhesion of human monocytes and the monocytic cell line U937. *Proceedings of the National Academy of Sciences of the United States of America,* vol. 87, No 3, (Feb 1990), pp 904-908, ISSN 1091-6490

Fuhrman B, Koren L, Volkova N, Keidar S, Hayek T, Aviram M. (2002) Atorvastatin therapy in hypercholesterolemic patients suppresses cellular uptake of oxidized-LDL by differentiating monocytes. *Atherosclerosis,* vol. 164, No. 1, (Sep 2002), pp 179-185, ISSN 0021-9150

Giroux LM, Davignon J, Naruszewicz M. (1993) Simvastatin inhibits the oxidation of low-density lipoproteins by activated human monocyte-derived macrophages. *Biochimica et Biophysica Acta,* vol. 1165, No. 3, (Jan 1993), pp 335-338, ISSN 0006-3002

Harrison DG, Freiman PC, Armstrong ML, Marcus ML, Heistad DD. (1987) Alterations of vascular reactivity in atherosclerosis. *Circulation Research,* vol. 61, No. 5 Pt 2, (Nov 1987), pp. II74-1180, ISSN 0009-7300

Hogue JC, Lamarche B, Tremblay AJ, Bergeron J, Gagne C, Couture P. (2008) Differential effect of atorvastatin and fenofibrate on plasma oxidized low-density lipoprotein, inflammation markers, and cell adhesion molecules in patients with type 2 diabetes mellitus. *Metabolism,* vol. 57, No. 3, (Mar 2008), pp 380-386, ISSN 0026-0495

Hokanson JE, Autsin MA. (1996) Plasma triglyceride level is a risk factor for cardiovascular disease independent of high–density lipoprotein cholesterol level: a meta–analysis of population–based prospective studies. *Journal of Cardiovascular Risk,* vol. 3, No. 2, (Apr 1996), pp. 213–219, ISSN 1350-6277

Holvoet P, Donck J, Laneloos M, Brouwers EK, Arnout J, Lesaffre E, Vanrenterghem Y, Collen D. (1996) Correlation between oxidized low density lipoproteins and von Willebrand factor in chronic renal failure. *Journal of Thrombosis and Haemostasis,* vol. 76, No. 5, (Nov 1996), pp. 663-669, ISSN 1538-7933

Holvoet P, Collen D, Van de Werf F. (1999) Malondialdehyde-modified LDL as a marker of acute coronary syndromes. *JAMA,* vol. 281, No. 18, (May 1999), pp. 1718-1721, ISSN 0098-7484

Hulthe J, Fagerberg B. (2002) Circulating oxidized LDL is associated with subclinical atherosclerosis development and inflammatory cytokines (AIR Study). *Arteriosclerosis, Thrombosis, and Vascular Biology,* vol. 22, No. 7 (Jul 2002), pp 1162-1167, ISSN 1079-5642

Imanishi T, Hano T, Matsuo Y, Nishio I. (2003) Oxidized low-density lipoprotein inhibits vascular endothelial growth factor-induced endothelial progenitor cell differentiation. *Clinical and Experimental Pharmacology and Physiology,* vol. 30, No. 9, (Sep. 2003), pp. 665-670, ISSN 0305-1870

Järvisalo MJ, Toikka JO, Vasankari T, Mikkola J, Viikari JS, Hartiala JJ, Raitakari OT. (1999) HMG CoA reductase inhibitors are related to improved systemic endothelial function in coronary artery disease. *Atherosclerosis,* vol.147, No. 2, (Dec 1999), pp. 237-242, ISSN 0021-9150

Katsouras CS, Karabina SA, Tambaki AP, Goudevenos JA, Michalis LK, Tsironis LD, Stroumbis CS, Elisaf MS, Sideris DA, Tselepis AD. (2001) Serum lipoprotein (a) concentrations and apoprotein (a) isoforms: association with the severity of clinical presentation in patients with coronary heart disease. *Journal of Cardiovascular Risk,* vol. 8, No. 5, (Oct 2001), pp. 311–317, ISSN 1350-6277

Keaney JF, Jr., Guo Y, Cunningham D, Shwaery GT, Xu A, Vita JA. (1996) Vascular incorporation of alpha-tocopherol prevents endothelial dysfunction due to oxidized LDL by inhibiting protein kinase C stimulation. *The Journal of Clinical Investigation,* vol. 98, No. 2, (Jul 1996), pp. 386-394, ISSN 0021-9738

Kwak BR, Mach F. (2001) Statins inhibit leukocyte recruitment: new evidence for their anti-inflammatory properties. *Arteriosclerosis, Thrombosis, and Vascular Biology,* vol. 21, No. 8, (Aug 2001), pp. 1256-1258, ISSN 0276-5047

Ky B, Burke A, Tsimikas S, Wolfe ML, Tadesse MG, Szapary PO, Witztum JL, FitzGerald GA, Rader DJ. (2008) The influence of pravastatin and atorvastatin on markers of oxidative stress in hypercholesterolemic humans. *Journal of the American College of Cardiology,* vol. 51, No. 17, (Apr 2008), pp. 1653-1662, ISSN 0735-1097

Li D, Chen H, Romeo F, Sawamura T, Saldeen T, Mehta JL. (2008) Statins modulate oxidized low-density lipoprotein-mediated adhesion molecule expression in human coronary artery endothelial cells: role of LOX-1. *Journal of Pharmacology and Experimental Therapeutics,* vol. 302, No. 2, (Apr 2002), pp. 601-605, ISSN 0022-3565

Li DY, Chen HJ, Mehta JL. (2001) Statins inhibit oxidized-LDL-mediated LOX-1 expression, uptake of oxidized-LDL and reduction in PKB phosphorylation. *Cardiovascular Research,* vol. 52, No. 1, (Oct 2001), pp. 130-135, ISSN 0008-6363

Li H, Freeman MW, Libby P. (1995) Regulation of smooth muscle cell scavenger receptor expression in vivo by atherogenic diets and in vitro by cytokines. *The Journal of Clinical Investigation,* vol. 95, No. 1, (Jan 1995), pp. 122-133, ISSN 0021-9738

Liu ML, Ylitalo K, Salonen R, Salonen JT, Taskinen MR. (2004) Circulating oxidized low-density lipoprotein and its association with carotid intima-media thickness in asymptomatic members of familial combined hyperlipidemia families. *Arteriosclerosis, Thrombosis, and Vascular Biology,* vol. 24, No. 8, (Aug 2004), pp. 1492-1497. ISSN 0276-5047

Mason RP, Walter MF, Jacob RF, (2004) Effects of HMG-CoA reductase inhibitors on endothelial function: role of microdomains and oxidative stress. *Circulation,* vol. 109, 21 Suppl. 1, (Jun 2004), pp. II34-41, ISSN 0009-7322

Mehta A, Yang B, Khan S, Hendricks JB, Stephen C, Mehta JL, (1995) Oxidized low-density lipoproteins facilitate leukocyte adhesion to aortic intima without affecting endothelium-dependent relaxation. Role of P-selectin. *Arteriosclerosis, Thrombosis, and Vascular Biology,* vol. 15, No 11, (Nov 1995), pp. 2076-2083, ISSN 0276-5047

Miyagishima K, Hiramitsu S, Kato S, Kato Y, Kitagawa F, Teradaira R, Shinohara R, Mori K, Kimura H, Ueda T, Ohtsuki M, Morimoto S, Hishida H, (2007) Efficacy of atorvastatin therapy in ischaemic heart disease - effects on oxidized low-density lipoprotein and adiponectin. *Journal of International Medical Research,* vol. 35, No. 4, (Jul-Aug 2007), pp. 534-539, ISSN 0300-0605

Mulder DJ, van Haelst PL, Wobbes MH, Gans RO, Zijlstra F, May JF, Smit AJ, Tervaert JW, van Doormaal JJ, (2007) The effect of aggressive versus conventional lipid-lowering therapy on markers of inflammatory and oxidative stress. *Cardiovascular Drugs and Therapy,* vol. 21, No. 2, (Apr 2007), pp. 91-97, ISSN 0920-3206

Nishi K, Itabe H, Uno M, Kitazato KT, Horiguchi H, Shinno K, Nagahiro S, (2002) Oxidized LDL in carotid plaques and plasma associates with plaque instability. *Arteriosclerosis, Thrombosis, and Vascular Biology,* vol. 22, No 10, (Oct 2002), pp. 1649-1654, ISSN 0276-5047

Nissen SE, Tuzcu ME, Schoenhagen P, Brown GB, Ganz P, Vogel RA, Crowe T, Howard G, Cooper CJ, Brodie B, Grines CL, DeMaria AN, REVERSAL investigators. (2004) Effect of intensive compared with moderate lipid lowering therapy on progression of coronary atherosclerosis. A randomized controlled trial. *JAMA,* vol. 291, No. 9, (Mar 2004), pp. 1071-1080, ISSN 0098-7484

Orem C, Orem A, Uydu HA, Celik S, Erdol C, Kural BV, (2002) The effects of lipid-lowering therapy on low-density lipoprotein auto-antibodies: relationship with low-density lipoprotein oxidation and plasma total antioxidant status. *Coronary Artery Disease,* vol. 13, No. 1, (Feb 2002), pp. 65-71, ISSN 0954-6928

Papathanasiou AI, Lourida ES, Tsironis LD, Goudevenos JA, Tselepis AD, (2008) Short- and long-term elevation of autoantibody titers against oxidized LDL in patients with acute coronary syndromes. Role of the lipoprotein-associated phospholipase A2 and the effect of atorvastatin treatment. *Atherosclerosis,* vol. 196, No. 1, (Jan 2008), pp. 289-297, ISSN 0021-9150

Penny WF, Ben-Yehuda O, Kuroe K, Long J, Bond A, Bhargava V, Peterson JF, McDaniel M, Juliano J, Witztum JL, Ross J Jr, Peterson KL, (2001) Improvement of coronary artery endothelial dysfunction with lipid-lowering therapy: heterogeneity of segmental response and correlation with plasma-oxidized low density lipoprotein. *Journal of the American College of Cardiology,* vol. 37, No. 3, (Mar 2001), pp. 766-774, ISSN 0735-1097

Puccetti L, Pasqui AL, Pastorelli M, Bova G, Cercignani M, Palazzuoli A, Angori P, Auteri A, Bruni F, (2002) Time-dependent effect of statins on platelet function in hypercholesterolaemia. *European Journal of Clinical Investigation,* vol. 32, No. 12, (Dec 2002), pp. 901-908, ISSN 0014-2972

Puccetti L, Sawamura T, Pasqui AL, Pastorelli M, Auteri A, Bruni F, (2005) Atorvastatin reduces platelet-oxidized-LDL receptor expression in hypercholesterolaemic patients. *European Journal of Clinical Investigation,* vol. 35, No. 1, (Jan 2005), pp. 47-51, ISSN 0014-2972

Robbesyn F, Salvayre R, Negre-Salvayre A, (2004) Dual role of oxidized LDL on the NF-kappaB signaling pathway. *Free Radical Research,* vol. 38, No. 6, (Jun 2004), pp. 541-551, ISSN 1071-5762

Robinson JG, Smith B, Maheshwari N, Schrott H. (2005) Pleiotropic effects of statins: benefit beyond cholesterol reduction? A meta-regression analysis. *Journal of the American College of Cardiology,* vol. 46, No. 10, (Nov 2005), pp. 1855-1862, ISSN 0735-1097

Ross R. (1999) Atherosclerosis--an inflammatory disease. *New England Journal of Medicine,* vol. 340, No. 2, (Jan 1999), pp. 115-126, ISSN 0028-4793

Rothe G, Herr AS, Stohr J, Abletshauser C, Weidinger G, Schmitz G, (1999) A more mature phenotype of blood mononuclear phagocytes is induced by fluvastatin treatment in hypercholesterolemic patients with coronary heart disease. *Atherosclerosis,* vol. 144, No. 1, (May 1999), pp. 251-261, ISSN 0021-9150

Sakabe K, Fukuda N, Wakayama K, Nada T, Shinohara H, Tamura Y, (2003) Effects of atorvastatin therapy on the low-density lipoprotein subfraction, remnant-like particles cholesterol, and oxidized low-density lipoprotein within 2 weeks in hypercholesterolemic patients. *Circulation Journal,* vol. 67, No. 10, (Oct 2003), pp 866-870, ISSN 1738-5520

Sasaki S, Kuwahara N, Kunitomo K, Harada S, Yamada T, Azuma A, Takeda K, Nakagawa M. (2002) Effects of atorvastatin on oxidized low-density lipoprotein, low-density lipoprotein subfraction distribution, and remnant lipoprotein in patients with mixed hyperlipoproteinemia. *The American Journal of Cardiology,* vol. 89, No. 4, (Feb 2002), pp. 386-389, ISSN 0002-9149

Sawamura T, Kume N, Aoyama T, Moriwaki H, Hoshikawa H, Aiba Y, Tanaka T, Miwa S, Katsura Y, Kita T, Masaki T, (1997) An endothelial receptor for oxidized low-density lipoprotein. *Nature,* vol. 386, No. 6620, (Mar 1997), pp. 73-77, ISSN 0028-0836

Schönbeck U, Gerdes N, Varo N, Reynolds RS, Horton DB, Bavendiek U, Robbie L, Ganz P, Kinlay S, Libby P, (2002) Oxidized low-density lipoprotein augments and 3-hydroxy-3-methylglutaryl coenzyme A reductase inhibitors limit CD40 and CD40L expression in human vascular cells. *Circulation,* vol. 106, No. 23, (Dec 2002), pp. 2888-2893, ISSN 0009-7322

Simon BC, Cunningham LD, Cohen RA. (1990) Oxidized low density lipoproteins cause contraction and inhibit endothelium-dependent relaxation in the pig coronary artery. *Journal of Clinical Investigation,* vol. 86, No. 1, (Jul 1990), pp. 75-79, ISSN 0021-9738

Steinberg D, Parthasarathy S, Carew TE, Khoo JC, Witztum JL. (1989) Beyond cholesterol. Modifications of low-density lipoprotein that increase its atherogenicity. *New England Journal of Medicine,* vol. 320, No. 14, (Apr 1989), pp. 915-924, ISSN 0028-4793

Steinberg D. (1997) Low density lipoprotein oxidation and its pathobiological significance. *The Journal of Biological Chemistry,* vol. 272, No. 34, (Aug 1997), pp. 20963-20966, ISSN 0021-9258

Tani S, Dimayuga PC, Anazawa T, Chyu KY, Li H, Shah PK, Cercek B, (2004) Aberrant antibody responses to oxidized LDL and increased intimal thickening in apoE-/- mice exposed to cigarette smoke. *Atherosclerosis,* vol. 175, No. 1, (Jul 2004), pp. 7-14, ISSN 0021-9150

Steinbrecher UP, Parthasarathy S, Leake DS, Witztum JL, Steinberg D. (1984) Modification of low density lipoprotein by endothelial cells involves lipid peroxidation and degradation of low density lipoprotein phospholipids. *Proceedings of the National Academy of Sciences of the United States of America,* vol. 81, No. 12, (Jun 1984), pp. 3883-3887, ISSN 1091-6490

Toshima S, Hasegawa A, Kurabayashi M, Itabe H, Takano T, Sugano J, Shimamura K, Kimura J, Michishita I, Suzuki T, Nagai R. (2000) Circulating oxidized low density lipoprotein levels. A biochemical risk marker for coronary heart disease. *Arteriosclerosis, Thrombosis, and Vascular Biology,* vol. 20, No. 10, (Oct 2000), pp. 2243-2247, ISSN 0276-5047

Holvoet P, Harris TB, Tracy RP, Verhamme P, Newman AB, Rubin SM, Simonsick EM, Colbert LH, Kritchevsky SB. (2003) Association of high coronary heart disease risk status with circulating oxidized LDL in the well-functioning elderly: findings from the Health, Aging, and Body Composition study. *Arteriosclerosis, Thrombosis, and Vascular Biology,* vol. 23, No. 8, (Aug 2003), pp. 1444-1448, ISSN 0276-5047

Tsimikas S, Witztum JL, Miller ER, Sasiela WJ, Szarek M, Olsson AG, Schwartz GG; Myocardial Ischemia Reduction with Aggressive Cholesterol Lowering (MIRACL) Study Investigators, (2004) High-dose atorvastatin reduces total plasma levels of oxidized phospholipids and immune complexes present on apolipoprotein B-100 in patients with acute coronary syndromes in the MIRACL trial. *Circulation,* vol. 110, No. 11, (Sep 2004), pp. 1406-1412, ISSN 0009-7322

van den Akker JM, Bredie SJ, Diepenveen SH, van Tits LJ, Stalenhoef AF, van Leusen R, (2003) Atorvastatin and simvastatin in patients on hemodialysis: effects on lipoproteins, C-reactive protein and in vivo oxidized LDL. *Journal of Nephrology,* vol. 16, No. 2, (Mar-Apr 2003), pp. 238-244, ISSN 1121-8428

Van Himbergen T, Roest M, De Waart F, De Graaf J, Voorbij H, Van Tits L, Stalenhoef A. (2004) Paraoxonase genotype, LDL-oxidation and carotid atherosclerosis in male life-long smokers. *Free Radical Research,* vol. 38, No. 6, (Jun 2004), pp. 553-560, ISSN 1071-5762

van Tits LJ, Smilde TJ, van Wissen S, de Graaf J, Kastelein JJ, Stalenhoef AF. (2004) Effects of atorvastatin and simvastatin on low-density lipoprotein subfraction profile, low-density lipoprotein oxidizability, and antibodies to oxidized low-density lipoprotein in relation to carotid intima media thickness in familial hypercholesterolemia. *Journal of Investigative Medicine,* vol 52, No. 3, (Apr 2004), pp. 177-184, ISSN 1080-5589

van Tits LJ, van Himbergen TM, Lemmers HL, de Graaf J, Stalenhoef AF. (2006) Proportion of oxidized LDL relative to plasma apolipoprotein B does not change during statin therapy in patients with heterozygous familial hypercholesterolemia. *Atherosclerosis,* vol. 185, No. 2, (Apr 2006), pp. 307-312, ISSN 0021-9150

Vasankari T, Ahotupa M, Toikka J, Mikkola J, Irjala K, Pasanen P, Neuvonen K, Raitakari O, Viikari J. (2001) Oxidized LDL and thickness of carotid intima-media are associated with coronary atherosclerosis in middle-aged men: lower levels of oxidized LDL with statin therapy. *Atherosclerosis,* vol. 155, No. 2, (Apr 2001), pp. 403-412, ISSN 0021-9150

Vasankari T, Ahotupa M, Viikari J, Nuotio I, Vuorenmaa T, Strandberg T, Vanhanen H, Tikkanen MJ. (2005) Effects of statin therapy on circulating conjugated dienes, a measure of LDL oxidation. *Atherosclerosis,* vol. 179, No. 1, (Mar 2005), pp. 207-209, ISSN 0021-9150

Weber C, Erl W, Weber KS, Weber PC, (1997) HMG-CoA reductase inhibitors decrease CD11b expression and CD11b-dependent adhesion of monocytes to endothelium and reduce increased adhesiveness of monocytes isolated from patients with hypercholesterolemia. *Journal of American College of Cardiology,* vol. 30, No. 5, (Nov 1997), pp. 1212-1217, ISSN 0735-1097

Witztum JL, Steinberg D. (1991) Role of oxidized low density lipoprotein in atherogenesis. *Journal of Clinical Investigation,* vol. 88, No. 6, (Dec 1991), pp. 1785-1792, ISSN 0021-9738

Zhao SP, Zhang DQ, (2004) Atorvastatin enhances cellular uptake of oxidized LDL in adipocytes from hypercholesterolemic rabbits. *Clinica Chimica Acta,* vol. 339, No. 1-2, (Jan 2004), pp. 189-194, ISSN 0009-8981

Zhu Q, McMaster J, Mymin D, Dembinski T, Hatch G, Choy PC, Kroeger EA, (2000) Effects of atorvastatin treatment on the oxidatively modified low density lipoprotein in hyperlipidemic patients. *Molecular and Cellular Biochemistry,* vol. 207, No. 1-2, (Apr 2000), pp. 9-17, ISSN 0300-8177

Part 3

Treatment for Coronary Artery Disease

9

Evaluation of Anti-Ischemic Therapy in Coronary Artery Disease: A Review

Marwan S.M. Al-Nimer
College of Medicine, Al-Mustansiriya University, Baghdad, Iraq

1. Introduction

Myocardial ischemia, or lack of oxygen, is caused by an imbalance between oxygen supply and oxygen demand in the heart. This imbalance is usually due to an inability to increase coronary blood flow in response to increased myocardial oxygen consumption. The inability to increase coronary blood flow is often related to atherosclerosis of the large coronary arteries, which leads to a progressive narrowing of the blood vessel lumen and a reduction in coronary blood flow. Coronary blood flow may also be restricted by either focal or generalized intense vasoconstriction (i.e. vasospasm) in the major coronary arteries. Antianginal drugs may effectively relieve or prevent acute ischemic episodes by increasing myocardial oxygen supply, decreasing myocardial oxygen demand, or both.

2. Conventional antianginal

2.1 Nitrates (short and long acting) and nitrites

Sir Thomas Lauder Brunton first used amyl nitrite in the treatment of angina pectoris in 1867. As a medical student, Brunton had became aware of prior clinical findings of Benjamin Ward Richardson that inhaled amyl nitrite rapidly increased the action of the heart (Richardson, 1864), and also the unpublished observations of Arthur Gamgee demonstrating that amyl nitrite greatly lessened 'arterial tension' in both animals and man (Brunton, 1867). **At the same time** William Murrell, began using the organic nitrate; glyceryl trinitrate (GTN), in the treatment of angina pectoris (Murrell, 1879). With GTN therapy, patients would obtain relief from angina with some patients also reporting that their angina could be aborted by taking the drug at the onset of symptoms. In the 1920s, Richard Bodo used the Starling's heart–lung preparation to determine the effects of two nitrite preparations on coronary flow (Bodo, 1928) as earlier work in myocardial studies demonstrated that nitrite preparations produced vasorelaxation (Francois-Frank, 1903; Schloss, 1913; Cow, 1910). By the 1930s, nitrites and nitrate esters were established treatments for angina and hypertension. Contro and colleagues observed a paradoxical action following inhalation of amyl nitrite in patients with coronary artery disease, in that electrocardiograph changes resembling myocardial ischemia would occur after administration of amyl nitrite due to a sudden drop in blood pressure followed by coronary insufficiency (Contro et al., 1952). Finally, the authors suggested that the nitrite could be used as a diagnostic test in patients with borderline or questionable history of coronary artery disease. The nitrites/nitrates are classified as agents that directly relax vascular smooth muscle, but can also relax other smooth muscles such as bronchial, ureteral, and uterine smooth muscle (Chen et al., 2001; Dong et al., 1998; Facchinetti et al., 1996; Yallampalli et al., 1993).

2.1.1 Mechanisms of action

It is generally believed that the therapeutic effect of these drugs involves the release of nitric oxide (NO) from nitrite, the activation of guanylyl cyclase, and relaxation of blood vessels. Interactions with nitroglycerin (GTN) and sulfhydryl-containing receptors are necessary for vascular smooth muscle relaxation and repeated administration of GTN produces sulfhydryl depletion and the development of tolerance. Subsequent studies have demonstrated the release of NO following the decomposition of an intermediate S-nitrosothiol. Additional studies suggest that an enzymatic mechanism may be responsible for the bio-activation of GTN.

2.1.2 Cardiovascular pharmacological effects

The most commonly nitrites and nitrates agents at this time include isosorbide dinitrate, isosorbide-5-mononitrate, and GTN which are effective in reducing ventricular preload by increasing peripheral venous capacitance. These drugs can also decrease pulmonary and systemic vascular resistances, but require higher doses than those needed for the increase in venous capacitance. These agents can reduce ventricular filling pressure, wall stress and myocardial oxygen consumption, and may also improve systolic and diastolic ventricular function by improving coronary flow in patients with ischemic cardiomyopathy. However, there is, as yet, no convincing evidence that organic nitrates improve mortality in patients with acute myocardial infarction. The limitations of this class of agents are well known and potentially include adverse hemodynamic effects, drug tolerance, lack of selectivity, and limited bioavailability. Nitrates are recommended by the ACC/AHA guidelines as part of the initial management of ST elevation myocardial infarction (STEMI) and unstable angina (UA)/non-ST elevation myocardial infarction (NSTEMI). Nitrates can provide symptomatic relief in acute coronary syndrome (ACS) but are not associated with a survival benefit in younger ACS patients. However, nitrate use in the elderly ACS patients is associated with a reduction in mortality, heart failure, and left ventricular dysfunction at 6 months follow-up. The antianginal properties of nitrates can be attributed to the augmentation of coronary flow and to the decrease in the heart's oxygen consumption that they cause. Nitrates induce coronary vasodilatation, leading to better myocardial perfusion. They also produce venodilatation, leading to decreased venous return, and thus to reduced cardiac preload. Glyceryl trinitrate also exerts antiplatelet effects in patients with stable angina pectoris. Short-acting GTN is used sublingually to relieve symptoms of angina. Long-acting nitrates can be used in combination with a beta blocker if monotherapy has proven unsuccessful or in combination with calcium channel antagonist if beta blockade leads to unacceptable adverse drug reactions. During exercise, nitrates increase the delay before the onset of angina and the time to 1 mm ST segment depression (TST), but their effects are improved when used in combination with another antianginal agent. Nitrates should be administered intermittently, with 8 to 12 hours of nitrate-free intervals, to prevent pharmacologic tolerance. However, a rebound phenomenon with anginal symptoms is possible during these intervals. Short acting nitrates control angina most effectively when administered in the morning. In contrast, long acting nitrates are designed for once per day dosing and should normally be administered at bedtime to maintain a therapeutic concentration in the plasma throughout the night and the subsequent vulnerable morning hours. The most frequent side effect of nitrates is headache, reported by up to 82% of patients in placebo-controlled trials in a dose-related fashion, with about 10% of patients reporting severe symptoms leading to discontinuation of the treatment (Thadani & Rodgers, 2006). Hypotension is frequent and usually asymptomatic, although syncope can rarely occur. The tolerance phenomenon associated with the chronic use of long-acting nitrates imposes the need for an 8–12 hour nitrate-free interval every day, which can occasionally lead to angina attacks at night during this period. Nitrates are contraindicated in patients with severe aortic stenosis or hypertrophic obstructive cardiomyopathy. Furthermore, concomitant use of nitrates and sildenafil can provoke severe potentially life-threatening hypotension, making this combination an absolute contraindication. Indeed, patients should be warned never to use sildenafil within 24 hours of nitrate consumption.

2.2 β-adrenoceptor blockers

β-blockers differ in physicochemical, pharmacokinetic and pharmacodynamic properties. Current drugs vary in their selectivity for β_1-, β_2- and β_3-adrenoceptors, and some, such as carvedilol and labetalol, are also α_1-adrenoceptor antagonists. Some have partial agonist activity or intrinsic sympathetic activity (ISA), local anaesthetic properties (membrane-stabilising activity), potassium (K^+) channel blocking activity or antioxidant properties. The number of β-blockers available rapidly increased and became the major first-line therapy for hypertension. Improvements in the symptomatic management of angina were followed by improvements in mortality in acute myocardial infarction and long-term when given post-myocardial infarction. β-blockers also reduce arrhythmias after both cardiac and non-cardiac surgery. Thus, β-blockers now have important role in improving both mortality and symptom control in ischaemic heart disease, arrhythmias and hypertension (Table 1) (Hollenberg, 2005). In patients with stable angina who also manifest congestive heart failure symptoms with reduced left systolic function, β-blockers are particularly beneficial and reduce heart failure related mortality by approximately 35% (Klein et al., 2003).

2.2.1 Properties of β-blockers

1. Subtype selectivity. The prototypical β-blocker propranolol has similar affinity for β1- and β2- adrenoceptors and lower affinity for β3-adrenoceptors. However, even the 'cardioselective' β-blockers, a nomenclature based on their selectivity for β1-adrenoceptors, are not, because none in clinical use are that selective (13-fold at most) (Baker, 2005; Schnabel, 2000). Although bisoprolol and nebivolol are the most β_1-selective and carvedilol having slight β_2-selectivity, it is not possible to predict what level of selectivity. Most currently available β-blockers (including propranolol) have low affinity for the β_3-adrenoceptor. There are, however, a subset of drugs comprising oxprenolol, carazolol, pindolol, nadolol, tertatolol, carteolol, arotinolol and nebivolol that have agonist effects at the β_3-adrenoceptor that could be responsible for the nitric oxide (NO)-mediated vasodilator properties observed with nebivolol (Baker, 2010). Even SR59230A, claimed to be selective for β_3-adrenoceptors, has a similar potency at all 3 subtypes (Baker, 2010, Michel, 2010).

2. Intrinsic sympathomimetic activity (ISA) and partial agonism. Some β-blockers are traditionally described as having ISA (Table 2). These drugs block the stimulatory effects of high-efficacy agonists, such as catecholamines, but stimulate agonist responses of their own. This is evident at both the cellular and tissue level with acebutolol, carteolol, penbutolol, pindolol, bucindolol and xamoterol, for which it is claimed that bradycardia and bronchoconstriction are less than for other β-adrenoceptor antagonists. However, drugs with ISA are less advantageous in the management of heart failure and migraine.
3. Low-affinity state of the β_1-adrenoceptor. Some β-adrenoceptor antagonists stimulate β_1-adrenoceptor function by interacting with a low-affinity state of the β_1-adrenoceptor (Molenaar, 2003) and the β_3-adrenoceptor (Baker, 2003). Activation of this low-affinity state of the β_1-adrenoceptor has been demonstrated in whole animals (Cohen, 2000) and humans (Kaumann and Molenaar, 1997). β-adrenoceptor antagonists with similar properties include oxprenolol, alprenolol, carazolol, pindolol and carvedilol. These ligands either stimulate agonist responses at concentrations much higher than those required to fully occupy and block the conventional catecholamine β_1-adrenoceptor site, or have biphasic concentration–response curves. However, there is currently no therapeutic use for this property of β-adrenoceptor antagonists.
4. Inverse agonism. Many β-adrenoceptor antagonists, at least at the β_2-adrenoceptor, are in fact inverse agonists (i.e. rather than just occupying the binding site and thus blocking the actions of agonists, they are associated with conformations of the receptor that turn off signalling) (Swaminath, 2005).
5. Other properties of β-blockers. Local anaesthetic or membrane-stabilising activity is shown by some β-adrenoceptor antagonists, notably propranolol and acebutolol and to a lesser extent pindolol and labetalol. This property is unlikely to be important in the therapeutic effects of β-blockers because it occurs at much higher concentrations than those normally encountered clinically. Individual (rather than class effect) properties of certain β-blockers include lipophilicity, K^+ channel blockade and antioxidant properties. Propranolol, timolol and metoprolol are somewhat lipophilic. Sotalol can block K^+ channels independently of its β-blocking properties. Carvedilol blocks α_1- and β-adrenoceptors, inhibits apoptosis and possesses antioxidant and free-radical-scavenging actions. Nebivolol causes NO-dependent vasodilation. These properties might contribute to their efficacy in cardiac failure.

2.2.2 Hemodynamic effects of β-blockers

β-adrenoceptor antagonists competitively inhibit the binding of endogenous catecholamines to β_1-adrenoceptors in the heart and most evidence strongly suggests that their anti-ischemic effects are due to cardiac depression. Myocardial oxygen demand is determined in large part by heart rate and cardiac contractility. Increased heart rate and contractility result in increased myocardial oxygen consumption and, conversely, reductions in heart rate and contractility lead to a decrease in oxygen consumption. By inhibiting the actions of norepinephrine and epinephrine on the heart, the β-adrenoceptor antagonists exert their negative dromotropic and intropic effects, and thereby attenuate the myocardial response to sympathetic nervous system stimulation that occurs, for example, with increased stress or exercise. Though most β-adrenoceptor antagonists lower resting heart rate to some extent, the effect on exercise-induced tachycardia is much more pronounced. Thus, for a given degree of physical activity, myocardial oxygen consumption is diminished. It is important to note that the β-adrenoceptor antagonists do not change the point of imbalance between myocardial oxygen supply and consumption at which angina occurs; rather, they reduce the likelihood that this point is reached. By mechanisms that remain poorly understood, β-adrenoceptor antagonists also decrease peripheral vascular resistance, which leads to a reduction in arterial blood pressure and afterload (Hoffman, 2007). Reduced afterload results in decreased left ventricular wall tension, which is another major determinant of myocardial oxygen demand. This beneficial effect of the β-adrenoceptor antagonists may be partially offset, however, by an increase in left ventricular end-diastolic volume that occurs due to increased cardiac filling during diastole, but the net effect is to lessen oxygen demand. On the other hand myocardial oxygen supply is a function of both oxygen delivery (the heart is almost exclusively dependent on aerobic metabolism and an adequate supply of oxygen is critical to sustained cardiac activity) and oxygen extraction from the blood. Since oxygen extraction from coronary blood is near maximal at rest, there is little reserve to meet increased demand due to increased cardiac activity (Tune et al., 2004). Thus, the most important determinant of myocardial oxygen supply is total coronary blood flow. β-adrenoceptor antagonists have little propensity to increase coronary blood flow and myocardial oxygen supply, in fact β-adrenoceptor antagonists may increase coronary vascular resistance by inhibiting the β_2-adrenoceptor-mediated vasodilator effects of endogenous catecholamines and leaving α-adrenoceptor-mediated vasoconstriction unopposed. Thus, the anti-ischemic effects of the β-adrenoceptor antagonists are largely due to their ability to reduce myocardial workload and decrease oxygen consumption, rather than to improve myocardial oxygen supply.

Propranolol	Hypertension, ischaemic heart disease, arrhythmias, portal hypertension, anxiety, essential tremor, migraine, thyrotoxicosis
Acebutolol	Hypertension, ischaemic heart disease, arrhythmias
Atenolol	Hypertension, ischaemic heart disease, arrhythmias, migraine
Betaxolol	Glaucoma
Bisoprolol	Hypertension, ischaemic heart disease, heart failure
Carteolol	Glaucoma
Carvedilol	Hypertension, ischaemic heart disease, heart failure
Celiprolol	Hypertension
Esmolol	Arrhythmias (short-term)
Labetolol	Hypertension
Levobunolol	Glaucoma
Metipranolol	Glaucoma
Metoprolol	Hypertension, ischaemic heart disease, arrhythmias, migraine
Nadolol	Hypertension, ischaemic heart disease, arrhythmias, migraine, thyrotoxicosis
Nebivolol	Hypertension, heart failure
Oxprenolol	Hypertension, ischaemic heart disease, arrhythmias, anxiety
Pindolol	Hypertension, ischaemic heart disease
Sotalol	Arrhythmias
Timolol	Glaucoma, hypertension, ischaemic heart disease, migraine

Table 1. Current indications for β-blockers from the British National Formulary September 2010 (www.bnf.org)

Generation	Drugs	Specifications
First	Propranolol, Timolol	Non-cardioselective
Second	Metoprolol	Cardioselective, short acting
	Atenolol, Bisoprolol, Betaxolol	Cardioselective, sustained release
Third	Labetalol	Non-cardioselective, vasodilation (Higher affinity for α_1 receptor (α_1 receptor blockade) than β_1 and β_2)
	Carvedilol	Cardioselective, vasodilation (β_1 selective, decerased selectivity at higher doses, α_1 receptor blockade, increases insulin sensitivity, antioxidant properties)
	Nebivolol	Cardioselective, vasodilation (Higher β_1 selectivity; endothelium-dependent vasodilation *via* the L-arginine/nitric oxide pathway)

Table 2. Classification of beta blockers that used for treatment of chronic stable angina

2.2.3 Clinical application of β-blockers in angina

β-adrenoceptor antagonists are a mainstay in the treatment of chronic stable angina. While coronary blood flow (i.e. oxygen supply) may be sufficient to meet myocardial oxygen requirements at rest in patients with fixed atherosclerotic lesions, the obstruction prevents blood flow from increasing during periods of increased oxygen demand. Under these conditions coronary blood flow is already at a maximal level in most patients, thus any increase in myocardial work can trigger an episode of acute angina. Precipitating factors include physical exertion, emotional stress or excitement, and temperature extremes. By decreasing heart rate, myocardial contractility, and afterload, β-adrenoceptor antagonists reduce myocardial workload and oxygen consumption at rest as well as during periods of exertion or stress. Oral β-adrenoceptor antagonists are widely used in long-term maintenance therapy to prevent acute ischemic episodes. Prophylactic use of these agents reduces the frequency and severity of acute anginal attacks. Because of their slow onset of action, oral β-adrenoceptor antagonists are not appropriate for terminating an acute attack of angina once it has begun; sublingual nitroglycerin is the agent most frequently used under these conditions. Several β-adrenoceptor antagonists, including propranolol, metoprolol, and atenolol, have cardioprotective effects and have been shown to decrease mortality after myocardial infarction (Bunch et al., 2005). In patients with variant (Prinzmetal's) angina, the major underlying cause of angina is vasospasm of one or more coronary arteries. Intense vasoconstriction decreases coronary blood flow, thereby reducing myocardial oxygen supply. Coronary vasospasm can occur in arteries with little or no atherosclerotic plaque and is not associated with an increase in myocardial oxygen demand. Indeed, variant angina may strike at any time of the day or night, including during periods of rest or sleep. In contrast to stable angina, variant angina is most often the result of an abrupt decrease in myocardial oxygen supply (i.e. coronary blood flow) rather than an increase in myocardial oxygen demand. Unlike nitrates and calcium channel blockers, β-adrenoceptor antagonists do not directly dilate coronary arteries to increase coronary blood flow. Moreover, blockade of vascular β-adrenoceptors inhibits the vasodilator actions of endogenous catecholamines and may exacerbate α-adrenoceptor-mediated vasoconstriction in coronary arteries. Thus, β-adrenoceptor antagonists may worsen coronary vasospasm and are not indicated for treatment of vasospastic angina. β-adrenoceptor antagonists may reduce the risk of progression to acute myocardial infarction in patients with unstable angina (Braunwald et al., 2002).The pathophysiology of this condition is often complex and may involve several underlying factors superimposed upon one another, including rupture of atherosclerotic plaques and thrombus formation, constriction of coronary arteries, and increased myocardial oxygen demand. In these patients, the beneficial effects of the β-adrenoceptor antagonists are likely due to a reduction in myocardial oxygen consumption. If coronary vasospasm is the major underlying problem, nitrates or calcium channel blockers would be more effective and β-adrenoceptor antagonists should be used with caution. When used concurrently, β-adrenoceptor antagonists can inhibit the baroreceptor-mediated reflex tachycardia and positive inotropic effects that may sometimes occur with organic nitrates. Alternatively, organic nitrates increase venous capacitance and can thereby offset β-adrenoceptor antagonist-mediated increases in left ventricular end-diastolic volume. Moreover, organic nitrates are coronary vasodilators and, as such, may prevent the increase in coronary vasomotor tone that may potentially result from blockade of vascular β-adrenoceptors. Dihydropyridine calcium channel blockers are also potent coronary vasodilators and provide similar advantages with regard to coronary vascular resistance in patients treated simultaneously with β-adrenoceptor antagonists. As with nitrates, dihydropyridines may also cause reflex tachycardia that can be alleviated by β-adrenoceptor antagonists. Concurrent use of β-adrenoceptor antagonists with the non-dihydropyridine calcium channel blockers, verapamil and diltiazem, is much more limited due to the potential for severe cardiac depression and must be used with great caution. In the long-term management of ischemic heart disease, β-adrenoceptor antagonists, with their antianginal effects, may also be combined with vasculoprotective drugs such as anti-platelet agents (aspirin, clopidogrel), angiotensin-converting enzyme inhibitors, and HMG-CoA reductase inhibitors to reduce the risk of ischemic vascular events.

2.3 Calcium entry blockers (CEBs)

The mode of action of most conventional antianginal agents involves hemodynamic changes, such as a reduction in systemic vascular resistance or coronary vasodilatation or negative inotropism, which improve the imbalance in myocardial oxygen supply and demand. CEBs bind to and inhibit L-type calcium channels, reducing calcium influx into cells. Intracellular calcium deprivation relaxes smooth muscle cells, causing vasodilation in the peripheral and coronary beds and increased coronary blood flow. The less selective, nondihydropyridine (DHP) CEBs, verapamil and diltiazem, also slow sinoatrial (SA) and atrioventricular (AV) nodal conductions to lower heart rate and depress contractility under physiological conditions. All the CEBs are effective coronary vasodilators. DHPs lower blood pressure and myocardial wall tension to reduce myocardial oxygen consumption. A rise in coronary blood flow further contributes to correct myocardial oxygen imbalance. These drugs lower the frequency of angina, reduce the need for nitrates, extend treadmill walking time, and improve ischemic ST-segment changes on exercise testing and electrocardiographic monitoring. Amlodipine, in particular, may have some independent action in relieving diastolic dysfunction other than a reduction in blood pressure. CEBs find clinical use in patients who cannot tolerate β-blockers, when they are ineffective, and in combination for additive anti-ischemic effects. Although they are effective antianginal agents, they do not modify the natural progression of the disease. The large International Verapamil-Trandolapril Study (INVEST) trial reported a reduction in number of patients with angina from about 65%-25% using verapamil as compared with atenolol, with no difference in mortality over a 2-year period (Pepine et al., 2003). When DHPs are used in combination with β-blockers, reflex tachycardia from the CCBs is blunted. Long-acting DHPs are preferred. If clinically needed, verapamil or diltiazem may be used with caution to lower heart rate or slow AV conduction further when ventricular function is preserved. In patients with stable angina and hypertension, β-blockers in combination with amlodipine and long-acting nifedipine, nicardipine, isradipine, or felodipine offer an advantage. Of all agents available, the greatest clinical experience has been with amlodipine and felodipine. Short-acting nifedipine has been linked to an increase in myocardial infarction (MI) and should be avoided in unstable angina or ACS. The A Coronary Disease Trial Investigating Outcome with Nifedipine GITS (ACTION) study showed that long-acting nifedipine (gastrointestinal therapeutic system) safely relieved angina and prolonged event-free survival in patients with stable angina and hypertension (Poole-Wilson et al., 2004; Sierra and Coca, 2008). Verapamil acts chiefly through a negative inotropic action, with less associated reflex tachycardia; diltiazem has greater vasodilatory actions than verapamil. Both verapamil and diltiazem are contraindicated in patients with uncompensated heart failure (HF) because of their negative inotropic effects; amlodipine and felodipine appear safe when left ventricle (LV) dysfunction is compensated. Use of non-DPHs after complex MIs should be avoided because of the possibility of HF as well (Packer et al., 1996; Goldstein et al., 1991). DHPs, particularly nifedipine, are effective in managing Prinzmetal's variant angina along with long-acting nitrates. Although CCBs are effective anti-ischemic agents, in patients with UA/ STEMI, they do not improve mortality. Diltiazem and verapamil are contraindicated in patients with STEMI accompanied by systolic LV dysfunction and HF. Immediate release forms of DHPs-CCBs are contraindicated in STEMI because reflex tachycardia increases myocardial oxygen demand and hypotension potentially lowers coronary perfusion pressure. Also, they should not be used in UA/STEMI without a β-blocker. Common side effects of headache, dizziness, flushing, and edema are due to vasodilation. Interaction with other negative chronotropic or inotropic agents to produce bradycardia, heart block, or HF has been reported. CCBs may also suppress lower esophageal sphincter contraction and worsen symptoms of gastroesophageal reflux disease. CEBs inhibit the CYPA4 enzyme in the liver and, therefore, may raise levels of statins and many other drugs, which may be overlooked (Kones, 2010). Cimetidine and grapefruit juice may raise the effective level of CEBs. Since magnesium is a calcium antagonist, magnesium supplements may enhance the actions of CEBs, particularly nifedipine. **Chronotherapy** with CCBs has been designed to achieve the highest plasma concentration during the most vulnerable time period while maintaining an adequate therapeutic dose throughout the remainder of the 24 hour period and has been marketed in the US since 1996. A variety of CCBs delivery formulations (e.g., with controlled-onset and/or extended release) have been approved by the FDA, and may be beneficially prescribed to lower blood pressure, heart rate and rate-pressure product between 6:00 A.M. and noon depending on the time of administration. Another study demonstrated an improvement in the duration of exercise with evening doses of this diltiazem preparation *versus* morning dosing.

3. Novel antianginal

New drugs based on novel mechanisms of action have emerged (Chaitman, 2005).

3.1 Ranolazine

Ranolazine (approved by the US Food and Drug Administration) is a unique anti-ischaemic drug that does not significantly affect haemodynamic parameters (Siddiqui et al., 2006). It was originally believed to modify the use of substrate by the ischaemic myocardium from lipids to glucose, thereby increasing metabolic efficiency. However, recent studies suggest that it inhibits the late sodium current (I_{NA}) and the accumulation of intracellular sodium and congruent cellular calcium overload *via* the sodium/calcium exchanger. As opposed to treatment with calcium channel antagonists and β-blockers, the ranolazine-induced improvement in diastolic function occurs without a decrease in systolic function. Clinical studies of the anti-ischaemic effect of ranolazine monotherapy in patients with stable angina showed a significant increase in exercise duration and an improved 1 mm ST-segment depression compared with atenolol. As an adjunct to standard doses of anti-ischaemia drugs (atenolol, amlodipine, diltiazem), ranolazine had an additional antianginal and anti-ischaemic effect, without causing significant hemodynamic changes. The ERICA study addressed the incremental benefit of adding ranolazine to maximal amlodipine regimen. Ranolazine significantly reduced the frequency of angina and GTN consumption compared with placebo. It also has another potentially favorable effect-namely, a dose-related reduction in haemoglobin (Hb_{A1c} %) concentrations in diabetic patients. More comparative trials of ranolazine with other antianginal agents and studies of its effects on long-term morbidity and mortality are needed. So far, results indicate that ranolazine may serve as a useful alternative or adjunct to conventional antianginal treatment. Adverse effects include constipation, nausea, and dizziness. Postural hypotension due to α-adrenergic receptor blocking has also been reported. Increases in QT- interval were observed but not associated *torsade de points*.

3.2 Trimetazidine

Trimetazidine (1-[2,3,4-trimethoxybenzyl] piperazine dihydrochloride) selectively inhibits the mitochondrial long chain 3-ketoacyl coenzyme A thiolase. It is widely used for the prophylactic treatment of episodes of angina pectoris at recommended daily doses ranging from 40–60 mg. Trimetazidine is a pure metabolic agent that induces the myocardium to shift from free fatty acids to predominantly glucose utilisation in order to increase adenosine triphosphate (ATP) generation per unit oxygen consumption. The antianginal properties of trimetazidine were previously shown in acute and chronic experimental conditions in which the cardioprotective effects were related to the positive effects on energy metabolism, hydroionic balance, coronary microcirculation, and oxidative stress. Efficacy studies reported that trimetazidine reduced ischemia during exercise stress tests, but there was no improvement in outcome. In a Cochrane meta-analysis of 23 studies including 1378 patients, trimetazidine was associated with a significant reduction in weekly angina episodes and improved exercise time to 1 mm ST-segment depression compared to placebo (Ciapponi et al., 2005). In patients with stable angina who experienced concomitant erectile dysfunction, trimetazidine plus sildenafil was both safe and more effective in controlling episodes of ischaemia during sexual activity than nitrates alone. These data indicate that trimetazidine is safe and effective for the treatment of symptoms of stable angina, either as monotherapy or adjunctive treatment. The Di Napoli study (2005) indicated that trimetazidine added to usual treatment improved the functional status of patients with ischaemic dilated cardiomyopathy, as shown by their distribution in the NYHA class after 18 months of treatment. Compared with control patients maintained with their usual treatment, trimetazidine treated patients' functional improvement was associated with a significant increase in left ventricle ejection fraction and a significant effect on ventricular remodelling. These effects were significant starting from 12 months and were maintained after 18 months of treatment. Bonello et al., (2007) demonstrates that pretreatment with a 60 mg acute oral loading dose of trimetazidine before elective percutaneous coronary intervention limits myocardial damage, as shown by a lower total amount of troponin (cTnI) release after coronary angioplasty.

3.3 Ivabradine

Few agents were developed for I_f inhibition in the past; the first of which is Alinidine, a clonidine derivative, that was soon abandoned due to its relative inotropic action (Ogiwara et al., 1988). Later, zetabradine, a benzazepinone derivative also went out of contention due to unacceptable ocular side effects and QTc prolongation (Frishman et al., 1995; Frishman et al., 2003). Ivabradine, a unique specific I_f current inhibitor, was first described by Thollon et al., more than two decades ago (Thollon et al., 1994). The I_f current inhibitor ivabradine was approved for the treatment of stable angina pectoris by the European Medicines Agency (EMEA) in 2005. Ivabradine is an inhibitor of the selective cardiac pacemaker hyperpolarized-activated I_f current, one of the most important pacemaker currents in the sinoatrial node (DiFrancesco & Camm 2004; Zaza & Rocchetti 2005). Ivabradine has no negative inotropic or hypotensive effects and is therefore a pure heart rate-lowering agent, in contrast to beta blockers. The pure heart rate-reducing effect of ivabradine offers the advantage of not disturbing hemodynamic parameters or left ventricular systolic and diastolic functions. Moreover, the increase in the duration of diastole is greater with ivabradine than with atenolol for a given heart rate (Colin et al. 2003), a beneficial phenomenon considering that most of the coronary perfusion occurs during diastole. Double-blind trials showed that ivabradine treatment increased exercise time to 1 mm ST-segment depression and limited angina compared to placebo, and had similar clinical effects to atenolol or amlodipine—namely, a two-third reduction in the number of anginal episodes and an increase in total exercise duration. Ivabradine offers clear therapeutic benefit for a whole range of patients with stable angina, including those with contraindication or intolerance to β-blockers; however, its effect on survival remains to be explored. Visual symptoms and sinus bradycardia are the main adverse reactions observed with the use of ivabradine. The visual symptoms are mainly ***phosphenes,*** which are episodes of enhanced brightness in limited areas of the visual field frequently triggered by abrupt changes in light intensity. They include photopsia, stroboscopic effect, and non-typical blurred vision, among others. However, the symptoms are generally transient, mild, and do not affect daily living activities. The visual symptoms are probably caused by the interaction of ivabradine with retinal hyperpolarization-activated *h* channels, responsible for responses to bright light stimuli, which are similar to the *f* ion channel located in the sinoatrial node (Demontis et al. 2002; Savelieva & Camm 2006). Sinus bradycardia has been reported by 4.6% of patients treated with ivabradine 7.5 mg twice daily (Tardif et al. 2005; Ruzyllo et al. 2007). Severe bradycardia (defined as a heart rate less than 40 beat/minute) has been shown to occur in 0.1% of patients. The QTc-interval was not increased in ivabradine recipients compared with atenolol.

3.4 Fasudil hydrochloride

[1-(5-isoquinolinesulfonyl)-homopiperazine] is a potent Rho-kinase (an intracellular signalling molecule involved in the vascular smooth muscle contractile response) inhibitor and vasodilator, used for the treatment of cerebral vasospasm, which is often due to subarachnoid hemorrhage, as well as to improve the cognitive decline seen in stroke victims. It has been found to be effective for the treatment of pulmonary hypertension. It was demonstrated in February 2009 that Fasudil could also be used to enhance memory and improve the prognosis of Alzheimer's patients. In patients with stable angina, fasudil treatment led to a significantly greater time to >1 mm ST-segment depression, but showed no difference from placebo in decreasing the time to angina, frequency of angina, or GTN use. In phase 2 dose-finding trials conducted in Japanese patients with stable effort angina, fasudil monotherapy at doses ranging from 5 mg three times daily to 40 mg three times daily increased maximum exercise time and time to the onset of ≥ 1 mm ST-segment depression compared with baseline. Fasudil was well tolerated, with minimal effects on blood pressure or heart rate at rest or during exercise (Shimokawa et al., 2002). Intracoronary fasudil ameliorate myocardial ischemia induced by intracoronary injection of acetylcholine in patients with cardiac syndrome X or microvascular angina (angina with normal coronary arteriogram) (Mohri et al., 2003).

3.5 Molsidomine

Molsidomine is a nitric oxide donating vasodilator. When compared with placebo, it reduced the incidence of anginal attacks and use of sublingual nitrates, and increased exercise capacity, in patients with stable angina. Higher doses provided better protection from angina, although hypotension was a side effect. These new drugs are not yet in routine clinical use; however, they may serve as useful alternatives or adjuncts to conventional antianginal treatment. Further studies and longer follow-up will determine their place in preventing death or myocardial infarction.

3.6 Potassium channel openers (KCOs)

Potassium-ATP (K_{ATP}) channels serve as endogenous homeostatic transducers balancing cellular resources in response to altered demand. In the heart, K_{ATP} channels protect against the metabolic insult of ischemia, and contribute as molecular mediators in the adaptive response to distress. Moreover, K_{ATP} channels regulate vascular tone, and thereby the delivery of metabolic resources to match demand.The possible smooth muscle relaxation mechanisms associated with K_{ATP} channels in the coronary artery are; in the endothelial cells the K_{ATP} channels are activated by adenosine and α_2-adrenoceptor stimulation and contribute to generation of nitric oxide, in the sympathetic neurons opening of presynaptic

K_{ATP} channels attenuates noradrenaline release. KCOs would enhance these exo-smooth muscle actions of the K_{ATP} channels and dilate the coronary artery. KCOs are chemically diverse, and belong to a number of structural classes. These include:

- Benzopyrans (levcromakalim, bimakalim)
- Benzothiadiazines (diazoxide)
- Cyanoguanidines (pinacidil)
- Cyclobutenediones (WAY-151616)
- Nicotinamides (nicorandil)
- Pyrimidines (minoxidil)
- Tertiary carbonoles (ZD-6169)
- Thioformamides (aprikalim)
- Dihydropyridine-like structures (ZM-244085)

3.7 Nicorandil

Nicorandil exerts dual actions: it increases the opening of ATP-gated K^+ channels, thereby relaxing smooth muscle and contributing to coronary vasodilatation; and it has a nitrate-donating moiety. As well as anti-ischaemic effects, nicorandil may have a cardioprotective action. Nicorandil may mimic the natural process of ischemic preconditioning, which involves ATP-dependent potassium channels. Several small randomized trials of patients with stable angina have shown that nicorandil prolongs the time to onset of ST-segment depression and exercise duration during stress testing and improves myocardial perfusion at rest and with exercise. In patients, nicorandil has been shown to be useful in the management of both stable and unstable angina with minimum adverse effects (Simpson et al., 2004). Nicorandil attenuated rest and effort angina, prolonged the duration of exercise and the time to onset of angina or ischemic ST-T changes (Markham et al., 2000). Long-term use of nicorandil was associated with reduction in cardiovascular events and the combined endpoints of death, myocardial infarction and hospitalization due to chest pain in patients with stable angina [The IONA Study Group, 2001]. Nicorandil is an effective anti-anginal agent at a dose of 10 to 40 mg twice a day, controlling stable chronic angina in 70 to 80 percent of patients (Simpson et al., 2004). The response to nicorandil is maintained for 12 hours, with an efficacy that compares favorably with that of nitrates, β-adrenoceptor and CEBs. In patients with unstable angina, nicorandil, when added to aggressive anti-anginal treatment, reduces transient myocardial ischemia, and arrhythmias when compared to placebo (Patel et al., 1999). In vasospastic angina, nicorandil, with potent vasospasmolytic activity, relieves both ergonovine-evoked and spontaneous coronary spasm, attenuates episodes of variant angina, suppresses ST-segment changes and improves perfusion defects. In MI, nicorandil improves ischemia-induced regional wall motion abnormalities, and perfusion in infarct-related areas. In the IONA trial of 5126 patients, the administration of nicorandil in addition to standard treatments reduced the primary end point (coronary death, MI, or hospitalisation for angina) by 17% after a mean follow-up of 1.6 years. There was also a significant reduction in the incidence of ACS and all cardiovascular events (IONA Study Group et al., 2002). In patients undergoing angioplasty, nicorandil preconditions the heart, improves coronary hemodynamics, dilates stenotic and non-stenotic segments, and ameliorates the "no-reflow" phenomenon (Yasuda et al., 2001). Intravenous nicorandil, in conjunction with coronary angioplasty, preserves microvascular integrity and myocardial viability in patients with acute myocardial infarction (Simpson et al., 2004). Nicorandil also reduces preload and afterload, enhances cardiac endothelial nitric oxide synthase expression and has antiplatelet, fibrinolytic and antioxidant properties (Simpson et al., 2004). Unlike GTN, no development of tolerance to the antianginal effect of nicorandil has been reported (Simpson et al., 2004). Main side-effects include headache, gastrointestinal disturbances and dizziness, mucosal ulceration, including stomatitis and mouth and anal ulcerations. No evidence of proarrhythmia, conduction disturbance, exacerbation of myocardial ischemia, infarction, abrupt withdrawal syndrome, symptomatic decrease in blood pressure or change in heart rate has been observed (Simpson et al., 2004;The Lona Study Group, 2001). Also, no adverse interaction has been reported in patients on oral anticoagulants or hypoglycemic agents. The pharmacokinetics of nicorandil is unaltered in the elderly or patients with renal or hepatic insufficiency (Simpson et al., 2004). Other KCOs like **Levcromakalim, aprikalim and KRN4884** relax conduit arteries (internal mammary and gastroepiploic arteries) used as coronary artery bypass grafts and could be useful in preventing spasm of bypass grafts in patients undergoing surgery for atherosclerotic heart disease.

3.8 Antiplatelets

Antiplatelet agents are the cornerstone of treatment for patients with ACS undergoing percutaneous coronary intervention (PCI).

3.8.1 Acetylsalicylic acid (Aspirin)

Platelet activation and aggregation after vulnerable plaque rupture with resultant thromboses of varying degrees are key components in the pathophysiology of ACS. Acetylsalicylic acid (ASA), causes irreversible acetylation of serine 529 of cyclooxygenase (COX-1) in platelets and the endothelium, thereby preventing thromboxane A_2 (TXA_2) production and resultant platelet aggregation. Studies have shown that ASA reduces the risk of angina, death, or MI by approximately 30% in patients with coronary artery disease (Collaborative overview of randomised trials of antiplatelet therapy-I, 1994; Antithrombotic Trialists' Collaboration, 2002). Although ASA is beneficial for preventing and treating vascular disease, ASA does not prevent all thrombotic events from recurring. Patients who have an ischemic event and are taking aspirin actually may have worse outcomes than do patients who are not taking aspirin (Alexander et al., 1999). This observation that led to the concept of "aspirin resistance (Bhatt and Topol, 2003; Patrono, 2003), a term that has been used when ASA is ineffective for protecting patients from thrombotic complications, for prolonging bleeding times, or for decreasing TXA_2 production. Potential causes of aspirin resistance include inadequate dosing, drug interactions, genetic polymorphisms of COX-1 and other genes involved in TXA_2 production, and upregulation of non-platelet sources of TXA_2 production (Hankey and Eikelboom, 2006). Unfortunately, the optimal treatment for aspirin resistance, if any, is unknown. The Altering aspirin therapy after a laboratory finding of aspirin resistance could be both safe and helpful (Michelson et al., 2005). Aspirin has been shown to be beneficial in the primary prevention, secondary prevention, and treatment of ACS because of the important role of platelets in thrombus formation. One study suggested that prior aspirin use by those who develop an ACS may actually predispose to worse outcomes than those not previously taking aspirin (i.e. **aspirin paradox**) (Santopinto et al., 2001).

From the Thrombolysis In Myocardial Infarction (TIMI) trials database of 66,443 patients, Rich et al., (2010) demonstrated that prior aspirin use is associated with a high-risk cohort of patients but not associated with increased mortality after an ACS, emphasizing that it is likely more a marker as opposed to a pathophysiologic factor related to an increased risk. Prior aspirin use was associated with an increase in the risk of recurrent myocardial infarction and the composite end point of death/recurrent myocardial infraction/ischemia requiring urgent revascularization/recent ischemia requiring hospitalization/stroke. This may be attributable to confounders that cannot be corrected for, aspirin resistance, or both.

3.8.2 Thienopyridines

Thienopyridines, such as **ticlopidine, clopidogrel**, and the newer agent **prasugrel**, block P2Y12 receptor signaling to prevent production of adenyl cyclase, thereby inhibiting platelet activation through adenosine diphosphate (ADP). They also limit ADP-mediated conversion of glycoprotein receptor (GPIIb/IIIa) to its active form. Their mechanism of action is independent of and complementary to that of aspirin, and the combination of agents is superior to aspirin alone. Because thienopyridines take longer than aspirin to cause irreversible antiplatelet effects, a loading dose usually is administered. The thienopyridines are prodrugs that must be metabolized *in vivo* into active form. Both prasugrel and clopidogrel require CYP450 metabolism for the generation of active metabolites, but the pathways leading to conversion to the active metabolites differ between the prodrugs.

3.8.2.1 Ticlopidine

A 1st-generation thienopyridine, in combination with ASA, is associated with reducing rates of vascular death and MI by 46% in NSTEMI patients (Balsano et al., 1990). It has also been shown to be superior to oral anticoagulants in preventing thrombotic complications after coronary stent placement (Urban et al., 1998). However, it is used less frequently than the newer thienopyridines in current clinical practice because of its potential for side effects primarily rash, nausea, neutropenia, and thrombocytopenia (Love et al., 1998).

3.8.2.2 Clopidogrel

Second generation thienopyridine, is the most widely studied and used ADP-receptor-blocking agent. Initial data regarding clopidogrel are derived from the Clopidogrel versus Aspirin in Patients at Risk of Ischaemic Events (CAPRIE) study [1996] which reported a 9% relative risk reduction in adverse cardiovascular events (vascular death, MI, or ischemic stroke) without a significant increase in bleeding. Also this study showed that the risk of the primary composite endpoint (cardiovascular death, MI, or stroke) was reduced 20% with the use of clopidogrel compared to aspirin. Clopidogrel has demonstrated considerable success in reducing thrombotic complications of ACS and/or PCI compared to aspirin alone and is standard of care for the management of patients with ACS and when added in patients undergoing PCI. In elderly STEMI patients who receive thrombolytics, a loading dose of clopidogrel is not recommended due to increased risk of intracerebral hemorrhage. Loading dose of clopidogrel is recommended in elderly STEMI patients only if primary PCI is performed. In UA/NSTEMI patients with a history of gastrointestinal bleeding, ASA and clopidogrel should be given with other agents, such as proton pump inhibitors (PPIs) that minimize the risk of recurrent gastrointestinal bleeding. Clopidogrel therapy must also be stopped 4 to 7 days before elective coronary artery bypass grafting (CABG), to prevent excessive intraoperative and post-operative bleeding (Mehta et al., 2006; Chu et al., 2004). As a result, clinicians might have to delay giving clopidogrel to patients who are undergoing early coronary angiography (within 48 hr of hospital admission) until it is clear that these patients will not undergo a coronary artery bypass graft surgery (CABG) procedure within the next several days. However, there is growing evidence to support broad variability among individual patient responses to clopidogrel. This clopidogrel resistance is associated with a higher risk of recurrent ischemic complications (Serebruany et al., 2005). The mechanisms underlying the variability of response to clopidogrel may be related to poor patient compliance, differences in clopidogrel dosing, gastric absorption problems, and varying availability and clearance of the active metabolite (O'queli et al., 2007). Genetic factors including polymorphisms of hepatic CYP3A—have received special attention (Frere et al., 2008). There have been reports of concerns that proton pump inhibitors (PPIs) may interfere with clopidogrel's ability to inhibit platelet aggregation, thereby increasing the risk of rehospitalization or death in association with ACS (Li et al., 2004; Juurlink et al., 2009; Ho et al., 2009). Combined use of clopidogrel and PPIs was associated with an increased risk of death from or rehospitalization for ACS when compared with use of clopidogrel alone (Ho et al., 2009).

3.8.2.3 Prasugrel

It is an orally administered P2Y12 receptor antagonist that is more potent, more rapid in onset, and more consistent in its inhibition of platelet aggregation than clopidogrel. In clinical studies, prasugrel has consistently demonstrated greater and more rapid platelet inhibition than clopidogrel in healthy subjects, patients with stable coronary artery disease and acute coronary syndrome, and those undergoing percutaneous coronary intervention. In addition, subjects who are poor responders to clopidogrel respond adequately to prasugrel (Brandt et al., 2007; Weerakkody et al., 2007a; 2007b). In the Assess Improvement in Therapeutic Outcomes by Optimizing Platelet Inhibition with Prasugrel-Throm-bolysis in Myocardial Infarction (TRITON-TIMI 38) trial, prasugrel significantly reduced the composite endpoint of cardiovascular death, nonfatal MI, or non-fatal stroke by 19%, when compared with clopidogrel (Wiviott et al., 2007). Prasugrel also reduced MI by 24%, the need for urgent revascularization by 34%, and stent thrombosis by 52% (Wiviott et al., 2008). However, the beneficial effect also was associated with a 0.5% absolute increase in non-CABG-related TIMI major bleeding and life-threatening bleeding and a 0.3% absolute increase in fatal bleeding (Wiviott et al., 2007). TRITON-TIMI 38 trial showed that patients with a history of transient ischemic attack or stroke, those who were 75 years or older, and those who weighed less than 60 kg were especially at risk of bleeding mainly during the maintenance phase (Wiviott et al., 2008; Murphy et al., 2008).

3.8.3 Nonthienopyridine antiplatelet agents

Cangrelor and Ticagrelor are direct and reversible inhibitors of the platelet P2Y12 receptor. **SCH 530348** is an oral protease-activated receptor-1 antagonist.

3.8.4 Glycoprotein IIb/IIIa inhibitors

The final common pathway of platelet activation and aggregation involves a conformational change of the GPIIb/IIIa receptors from a resting state to an active state. The activated

GPIIb/IIIa receptors undergo bivalent binding with soluble ligands, with fibrinogen, and, under high shear conditions, with von Willebrand factor, which leads to fibrinogen-mediated cross-linking of platelets; a key event in thrombus formation and thrombosis. GPIIb/IIIa inhibitors are potent inhibitors of platelet aggregation by all types of stimuli (for example, ADP, serotonin, collagen, and thrombin). Currently three types of GPIIb/IIIa inhibitors are used clinically: abciximab, tirofiban, and eptifibatide.

3.8.4.1 Abciximab

It is a recombinant human-murine chimeric Fab-fragment with a half-life of 10 minutes. Abciximab was initially studied in percutaneous trans-luminal coronary angioplasty (PTCA) trials, in the prestent era of the early 1990s. However, the advent of GPIIb/IIIa inhibitors revolutionized the use of catheter-based therapies in the treatment of peripheral artery disease, cerebrovascular atherosclerotic disease, and various forms of coronary artery disease, as well as stable angina, UA, NSTEMI, and STEMI. Results from the Evaluation of c7E3 for the Prevention of Ischemic Complications (EPIC) trial showed that in relatively high-risk patients (those with UA, evolving MI, or complex angiographic lesion morphology) who were given abciximab, there was a 35% reduction in the primary composite end-point (death, MI, or recurrent ischemia) compared with patients who received a placebo (EPIC investigation, 1994). The c7E3 Fab Antiplatelet Therapy in Unstable Refractory Angina (CAPTURE) trial [1997] showed a 30% relative reduction, within 30 days after PTCA, in the primary endpoint of death (any cause), myocardial infarction, or recurrent ischemia requiring urgent revascularization. Furthermore, abciximab reduced the rate of myocardial infarction before, during, and after PTCA, even in patients given nitrates and heparin. Also revealed that abciximab facilitated thrombus resolution and prevented recurrent ischemia, as measured by continuous electrocardiographic monitoring. The Global Use of Strategies to Open Occluded Coronary Arteries IV–Acute Coronary Syndrome (GUSTO IV-ACS) trial studied 7,800 UA/NSTEMI patients who were not scheduled to undergo early revascularization. The results of the study showed that abciximab administration provided no benefit, even in a subgroup of patients who had elevated troponin levels (Simoons et al., 2001).

3.8.4.2 Tirofiban hydrochloride

It is a low molecular weight nonpeptide derivative of tyrosine with a half-life of 1.3 hours. In the Platelet Receptor Inhibition in Ischemic Syndrome Management (PRISM) study (1998), 3,232 patients with UA were randomlyassigned to receive either heparin or tirofiban for 48 hours. Results showed a 32% reduction in the rate of death, MI, or refractory ischemia at 48 hours (3.8% with tirofiban *vs* 5.6% with heparin), but there was no significant difference in the composite endpoint at 30 days (15.9% in the tirofiban group vs 17% in the heparin group). In the Platelet Receptor Inhibition in Ischemic Syndrome Management in Patients Limited by Unstable Signs and Symptoms (PRISM-PLUS) trial (1998) 1,915 patients with UA and non-Q-wave MI were randomly assigned to receive heparin, tirofiban, or both. Patients also received ASA in the absence of any contraindications. The tirofiban only arm was stopped prematurely because of excess death at 7 days (4.6% *vs* 1.1% in the heparin-only arm). The greatest benefit was seen in the group receiving both heparin and tirofiban, for whom the frequency of the composite endpoint (7-day death, MI, or refractory ischemia) was reduced (17.9% *vs* 12.9% in the heparin-only arm). The observed benefit was sustained at 30 days (18.5% *vs* 22%) and at 6 months (27.7% *vs* 32%).

3.8.4.3 Eptifibatide

It is a cyclic heptapeptide that selectively inhibits the arginin-glycin-aspartate (RGD) motifs sequence of the GPIIb/IIIa receptors and has a half-life of 150 minutes. The Platelet Glycoprotein IIb/IIIa in Unstable Angina: Receptor Suppression Using Integrilin Therapy (PURSUIT) trial (1998) data showed that the administration of eptifibatide resulted in a 10% reduction in the relative risk of death and MI at 30 days in patients who had NSTEMI. Boersma and colleagues (2002) clarified the importance of GPIIb/IIIa inhibitors in the management of moderate to high-risk UA/NSTEMI patients. Boersma's meta-analysis pooled 31,402 patients from six GPIIb/IIIa trials for ACS. Results showed a 10.8% event rate in the GPIIb/IIIa inhibitor group (n=18,297), versus an 11.8% event rate in the placebo group (n=13,105), and a 9% reduction in the odds ratio of death or MI. The benefit was largest in a subset of patients who had evidence of myocardial necrosis, as suggested by elevated troponin levels. The magnitude of the treatment effect also was found to be greater in patients who underwent a PCI procedure within 5 days. The Early GPIIb/IIIa Inhibition in Non-ST-Segment-Elevation Acute Coronary Syndrome (EARLY ACS) trial (Giugliano et al., 2009) studied 9,494 high-risk NSTEMI patients undergoing an invasive procedure at study centers in 29 countries were randomly assigned to receive either eptifibatide ≥12 hours before angiography (the early eptifibatide group) or a matching placebo infusion with provisional use of eptifibatide after angiography (the delayed-eptifibatide group). Results showed no statistical difference in the primary efficacy endpoint of a composite of death, MI, or recurrent ischemia requiring urgent revascularization, or in the occurrence of a thrombotic complication during PCI (9.3% in the early-eptifibatide group *vs* 10% in the delayed-eptifibatide group). However, early use of eptifibatide was associated with an increased risk of nonfatal bleeding and the need for transfusion (Giugliano et al., 2009).

3.9 Anticoagulants

Anticoagulants are effective for reducing the occurrence of major ischemic events in patients with ACS. The principal adverse effect associated with their use is bleeding. Bleeding during anticoagulant therapy is independently associated with an increased risk of MI and death, which further offsets the clinical benefit (Eikelboom et al., 2006; Rao et al., 2004). In the treatment of non-ST elevation (NSTE) ACS, enoxaparin, a low-molecular-weight heparin (LMWH), reduces the odds of death or non-fatal MI by 16% compared with unfractionated heparin (UFH) (odds ratio [OR]: 0.84; $_{95\%}$ C.I: 0.76-0.92) but does not reduce death and increases the odds of major bleeding by 25% (OR: 1.25; $_{95\%}$ CI: 1.04-1.50) (Murphy et al., 2007). In the treatment of STEMI, enoxaparin compared with UFH reduces the odds of death or non-fatal MI by 22%, but increases the risk of bleeding by 45% and is not associated with a mortality benefit. Another LMWH, reviparin, reduces both reinfarction and mortality among patients with acute STEMI compared with standard treatment, but increases the risk of life-threatening bleeding (Yusuf et al., 2005).

3.9.1 Unfractionated heparin (UFH)

Unfractionated heparin is a glycosaminoglycan comprising multiple different polysaccharide chain lengths of varying molecular weights. It exerts its anticoagulative effect by activating and accelerating the proteolytic activity of plasma cofactor antithrombin (AT). Heparin binds to the lysine site on AT, producing a conformational change at the arginine-reactive site that converts AT from a slow, progressive thrombin (factor IIa) inhibitor to a rapid inhibitor of thrombin and factor Xa thereby preventing thrombus propagation. Only one third of any given dose of heparin actually binds to AT and exerts its anticoagulative effect. Heparin also binds to a number of different circulating plasma proteins (acute phase reactants), blood cells, and endothelial cells, which contributes to its differing anticoagulative effects in different patients. Therefore, close and frequent monitoring of the activated partial thromboplastin time is necessary to ensure that a safe therapeutic range is maintained. In a double-blind, randomized, placebo-controlled trial involving 479 UA/NSTEMI patients, the incidence of MI was reduced from 11.9% in the placebo group to 3.3% in the ASA group, 0.8% in the heparin group, and 1.6% in the heparin plus ASA group (Theroux et al., 1988). Similarly, the incidence of refractory angina was reduced from 22.9% in the placebo group to 16.5% in the ASA group, 8.5% in the heparin group, and 10.7% in the heparin plus ASA group. *The combination of heparin plus ASA was found to be no more beneficial than heparin alone.* Meta-analysis using data from 6 randomized trials that included 1,353 patients found that patients who received a combination of UFH and ASA had a 33% risk reduction in cardiovascular death and MI ($_{95\%}$ C.I, 2%–56%) than did patients who received a placebo (Oler et al., 1996). *The ACC/AHA Guidelines state that patients with NSTEMI should receive heparin, unless contraindicated.* Most trials of UFH involving UA/NSTEMI patients recommend heparin therapy for 2 to 5 days.

3.9.2 Low-molecular-weight heparin

Low-molecular weight heparin is derived from heparin by chemical or enzymatic depolymerization, which yields fragments approximately one third the size of heparin. Most of the fragments contain fewer than 18 saccharide units and catalyze the inactivation of factor Xa more than of factor IIa (UFH inhibits factors Xa and IIa equally) (Weitz, 1997). Compared with UFH, LMWH has lower plasma-protein binding and therefore, a more predictable anticoagulative effect, has a greater bioavailability, is conveniently administered in subcutaneous doses (once/day or twice/day), and requires less frequent laboratory monitoring. Because LMWH is cleared by the kidneys, dosing should be decreased to half in patients with creatinine clearances of <30 ml/min and avoided altogether in patients with severe renal insufficiency. LMWHs; **ardeparin, dalteparin, enoxaparin, nadroparin, reviparin, and tinzaparin** are now considered the mainstay of antithrombotic agents for the prophylaxis and treatment of venous thrombo-embolism (VTE). Dalteparin, enoxaparin, and tinzaparin are all approved by the FDA and currently available in the United States. The FDA-approved indications vary among the different LMWHs. Dalteparin and enoxaparin are indicated for VTE prophylaxis and ACS treatment, while enoxaparin and tinzaparin are indicated for treatment of VTE. As enoxaparin has been available since the early 1980s, it is the LMWH most widely studied, as reflected by its extended list of FDA-approved indications. Fast Revascularization during Instability in Coronary Artery Disease (FRISC) trial found that dalteparin (120 IU/kg with a maximal dose of 10,000 IU, twice daily) was associated with a 63% relative risk reduction in death or MI (1.8% in the treatment group *vs* 4.8% in the placebo group) in the first six days (Swahn and Wallentin, 1997). At 40 days, differences in the incidence of MI and death in patients receiving dalteparin persisted, although a sub-group analysis revealed that dalteparin's effect was mostly confined to patients who were nonsmokers. In the Efficacy and Safety of Subcutaneous Enoxaparin in Non-Q-wave Coronary Events (ESSENCE) trial found that the risk of death, MI, or recurrent angina in patients with UA/NSTEMA was significantly lower in the enoxaparin (1 mg/kg twice daily) patients than in the UFH patients (16.6% vs 19.8%). Even at 30 days, the benefit remained (19.8% *vs* 23%), but at the cost of increased minor bleeding (Cohen et al., 1997). There was no significant change in the incidence of major bleeding (6.5% *vs* 7%). The Thrombolysis In Myocardial Infarction 11B (TIMI 11B) trial found that enoxaparin may be more effective than UFH for reducing death and serious cardiac ischemic events during the acute management of UA/NSTEMI patients, without causing a significant increase in the rate of major bleeding (Antman et al., 1999). A meta-analysis of the approximately 22,000 UA/NSTEMI patients enrolled in six randomized trials comparing enoxaparin and UFH showed a relative risk reduction of 9% in the combined endpoint of death or MI at 30 days for patients receiving enoxaparin (10.1% *vs* 11% with UFH). There were no significant differences in major bleeding at 7 days (Petesern et al., 2004). *Enoxaparin was consistently beneficial when an early conservative strategy was implemented.* The Superior Yield of the New Strategy of Enoxaparin, Revascularization and Glycoprotein IIb/IIIa Inhibitors (SYNERGY) trial treat UA/NSTEMI patients with an early-invasive strategy taking the primary endpoint was all-cause death or nonfatal MI at 30-day follow-up (Ferguson et al., 2004). The primary endpoint occurred in 14.5% of patients receiving UFH and in 14% of patients receiving enoxaparin (a nonsignificant 3% risk reduction). Enoxaparin therapy was associated with a 20% increase in TIMI major bleeding in UA/NSTEMI patients undergoing invasive procedures, especially CABG procedures. Blazing et al., (2004) showed that the event rates in 3,987 patients receiving the GPIIb/IIIa inhibitor tirofiban were similar to those in patients receiving enoxaparin and those receiving UFH. The primary endpoint was a composite of death, new MI, or refractory ischemia within 7 days. However, the incidence of TIMI major bleeding not related to CABG revealed an event rate of 15% in the enoxaparin group compared with 4% in the UFH group. *Compared with UFH, enoxaparin appears to be superior in reducing ischemic events in UA/NSTEMI patients who are treated with early-conservative strategies.*

3.9.3 Factor X (prothrombinase enzyme) inhibitors

Fondaparinux is a synthetic sulfated pentasaccharide that binds to AT early in the coagulation cascade, thereby indirectly inhibiting factor Xa. Its specificity and selectivity, combined with its long half-life and 100% bioavailability, enables once-daily anticoagulation without the need to monitor the activated clotting time. Fondaparinux inhibits factor Xa within the clot itself without inhibiting platelet function, which prevents thrombus progression and enhances AT's effectiveness in a safe manner. The Organization to Assess Strategies for Ischemic Syndromes (OASIS) study showed that fondaparinux was statistically equivalent to enoxaparin with respect to the primary efficacy endpoint (death, MI, or refractory ischemia) at 9 days (5.8% *vs* 5.7%, respectively). The composite of death, MI, refractory ischemia, or major bleeding at 9 days occurred in 7.3% of fondaparinux patients vs 9% of enoxaparin patients. The efficacy was maintained for up to six months. Major bleeding at 9 days was significantly lower with fondaparinux than with enoxaparin (2.2% *vs* 4.1%). Results from MICHEL-ANGELO OASIS-5 Steering (2005) showed that fondaparinux increased the rate of guiding-catheter thrombus formation (29 episodes (0.9%]) with fondaparinux vs 8 episodes with enoxaparin (0.3%).

Bivalirudin is an FDA-approved direct thrombin inhibitor. The Bivalirudin Angioplasty Trial (BAT) compared bivalirudin to heparin and found that bivalirudin had superior clinical outcomes in terms of reducing the rate of death, MI, and revascularization (6.2% *vs* 7.9% for bivalirudin versus heparin). Also, bivalirudin was associated with a decreased frequency of hemorrhage compared with heparin (3.5% *vs* 9.3%) (Bittl et al., 2001). In a similar study (Comparison of Abciximab Complications with Hirulog Ischemic Events Trial [CACHET]), bivalirudin plus provisional abciximab was compared with heparin plus planned abciximab (Lincoff et al., 2002). Again, bivalirudin had superior clinical outcomes regarding death, MI, revascularization, and major hemorrhage at seven days (14.1% *vs* 3.5% for heparin versus bivalirudin). Bivalirudin is addressed in the guidelines as an option for invasive management of ACS. It was studied in 6010 low- to moderate-risk patients undergoing urgent or elective PCI in the REPLACE-2 trial (Lincoff et al., 2003). In that study, the primary composite endpoint (death, MI, urgent repeat revascularization, or in-hospital major bleeding) occurred in 9.2% of patients in the bivalirudin group *vs* 10% of those in the heparin plus GP IIb/IIIa group within 30 days of randomization. There was no significant difference between bivalirudin alone compared with heparin plus a GP IIb/IIIa inhibitor for the composite ischemia endpoint. In addition, bivalirudin alone was shown to have a significantly lower rate of major bleeding and reduced rate of the net clinical outcome (Stone et al., 2006).

3.10 Thrombolytics

All available fibrin-specific thrombolytic agents have the same general mechanism of fibrinolysis. They have the property of fibrin-enhanced conversion of plasminogen to plasmin. When introduced into systemic circulation at pharmacologic concentrations, they preferentially bind to fibrin in a thrombus and catalyze cleavage of entrapped plasminogen to plasmin. This begins local fibrinolysis with limited systemic proteolysis. These agents differ from the prototype streptokinase (nonfibrin-specific) in that they enzymatically cleave plasminogen to plasmin, whereas streptokinase causes an indirect conformational change in the plasminogen molecule, which then acts as plasmin. Examples of these agents include alteplase (rt-PA), reteplase (r-PA) and tenecteplase (TNK) which are approved for treatment of acute myocardial infarction. As measured by decreases in plasminogen and fibrinogen levels, r-PA, rt-PA, and TNK have increasing fibrin specificity. TNK, is a genetically engineered variant of rt-PA. Its name refers to the sites of amino acid modification (T103N, N117Q, KHRR 296-299 AAAA). This modification is believed responsible for the increased fibrin specificity compared with r-PA and rt-PA. TNK has improved resistance to inactivation by plasminogen activator inhibitor-1 (PAI-1) compared with rt-PA (Collen et al., 1994; Keyt et al., 1994). Plasminogen activator inhibitor-1 is an endogenous substance capable of rapidly binding and inhibiting both single-chain and two-chain endogenous tissue plasminogen activator (t-PA), and similarly inactivates r-PA and rt-PA (Nordt et al., 1998). Thrombolytic therapy reduced the mortality of patients with acute myocardial infarction. Survival benefit is documented with streptokinase, anistreplase, rt-PA, r-PA, and TNK. Thrombolysis trials showed thrombolytics to be beneficial in most patients; however, approximately 25% of patients eligible for therapy do not receive it, with those at highest risk for death least likely to be treated (Barron et al., 1998). The available data showed the efficacy fibrin-specific thrombolytic drugs in establishing the patency in an occluded coronary artery. These studies were specifically designed to measure patency rates, not mortality rates, as the primary outcome. Also r-pA-rt-PA and TNK improve the survival rate and provide similar combined mortality benefit after acute myocardial infarction. In all trials the most critical adverse event was bleeding. Intracranial hemorrhage occurred at a rate less than 1% with r-PA, rt-PA, and TNK, with higher frequency in patients older than 75 years. Other noncerebral major bleeding complication requiring blood transfusion occurred at a similar rate with r-PA and rt-PA, and was significantly less with TNK. No other adverse events have been reported. Unlike streptokinase, rechallenge with fibrin-specific agents does not produce an antigenic response. Contraindications for r-PA, rt-PA, and TNK include active internal bleeding; intracranial or intraspinal surgery or trauma within 2 or fewer months; intracranial neoplasm, arteriovenous malformation, or aneurysm; bleeding diathesis; and severe uncontrolled hypertension. Conditions that may increase the risk of bleeding (warnings) are recent major surgery (≤ 10 days), cerebrovascular disease, recent (≥ 10 days) gastrointestinal or genitourinary bleeding, recent (≤ 10 days) trauma, hypertension (≥ 180 mm Hg systolic, ≥ 110 mm Hg diastolic), acute pericarditis, subacute bacterial endocarditis, hemostatic defects secondary to severe hepatic or renal disease, significant liver dysfunction, pregnancy, retinopathy, current therapy with oral anticoagulants (warfarin), and septic thrombophlebitis. Although advanced age (> 75 yrs) increases the risk of bleeding, these patients still experience significant benefit from therapy.

3.11 Angiotensin converting enzyme inhibitors (ACEIs)

Angiotensin-converting enzyme inhibitors (ACEIs) have been shown to reduce the rate of mortality and to prevent cardiovascular events in patients with coronary artery disease, especially after acute myocardial infarction (The EUROPA, 2003; Pfeffer et al., 1995). The authors of the EUROPA (European Trial on Reduction of Cardiac Events With Perindopril in Stable Coronary Artery Disease) study showed a 14% reduction in total rate of mortality, nonfatal MI, unstable angina, and cardiac arrest. ACEIs, through the reduction of angiotensin II and increased bradykinin availability, explicate their cardioprotective proprieties on left ventricular afterload and remodeling, improving cardiac hemodynamics, and reducing ventricular mass (Okin et al., 2003). In addition to lowering blood pressure, ACEIs possess a vasculoprotective and anti-ischemic action through their antiatherosclerotic, antithrombotic, anti-inflammatory effects (Brasier et al., 2002).Long-term treatment with ACE inhibitors after myocardial infarction is associated with improved outcomes, especially in patients with left ventricular systolic ejection fraction less than 40%. Elderly ACS patients appear to derive greater benefit from ACE inhibitors than their younger counterparts. ARBs should be used as an alternative in ACE inhibitor intolerant patients. ACE inhibitors and angiotensin receptor blockers (ARBs) are not part of the initial management of ACS patients and should not be started until the patient is stabilized and is ready for hospital discharge. Renal function and electrolytes should be monitored closely, especially in elderly patients.

3.12 Lipid lowering agents; HMG-Co reductase inhibitors; Statins

Statins were initially identified as secondary metabolites of fungi. One of the first natural inhibitors of HMG-CoA reductase, ML-236B, was isolated as a metabolite from cultures of *Penicillium citrinum* and was shown to be an extremely potent competitive inhibitor of HMG-CoA reductase. Statins are either hydrophilic such as pravastatin and rosuvastatin or lipophilic statins e.g. atorvastatin and simvastatin. The beneficial effects of statins extend to patients regardless of age, sex, or baseline cholesterol levels. The pleiotropic (pleiotropy" comes from the Greek words *pleio*, which means many, and *trepein*, which means influencing) effects of statins include:

1. Improve endothelial function in patients with hypercholesterolemia and atherosclerosis *via* up-regulating eNOS.
2. Attenuate cytokine-mediated vascular smooth muscle cell (VSMC) proliferation in coronary artery smooth muscle cells and also inhibit pathological proliferation such as that observed in transplant-associated arteriopathy
3. Could inhibit cardiac hypertrophy through an antioxidant mechanism involving inhibition of Rac1 geranylgeranylation
4. Exert protective function against ischemic myocardial injury
5. Inhibit platelets aggregation
6. Modulate immune activation and to exert anti-inflammatory effects on the vascular wall by decreasing the number of inflammatory cells in atherosclerotic plaques
7. Contribute to plaque stability by reducing plaque size or by modifying the physiochemical properties of the lipid core
8. Protect the brain from Alzheimer's dementia

Statins very effective in the reduction of mortality and non-fatal cardiovascular events rates in both primary and secondary prevention of ischemic heart disease. Statins *via* their pleotropic effects inhibit the pathogenic pathways of coronary artery disease. They reduce total-and LDL-cholesterol accumulation in plaque, endothelial dysfunction, activation of inflammation and thrombus formation. An increasing number of observations demonstrate that statins may play a beneficial role not only in early secondary prevention but also directly in the therapy of ACS i.e. when statin treatment is started as first-line care in clinically unstable patient. The study of Ostadal et al., (2010) failed to demonstrate the beneficial effect of fluvastatin as first line therapy in acute coronary syndrome on the serum markers of inflammation and plaque instability; C-reactive protein, interleukin 6, pregnancy-associated plasma protein A (PAPP-A/proMBP). Statins is the most efficacious therapies for patients with established coronary disease, and evidences suggest that these agents are beneficial in the setting of ACS. Intensive lipid-lowering therapy reduces adverse clinical events, including death and MI, compared with moderate-dose therapy in patients with acute coronary syndrome (de Lemos et al., 2004). The best recognized and most commonly reported adverse effects of statins are muscle adverse effects and include muscle pain, fatigue and weakness as well as rhabdomyolysis. Fibrates, particularly gemfibrozil, amplify the risk of rhabdomyolysis on statins (most powerfully for cerivastatin), due to their effect of impeding statin metabolism and perhaps their additional lipid-modifying effects. Concurrent administration of statins with CYP3A4 inhibitors (e.g. cyclosporine, erythromycin, azole antifungal and antiretrovirals such as ritonavir.) may raise statin concentrations and risk of toxicity, including rhabdomyolysis. Grapefruit juice and perhaps pomegranate juice inhibit CYP3A4 and have been presumptively linked to statin rhabdomyolysis. Non muscle statin adverse effects include cognitive problems, gastrointestinal and neurological symptoms, psychiatric symptoms, sleep problems, glucose elevations.

4. Miscellaneous

Perhexiline has been used as an antianginal drug since the early 1970s (Armstrong et al., 1974) when its mode of action was thought to be *via* coronary artery vasodilatation mediated by calcium channel antagonism (Opie, 1980). Perhexiline is now thought to exert its anti-anginal action primarily by inhibiting the enzyme carnitine palmitoyltransferase (Kennedy et al., 1996). This inhibition reduces fatty acid metabolism in favour of carbohydrate metabolism which increases available energy for the same amount of oxygen. Perhexiline is relatively free of negative inotropic effects and does not increase airways resistance and is therefore not contraindicated in such situations. Perhexiline has been shown to be superior to β-adrenoceptor blockers in its ability to reduce the frequency of anginal attacks and in addition, because it has a different mode of action, it provides additional antianginal benefit when added to existing agents (Stewart et al., 1996). Its use declined in the mid 1970s (Horowitz, 1995) because of the occurrence of severe adverse effects during long-term therapy including neuropathy and hepatotoxicity (Cooper et al., 1985). The incidence of these adverse effects was noted to be related to plasma perhexiline concentration and it was observed that adverse effects could be prevented if plasma concentrations were kept below defined values (Pilcher et al., 1985; Horowitz., 1986).

l-carnitine

L-carnitine is a naturally occurring amino acid essential for the transport of fatty acids into the mitochondria. It involved in oxidation of long-chain fatty acids and stabilization of cellular membranes and is also a free-radical scavenger. Skeletal and cardiac muscle use fatty acids as main source of energy, therefore, carnitine deficiency mainly manifests as dysfunction of the above tissues. Carnitine depletion can also cause hypoglycemia, hyperammonemia, hypoketonemia, coma, seizures, and developmental disorders. Cardiac muscle contains very high levels of carnitine compared with other tissues. Myocardial ischemia has been shown to deplete carnitine levels in the myocardium. When combined with elevated levels of fatty acids during ischemia, this leads to elevation of toxic metabolites of fatty acid esterification. It has been suggested that depletion of free L-carnitine in the ischemic myocardium can impair the electrical and contractile activities of the heart. Carnitine may make cardiomyocytes more resistant to free radicals. Another proposed mechanism is through shifting the metabolism from fatty acid oxidation to glucose oxidation. Propionyl L-carnitine (PLC) is a carnitine derivative that may have enhanced beneficial effects compared with carnitine. Carnitine significantly reduced left ventricular end-diastolic, end-systolic pressures, and infarct size in patients presenting with acute myocardial infarction and reduced the mortality rate from heart failure (Iliceto et al., 1995; Singh et al., 1996). In patients with chronic stable angina, carnitine improved exercise tolerance; significant improvements in exercise duration and time needed for ST-segment changes to return to baseline (Iyer et al., 2000).

Ribose

Ribose is a pentose sugar that has been shown in numerous animal experiments to enhance ATP production and improve cardiac function. Ribose can enhance metabolism by entering the pentose phosphate pathway and bypassing the rate limiting enzymes of glucose-6-phosphate dehydrogenase and 6-phosphogluconate-dehydrogenase. It improves the time to ST-segment depression and time to moderate angina, and diastolic relaxation by restoring ATP levels (Pliml et al., 1992). Ribose supplementation improves diastolic heart function, increases exercise tolerance and enhances patient quality of life. These benefits are provided by the role ribose plays in increasing cardiac energy reserves that become depressed during ischemia or hypoxia associated with coronary artery disease or congestive heart failure.

Dichloracetate (DCA)

Dichloroacetate (DCA) can overcome fatty acid inhibition of glucose oxidation by stimulating the pyruvate dehydrogenase complex, the rate-limiting enzyme for glucose oxidation (Stacpoole et al., 1998). By this effect, DCA enhances contractile function during reperfusion and significantly improves cardiac efficiency. The beneficial effect of DCA in ischemia-reperfusion injury may be attributed to:

1. DCA reduces the proton production from glucose metabolism. This was associated with an increase in the rate of intracellular pH recovery as well as in improvement in cardiac efficiency (Liu et al., 1999).
2. DCA may exert its beneficial effects by influencing mitochondrial proton leak. Proton leak occurs when proton motive force is consumed without ATP synthesis (Brand et al., 1994).

In clinical studies, DCA has been shown to increase left ventricular stroke volume in patients with coronary artery disease and dramatically improve recovery of cardiac work following ischemia. DCA improves acidosis in critically ill patients and, likewise, improves myocardial hemodynamics in those with chronic coronary artery disease and congestive heart failure; however, its metabolism is variable and clinical data on its use in chronic ischemic heart disease are limited (Schofield and Hill, 2001). The use of DCA is limited by its low potency (blood levels need to approach millimolar levels) and short half-life.

Glucose Insulin Potassium (GIK)

Glucose-insulin-potassium (GIK) therapy is one of the most widely investigated approaches used in a clinical setting; it was first reported in 1962 with results from new trials continuing to be published. In the 1960's Sodi-Pallares refined the treatment by adding insulin and potassium to the infusion, and demonstrated that the treatment was effective for the arrhythmias and angina (Sodi-Pallares et al., 1962; 1963).

The beneficial effects of hyperglycemia and hyperinsulinemia could be due to:

1. An increase glycolytically derived ATP
2. An increase in pyruvate dehydrogenase enzyme activity due to decreased plasma FFA concentration and elevated insulin levels, resulting in less lactate and H^+ accumulation
3. Less accumulation of noxious fatty-acyl CoAs due to lower FFA levels.

Glucose and insulin infusion was also decrease infarct size and prevent the fall in creatine phosphate, ATP and pH in animal models of ischemia/reperfusion injury (Maroko et al., 1972; Opie and Owen, 1976). Clinical trials with glucose and insulin infusion following myocardial infarction) or coronary artery by-pass surgery (Gradinak et al., 1989) have generally been favorable. Although in general GIK therapy is found to improve outcome after acute myocardial infarction, this is not a uniform observation (Pache et al., 2004). The most frequently mechanism underlying the protection associated with increased myocardial glucose use are that it improves efficiency by decreasing oxygen consumption and improves the coupling between glucose oxidation and glycolysis, thereby reducing intracellular acidosis (Liu et al., 2002). Glucose and insulin infusions have been used to raise glycogen levels prior to cardiac surgery. In general, an infusion of glucose and insulin results in hyperglycemia (>10 mM), hyperinsulinemia (>80 μU/ml), and low plasma FFA levels (<0.3 mM) (Wisneski et al., 1990). Hyperglycemia and hyperinsulinemia result in an increase in glycogen synthesis. Studies in patients have shown that infusing glucose and insulin overnight prior to cardiac surgery results in a 50–70% increase in cardiac glycogen concentration and improved clinical outcome from cardiac surgery (Berggren et al., 1982). Coronary-artery-bypass graft patients with elevated preoperative myocardial glycogen levels had reduced serum levels of myocardial enzymes during the post-operative period and a lower incidence of arrhythmias.

Etomoxir

Etomoxir (ethyl 2-[6-(4-chlorophenoxy)hexyl]oxirane-2-carboxylate) is an inhibitor of carnitine palmitoyltransferase I enzyme (CPT I). It is of potential interest in the treatment of diabetes since inhibition of fatty acid oxidation should increase glucose utilization and decrease gluconeogenesis. By inhibiting fatty acid oxidation, fatty acid-induced inhibition of glycolysis may be overcome, thereby increasing glucose utilization. As a result of inhibition the CPT I the myocardial fatty acid oxidation is reduced and thereby relieves fatty acid inhibition of pyruvate dehydrogenase enzyme activity, and increases the oxidation of glucose and lactate. This has anti-ischaemic efficacy and improves cardiac function during the recovery from ischaemia. However, long-term administration of such agent has been found to be associated with toxicity problems, and in particular their causing cardiac hypertrophy (Rupp et al., 1995). In experimental animal model, etomoxir does not affect ventricular mass in rats with left ventricular hypertrophy following aortic banding, and actually prevents the impairment in contractile function in this model.

Diazeniumdiolates (NONOates)

The first of this class was diethylamine NONOate; DEA/NO synthesized in 1960. However, Diazeniumdiolates only became the focus of attention in the NO world in the 1990s when their NO donor properties were considered in biological settings (Maragos et al., 1991). An attractive feature of this class of compounds is that their decomposition is not catalysed by thiols or biological tissue, unless specifically designed to (see below) and, because NO release follows simple first-order kinetics, the rate of NO release can be accurately predicted. Subsequently, biological activity such as vasodilatation, inhibition of platelet aggregation, inhibition of blood coagulation and inhibition of VSMC proliferation closely correlate with the amount of NO generated *in vitro*. At present, NONOates not used clinically, although they have been tested frequently in experimental models of cardiovascular disease. The primary cardiovascular focus for NONOates has been in the prevention of thrombosis and neointimal formation following vascular injury, an inevitable result of interventional cardiology techniques, such as balloon angioplasty, bypass grafting or placement of stents.

S-Nitrosothiols

The *S*-nitrosothiol class of NO donors covers a vast array of different compounds which contain a single chemical bond between a thiol (sulphydryl) group (R-SH) and the NO moiety. Biological activity of *S*-nitrosothiols is highly influenced by the molecular environment of the parent thiol. It is important to acknowledge that a vast number of factors are capable of releasing NO from *S*-nitrosothiols, including light, heat, transition metals, thiols, superoxide and enzymes such as xanthine oxidase, superoxide dismutase, protein disulphide isomerase and various dehydrogenases. *S*-nitrosothiols have advantages over other classes of NO donors, such as the nitrates, as they have far less stringent metabolic requirements and this may be the reason that they do not induce tolerance with long-term use (Hanspal *et al.*, 2002). *S*-Nitrosothiols are not used clinically at present, but there are a large number of animal and clinical studies demonstrating their advantageous features, especially in the cardiovascular system.

Plants, herbs, and other natural resources

Several studies reported that some herbal medicines exert an effect on hemodynamic function in human. The effect of these natural plants and herbs are either directly or indirectly *via* their antioxidant properties. The use of such remedies is not free from serious adverse effect as well as adverse interactions with other drugs prescribed in acute coronary syndrome. The followings are the most common natural substances that exert certain pharmacological actions on the cardiovascular system.

Hawthorn

It also known as Crataegus laevigata or Crataegus monogyna, is an herb commonly found in Europe, western Asia, North America and North Africa. Modern medicinal extracts usually incorporate the leaves and flowers of the hawthorn tree, whereas traditional preparations use the fruit. Parts of the hawthorn tree contain flavonoids, which decrease the likelihood of blood vessel damage. Consuming hawthorn extract may improve angina patients' heart function and ability to exercise. It has been used for cardiac and circulatory disorders since the first century AD (Weihmayr and Ernst, 1996). Hawthorn berries, flowers and leaves of *Crataegus laevigata* (Poiret) have been used traditionally throughout Europe to treat cardiovascular diseases including hypertension, myocardial dysfunction, angina and tachycardia (Mills and Bone, 2000). In France, it is also used for insomnia and anxiety (British Herbal Medicine Association, 2003). Twentieth century German research revealed the efficacy of hawthorn for the treatment of cardiac failure (Pittler et al., 2003), and it is for this use that hawthorn is best known. The ethanolic extract of *Crataegus oxycantha* (COC) is traditionally used as a cardiotonic in China, India, and many European countries. COC contains oligomeric proanthocyanidins, flavonoids, and polyphenols which are well-known for their antioxidant properties (Svedstrom et al., 2002). Human subjects treated with COC extract after myocardial infarction have shown improvements in heart rate, reduction in blood pressure, and an increase in the left-ventricular ejection volume (Degenring et al., 2003; Walker et al., 2002). It has also been shown that an alcoholic extract of COC promoted improvement in tricarboxylic acid (TCA) cycle enzyme activity and protected the mitochondria against isoproteronol-induced cardiac injury (Jayalakshmi and Devaraj, 2004; Jayalakshmi et al., 2006). Recently COC extract may reduce the oxidative stress in the reperfused myocardium of isolated rat heart preparation, and play a significant role in the inhibition of apoptotic pathways (*via* upregulating the antiapoptotic proteins and downregulationg the proapoptotic proteins) to cardioprotection (Swaminathan et al.,2010). Hawthorn demonstrated numerous properties that may be beneficial in heart failure including anti-arrhythmic activities (Garjani et al., 2000; Chatterjee et al., 1997), and the ability to increase coronary blood flow (Occhiuto et al., 1986 (a,b), and cardiac output (Brixius et al., 1998). These effects may be mediated by inhibition of phosphodiesterase types

III and IV (Schussler et al., 1995), antioxidant activities (Bahorun et al., 2003) and anti-inflammatory effects (Chatterjee et al., 1997). A meta-analyses of clinical trials concluded that hawthorn may be a safe and effective treatment for chronic heart failure (Pittler et al., 2003). Crataegus extract (hawthorn), raises intracellular calcium, prolongs the action potential, and may improve exercise capacity in mild heart failure. It is widely used in Europe by heart failure patients as a "natural" remedy. Hawthorn contains no cardioactive glycosides. The principle active components are flavonoids: non-toxic phytochemicals that are widespread in fruit and vegetables and that have health benefits. It showed low toxicity in animal studies and minimal side effects in clinical trials (Mills and Bone, 2005). No drug–herb interaction has been reported in animal trials, and in a human study no interaction was observed between hawthorn and digoxin (Tankanow et al., 2003). Herbal practitioners use hawthorn for cardiovascular dysfunction, including mild manifestations in otherwise healthy people, without restriction on long-term use.

Cactus

Cactus (*Opuntia*) has been used for many years as a common vegetable and as medicine by the Native Americans and Mexicans (Cornett, 2000; Kay, 1996; Knishinsky, 1971; Tesoriere et al., 2004). Cactus contains a fruit known as cactus pear (*Opuntia ficus-indica*) and the plant is referred to as nopale (pad). Cactus pear contains pectin, carotenes, betalains, ascorbic acid, quercetina and quercetin derivatives all of which have antioxidant activity (Wang, 1988). In Chinese medicine, cactus fruit is considered a weak poison and used as medicine for treatment of inflammation and pain. It has also been used as a detoxification agent for snake bite. Opuntia ficus indica supplementation induced changes in heart rate variability in athletes in terms of increasing high and low frequency activities and reducing the heart rate (Schmitt et al., 2008). Cactus, also known as *Selenicereus grandiflorus*, may be effective for treating angina. Cactus can be used as a diuretic, cardiac stimulant and spinal and motor nerve stimulant. The principle action of cactus is upon the circular muscle fibers of the heart and arterioles, or tiny arteries, and that cactus is beneficial for cardiac incompetence, congestive heart failure, cardiac weakness, mitral insufficiency and angina. The succulent stem is the part of the cactus used for treating heart-related conditions. Overdose may cause arrhythmias, chest pain, pericarditis, confusion, headaches, vertigo and gastrointestinal symptoms.

***Ammi visnaga* (Khella, Khillah)**

Khella, also known as *Ammi visnaga*, may help treat angina. Khella is an African plant that contains spasm-relieving compounds, including khellin. In early studies, purified khellin demonstrated an ability to relieve angina-related symptoms, although it is unknown whether the whole herb would have similar effects. Khella improves blood supply to the myocardium, and increases efficiency of myocardial metabolism--two factors that could decrease angina-related pain or discomfort. Khella is often used to treat mild forms of angina, mild obstructive pulmonary disease and various problems of the urinary tract. As early as 1945 Anrep et al., demonstrated in physiological experiments that khellin is an effective coronary vasodilator in doses insufficient to cause any general fall in blood pressure. And in the preliminary clinical trial khellin has advantages over the nitrites and other reputed vasodilators in that it has a selective action on the coronary vessels, and effective doses need not, therefore, lower systemic blood pressure. Its action is slower but more prolonged than that of the nitrites. It may be given in the form of continuous treatment to abolish or reduce the frequency and severity of anginal attacks, or to relieve individual severe attacks of pain.

***Vaccinium myrtillus* (Bilberry)**

It is a member of the Ericaceous family found in the mountains and forests of Europe and North America. *Vaccinium myrtillus* extracts (VME) contained 15 different anthocyanins which possess potent antioxidant properties, stabilize collagen fibers, promote collagen biosynthesis and inhibit platelet aggregation. In experimental animal studies VME have demonstrated to be of benefit in improving vascular tone, blood flow and vasoprotection (Lietti et al., 1976; Colantuoni et al., 1991). In isolated rat heart preparation bilberry extract increases the coronary flow, decreases the lactic dehydrogenase enzyme release during reperfusion and shorten the duration of arrhythmias (Žiberna et al., 2009).

Co-Enzyme Q_{10}

Coenzyme Q_{10} (CoQ_{10}) is the predominant human form of endogenous ubiquinone. It synthesized in the mitochondrial inner membrane. CoQ_{10} and comprised of a ubiquinone head group attached to a tail of 10 five-carbon isoprenoid units that anchors the molecule to the mitochondrial membranes. It acts in the in the mitochondrial respiratory chain as electrons carrier from complex I and II to complex III. It is antioxidant and plays a role in the regulation of membranes physiochemical properties and modulates the endothelial function. Supplemental CoQ_{10} is known to reduce lipid peroxidation (Sugiyama et al., 1980). Good evidence supports its use in congestive heart failure, type 2 diabetes, atherosclerosis, migraine, and Parkinson disease (Bonakdar and Guarnieri, 2005). Coenzyme Q10 levels are reduced by statin therapy because it shares the hepatic mevalonate synthetic pathway with cholesterol (Jula et al., 2002). Patients with hypertension have reduced serum levels of CoQ_{10} (Yamagami and Shibata, 1975). A meta-analysis of 12 clinical trials of 352 patients concluded that CoQ_{10} lowers blood pressure therefore it would seem acceptable to add CoQ_{10} to conventional anti-hypertensive therapy (Rosenfeldt et al., 2007). CoQ10 supports the production of energy in the heart and supports the health of the cardiac muscle.

***Zingiber officinale* (Ginger)** also strong antioxidants that support the health of the blood vessel and help protect the heart and vessels from the damage of free radicals. It reduces the levels of triglycerides and low-density lipoprotein-cholesterol, and inhibits the blood platelet aggregation. The pharmacologic cardiac effects of ginger are based on its activity as hypolipemic agent, anticoagulant and hypotensive.

***Allium sativum* (Garlic)**

The health benefits of garlic have been known since at least 1500 B.C. when ancient Chinese and Indians used it as a blood-thinning agent. Hippocrates, the father of modern medicine, used garlic to treat cervical cancer. Subsequent studies found efficacy of garlic as a cardioprotective. Numerous studies documented the hypoglycemic, antiatherogenic and antiatherosclerotic properties of garlic (Elkayam et al., 2003; Agarwal, 1996; Banerjee and Maulik, 2002). Garlic was also found to be beneficial against ischemic heart disease (Tyrrell. 1979). A significant number of clinical trials found garlic to lower total as well as LDL cholesterol (Kwon et al., 2003) and recently it is useful for lowering high blood pressure (McMahon and Vargas, 1993). Many of the physiological effects of garlic are attributed to the volatile sulfur compounds like thiosulfinates, which are also responsible for its pungent aroma. Recently, the cardioprotective ability of garlic was attributed to s-allylcysteine (Perez-Severiano et al., 2004). Blood pressure reducing properties of garlic have been linked to its hydrogen sulphide production and allicin content - liberated from alliin and the enzyme alliinase which has angiotensin II inhibiting and vasodilating effects, as shown in animal and human cell studies. Bhatti et al (2008) demonstrated that garlic extract exaggerated the cardio protection offered by ischemic preconditioning and *per se* treatment with garlic extract also protects the myocardium against ischemia reperfusion induced cardiac injury. This effect is probably attributed to the inhibition of platelet aggregation, oxidative stress or to fibrinolytic properties.

Arjun (*Terminalia arjuna*) has demonstrated great promise for improving heart function and reducing angina. Arjun (*Terminalia arjuna*) is a tree common in Central and South India. Its bark has a long history of use in Ayurvedic medicine (the traditional medicine of India) for the treatment of heart problems, such as angina. Research demonstrates that arjun may in fact be very effective in reducing angina and improving heart function. A one-week, double-blind, placebo-controlled crossover trial of 58 people evaluated the effectiveness of arjun for angina by comparing it against placebo, isosorbide mononitrate (Bharani et al., 2002). The results indicated that the herb reduced anginal episodes and increased exercise capacity. A subsequent 3-month study compared the effectiveness of arjun against placebo in 40 people with a recent heart attack (Dwivedi et al., 2005). All participants in this study suffered from ischemic mitral regurgitation. The results showed that use of the herb improved heart function and reduced angina symptoms. Another study found benefits with an Ayurvedic herbal combination containing arjun (Antani et al., 1990).

Coleus forskohlii

Coleus forskohlii (CF) is a plant native to India. Since ancient times, plants of the *Coleus* species have been used as an herbal medicine to treat various disorders of the cardiovascular, respiratory, gastrointestinal, and central nervous systems. Forskolin has been isolated from the roots of the India-based *Coleus Forskohlii*. Forskolin is a diterpene that acts directly on adenylate cyclase leading to generate cAMP from ATP in the cell. cAMP regulates the body's thermogenic response to food, increases the body's basal metabolic rate, and increases utilization of body fat and stimulates lipolysis. cAMP stimulates the cardiac muscle and dilates the large blood vessels.

Vitamins

Ascorbic acid

It has a favorable redox couple that protects vitamin E and glutathione from oxidation. In clinical studies, ascorbic acid supplementation improves nitric oxide-dependent vasodilation in human subjects with coronary artery disease, hypertension, hypercholesterolemia, and diabetes mellitus (Taddei et al., 1998).

Vitamin E (alpha-tocopherol)

Vitamin E is a lipid soluble, chain-breaking radical scavenger family of eight related tocopherols and tocotrienols, and is considered the most important antioxidant in cell membranes (Herrera and Barbas, 2001). Of the various forms, alpha-tocopherol has the highest bioavailability and protects cell membranes against oxidation by reacting with lipid radicals produced during lipid peroxidation chain reactions (Herrera and Barbas, 2001). Despite an initial small study demonstrating a therapeutic benefit of vitamin E on reducing non-fatal myocardial infarction, more recent, placebo-controlled, large-scale trials of antioxidants have been disappointing and have found no clinically benefical effects of long term vitamin E supplementation (Brown et al., 2001; Lonn et al., 2005).

Vitamin D

Recently data demonstrated that vitamin D insufficiency/deficiency is significantly associated with all-cause mortality, at least in the American population. The NHANES III database clearly shows: 1) an increase in adjusted all-cause mortality as the serum 25-hydroxy calciferol (OHD) level falls to less than 30 ng/ml, especially in women; and 2) peak protection from death with a 25OHD level in the 35–40 ng/ml range. In fact, most of the increase in all-cause mortality can be attributed to cardiovascular disease deaths in this population. The prevalence of coronary artery disease, heart failure, and peripheral artery disease is significantly increased in a stepwise fashion as the serum 25OHD level drops to less than 30 and then 20 ng/ml (Kim et al., 2008).

Omega-3 polyunsaturated fatty acids

As early as 1944, Sinclair described the rarity of CHD in Greenland Eskimos despite their consumption of diet high in fat and cholesterol (Sinclair, 1953). Sinclair observed that the Eskimos had a tendency to bruise and to bleed easily, and subsequently Bang and Dyerberg demonstrated that the Eskimos had reduced platelet counts (50 000–80 000/mm^3 lower) and decreased platelet aggregation, resulting in prolonged bleeding times. Bang and Dyerberg (1972;1980) and Dyerberg et al.,(1975) in their study comparing Greenland Eskimos and Danish controls, found, as expected, that the Eskimos, who eat about 500 g of fish per person per day (compared with 10–20 g/d in Westernized societies), had considerably higher levels of omega-3 fatty acids and lower levels of arachidonic acid in plasma, platelets, and red blood cell membranes. Interestingly, in addition to reduced rates of coronary heart disease, the Greenland Eskimos also had a more favorable lipid profile and low levels of blood pressure. Coronary heart disease is also less prevalent in Japan, despite higher prevalence of hypertension and smoking, which may be partly due to the Japanese population's traditionally high consumption of fish compared to populations in the Western world. Even within Japan, the Japanese islanders, who eat three times more fish compared to the mainland population, have lower rates of hypertension, coronary heart disease, and all-cause mortality (Lavie et al., 1987; Lavie and Milani, 1996). The mechanism of actions of Omega-3 PUFA includes:

1. Significant reduction of triglycerides.
2. Antiarrhythmic effect. The level of long-chain n-3 fatty acids was significantly and inversely related to the risk of sudden coronary death
3. Significant reduction in mean blood pressure, systemic vascular resistance,
4. Omega-3 fatty acids may confer cardioprotection in part by improving autonomic sympathovagal balance.

5. Very high doses of omega-3 fatty acids (i.e. 8 g/d) provide anti-inflammatory effects. The anti-inflammatory properties may also play an important role in stabilization of unstable plaque in patients with ACS (Lee et al., 2008; Alaswad et al., 2002). Eicosapentaenoic acid competes with arachidonic acid for the cyclooxygenase, leading to decrease the synthesis of thromboxane A_2, which is a strong platelet agonist, and increases the synthesis of thromboxane A_3, which is relatively inactive, so the net effect of high doses of omega-3 fatty acids is platelet inhibition.

Observational studies have also reported inverse associations of cardiovascular disease with dietary intake or plasma concentrations of omega 3 fatty acids (mainly eicosapentanoic acid and docosahexaenoic acid), suggesting that supplementation with omega 3 fatty acids might exert protective effects on cardiovascular disease (Bucher et al., 2002; Kromhout, 1985). These fatty acids have been shown to have beneficial effects on several cardiovascular risk factors—including blood pressure, plasma triglyceride concentration, and markers of thrombosis and inflammation—and may also have antiarrhythmic effects (Wang et al., 2006). Although some trials involving patients with a history of cardiovascular diseases or with high levels of cardiovascular risk factors have reported positive effects of omega 3 fatty acids on cardiovascular events, other trials have reported no effects on arrhythmia or mortality (Brouwer et al., 2009; Burr et al., 2003).

5. Cardiovascular adverse effects of herbal remedies

Several natural remedies interact with known pharmacological agents that indicated in acute coronary syndrome. Among these:

Aloe vera may cause hypokalemia and inducing digitalis toxicity and cardiac arrhythmias in patients with heart failure

Butcher's broom is mainly indicated for circulatory disorder and it reduced the effect of α-adrenoceptor effects in patients with hypertension and heart failure

Capsicum which is indicated for shingles, trigeminal and diabetic neuralgia may elevate the blood pressure in patients treated with monoamine oxidase inhibitors

Fumitory used as hypotensive agent and enhances the effects of β-adrenoceptors, calcium entry blockers and glycosides.

Ginseng causes high blood pressure

Gossypol, a male contraceptive increases the effect of diuretics and causes hypokalemia

Grape fruit juice augments the cardiac effects of calcium entry blockers

Hawthorn potentiates the actions of glycosides and nitrite

Irish moss potentiates the antihypertensives effects

Kelp increases the effects of antihypertensives

Khella increases the cardiac actions of calcium entry blockers

Licorice increases the blood pressure and causes hypokelemia which potentiates the

Lily of the valley increases effects of β-aderenoceptor, calcium entry blockers, digitalis and quinidine

Ma-huang (ephedra) increases heart rate and blood pressure

Oleander increases the effect of angiotensin converting enzyme inhibitors, antiarrhythmics, β-adrenoceptor blockers, calcium entry blockers and cardiac glycosides.

St. John's wort induces arrhythmias, heart block, hyperkalemia and death

Strophanthus increases heart rate and blood pressure in patients treated ith monoamine oxidase inhibitors

Yohimbine increases heart rate and induces changes in blood pressure

6. References

A comparison of aspirin plus tirofiban with aspirin plus heparin for unstable angina. Platelet Receptor Inhibition in Ischemic Syndrome Management (PRISM) Study Investigators. *N Engl J Med* 1998; 338(21):1498-1505

A randomised, blinded, trial of clopidogrel versus aspirinin patients at risk of ischaemic events (CAPRIE). CAPRIESteering Committee. *Lancet* 1996; 348(9038): 1329-1339

Agarwal KC. Therapeutic actions of garlic constituents. *Med Res Rev* 1996; 16:111–124

Alaswad K., Lavie C. J., Milani R. V., O'Keefe J. H., Jr Fish oil in cardiovascular protection. *Ochsner J* 2002; 4:83–91

Alexander JH, Harrington RA, Tuttle RH, Berdan LG, Lincoff AM, Deckers JW, Simoons ML, Guerci A, Hochman JS, Wilcox RG, Kitt MM, Eisenberg PR, Califf RM, Topol EJ, Karsh K, Ruzyllo W, Stepinska J, Widimsky P, Boland JB, Armstrong PW. Prior aspirin use predicts worse outcomes in patients with non-ST-elevation acute coronary syndromes. PURSUIT Investigators. Platelet IIb/IIIa in Un-stable angina: Receptor Suppression Using Integrilin Therapy. *Am J Cardiol* 1999; 83: 1147-1151.

Anrep GV, Barsoum GS, Kenawy MR, Misrahy G. Ammi visnaga in the treatment of the anginal syndrome. *Br Heart J* 1946; 8: 171–177

Antani J, Kulkarni R, Antani N. Effect of Abana on: ventricular function in ischaemic heart disease. *Japanese Heart Journal* 1990; 31:829-835

Antithrombotic Trialists' Collaboration. Collaborative meta-analysis of randomised trials of antiplatelet therapy for prevention of death, myocardial infarction, and stroke in high risk patients. *BMJ* 2002; 324(7329): 71-86

Antman EM, McCabe CH, Gurf inkel EP, Turpie AG, Bernink PJ, Salein D, Bayes De Luna A, Fox K, Lablanche JM, Radley D, Premmereur J, Braunwald E. Enoxaparin prevents death and cardiac ischemic events in unstable angina/non-Q-wave myocardial infarction. Results of the thrombolysis in myocardial infarction (TIMI) 11B trial. *Circulation 1999*; 100:1593-1601

Armstrong ML, Brand D, Emmett AJ, Hodge JLR, Kelleway GSM, Mesitz P, Refman M, Wallace DC. A multicentre trial of perhexiline maleate, beta-blocker and placebo in angina pectoris. *Med J Aust* 1974; 2:389–393

Bahorun T, Aumjaud E, Ramphul H, Rycha M, Luximon-Ramma A, Trotin F, Aruoma OI. Phenolic constituents and antioxidant capacities of Crataegus monogyna (Hawthorn) callus extracts. *Nahrung* 2003; 47:191–198

Baker JG. The selectivity of β-adrenoceptor agonists at human β1-β2- and β3-adrenoceptors. *Br J Pharmacol* 2010; 160:1048–1061

Baker JG. The selectivity of β-adrenoceptor antagonists at the human β1 β2 and β3 adrenoceptors. *Br J Pharmacol* 2005; 144:317–322

Balsano F, Rizzon P, Violi F, Scrutinio D, Cimminiello C, Aguglia F, Pasotti C, Rudelli G. Antiplatelet treatment with ticlopidine in unstable angina. A controlled multicenter clinical trial. The Studio della Ticlopidina nell'Angina Instabile Group. *Circulation* 1990; 82:17-26

Banerjee SK, Maulik SK. Effect on garlic on cardiovascular disorders: A review. *Nutrition J* 2002; 1: 4

Bang H O, Dyerberg J. Lipid metabolism and ischemic heart disease in Greenland Eskimos. *Adv Nutr Res* 1980; 3: 1–22

Bang HO, Dyerberg J. Plasma lipids and lipoproteins in Greenlandic west coast Eskimos. *Acta Med Scand* 1972; 192:85–94

Barron HV, Bowlby LJ, Breen T, Rogers WJ, Canto JG, Zhang Y, Tiefenbrunn AJ, Weaver WD. Use of reperfusion therapy for acute myocardial infarction in the United States: data from the National Registry of Myocardial Infarction 2. *Circulation* 1998; 97:1150-1156

Berggren H., R. Ekroth, J. Herlit, A Hjalmarson, A. Waldenstrom, J. Waldensstrom, and G. William-Olsson. Improved myocardial protection during cold cardioplegia by means of increased myocardial glycogen stores. *Thorac Cardiovasc Surg* 1982; 30:389–392

Bharani A, Ganguli A, Mathur LK, Jamra Y, Raman PG. Efficacy of Terminalia arjuna in chronic stable angina: a double-blind, placebo-controlled, crossover study comparing Terminalia arjuna with isosorbide mononitrate. *Indian Heart J* 2002; 54:170-175

Bhatt DL, Topol EJ. Scientific and therapeutic advances in antiplatelet therapy. *Nat Rev Drug Discov* 2003; 2: 15-28

Bhatti R, Singh K, Ishar MPS, Singh J. The effect of *Allium sativum* on ischemic preconditioning and ischemia reperfusion induced cardiac injury. *Indian J Pharmacol* 2008; 40: 261–265

Bittl JA, Chaitman BR, Feit F, Kimball W, Topol EJ. Bivalirudin versus heparin during coronary angioplasty for unstable or postinfarction angina: final report reanalysis of the Bivalirudin Angioplasty Study. *Am Heart J* 2001; 142: 952-959

Blazing MA, de Lemos JA, White HD, Fox KA, Verheugt FW, Ardissino D, DiBattiste PM, Palmisano J, Bilheimer DW, Snapinn SM, Ramsey KE, Gardner LH, Hasselblad V, Pfeffer MA, Lewis EF, Braunwald E, Califf RM.; 'A to Z' Investigators. Safety and eff icacy of enoxaparin vs unfractionated heparin in patients with non-ST-segment elevation acute coronary syndromes who receive tirofiban and aspirin: a randomized controlled trial [published erratum appears in *JAMA* 2004; 292:1178, *JAMA* 2004; 292:55-64.

Bodo R. The effect of the 'heart tonics' and other drugs upon heart-tone and coronary circulation. *J Physiol* 1928; 64:356–387

Boersma E, Harrington RA, Moliterno DJ, White H, Theroux P, Van de Werf F, de Torbal A, Armstrong PW, Wallentin LC, Wilcox RG, Simes J, Califf RM, Topol EJ, Simoons ML. Platelet glycoprotein IIb/IIIa inhibitors in acute coronary syndromes: a meta-analysis of all major randomised clinical trials [published erratum appears in *Lancet* 2002; 359(9323):2120, *Lancet* 2002; 359(9302):189-198

Bonakdar A, Guarnieri E. Coenzyme Q10. *Am Fam Physician* 2005; 72:1065–70

Bonello L, Sbragia P, Amabile N, Com O, Pierre SV, Levy S, Paganelli F. Protective effect of an acute oral loading dose of trimetazidine on myocardial injury following percutaneous coronary intervention *Heart*. 2007; 93: 703–707

Brand MD, Chien L, Ainscow EK, Rolfe DFS, Porter RK. The causes and functions of mitochondrial proton leak. *Biochem Biophys Acta* 1994; 1187:132–139

Brandt JT, Payne CD, Wiviott SD, Weerakkody G, Farid NA, Small DS, Jakubowski JA, Naganuma H, Winters KJ. A comparison of prasugrel and clopidogrel loading doses on platelet function: magnitude of platelet inhibition is related to active metabolite formation. *Am Heart J* 2007; 153:66.e9–e16

Brasier A, Recinos A, Eledrisi MS. Vascular inflammation and the renin-angiotensin system. *Atherioscler Thromb Vasc Biol* 2002; 22:1257-1266

Braunwald E, Antman EM, Beasley JW, Califf RM, Cheitlin MD, Hochman JS, Jones RH, Kereiakes D, Kupersmith J, Levin TN, Pepine CJ, Schaeffer JW, Smith EE 3rd, Steward DE, Theroux P, Gibbons RJ, Alpert JS, Faxon DP, Fuster V, Gregoratos G, Hiratzka LF, Jacobs AK, Smith SC Jr; American College of Cardiology; American Heart Association. Committee on the Management of Patients With Unstable Angina. American College of Cardiology/American Heart Association (ACC/AHA) 2002 guideline update for the management of patients with unstable angina and non-ST-segment elevation myocardial infarction–summary article: a report of the American College of Cardiology/American Heart Association task force on practice guidelines (Committee on the Management of Patients With Unstable Angina) *J Am Coll Cardiol* 2002; 40:1366–1374

British Herbal Medicine Association. A guide to traditional herbal medicines: a source book of accepted traditional uses of medicinal plants within Europe. Bournemouth: BHMA; 2003

Brixius K, Frank K, Munch G, Muller-Ehmsen J, Schwinger RHG. WS 1442 (Crataegus-Special Extract) increases contractile force in the myocardium of humans with congestive heart failure. *Herz-Kreislauf* 1998; 30:28–33

Brouwer IA, Raitt MH, Dullemeijer C, Kraemer DF, Zock PL, Morris C, Katan MB, Connor WE, Camm JA, Schouten EG, McAnulty J. Effect of fish oil on ventricular tachyarrhythmia in three studies in patients with implantable cardioverter defibrillators. *Eur Heart J* 2009; 30:820-826

Brown BG, Zhao XQ, Chait A, Fisher LD, Cheung MC, Morse JS, Dowdy AA, Marino EK, Bolson EL, Alaupovic P, Frohlich J, Albers JJ. Simvastatin and niacin, antioxidant vitamins, or the combination for the prevention of coronary disease. *N Engl J Med* 2001; 345: 1583–1592

Brunton TL. On the use of nitrite of amyl in angina pectoris. *Lancet* 1867; 2: 97–98

Bucher HC, Hengstler P, Schindler C, Meier G. N-3 polyunsaturated fatty acids in coronary heart disease: a meta-analysis of randomized controlled trials. *Am J Med* 2002; 112: 298-304

Bunch TJ, Muhlestein JB, Bair TL, Renlund DG, Lappe DL, Jensen KR, Horne BD, Carter MA, Anderson JL. Intermountain Heart Collaborative Study Group. Effect of beta-blocker therapy on mortality rates and future myocardial infarction rates in patients with coronary artery disease but no history of myocardial infarction or congestive heart failure. *Am J Cardiol* 2005; 95:827–831

Burr ML, Ashfield-Watt PA, Dunstan FD, Fehily AM, Breay P, Ashton T, Zotos PC, Haboubi NA, Elwood PC. Lack of benefit of dietary advice to men with angina: results of a controlled trial. *Eur J Clin Nutr* 2003; 57: 193-200

Chaitman B R. Pharmacological approaches to the symptomatic treatment of chronic stable angina: a historical perspective and future directions. *Can J Cardiol* 2005; 21:1031–1034

Chatterjee SS, Koch E, Jaggy H, Krzeminski T. In vitro and in vivo studies on the cardioprotective action of oligomeric procyanidins in a Crataegus extract of leaves and blooms. *Arzneimittel-Forschung* 1997; 47:821–825

Chen CF, Yeh SU, Chien CT, Wu MS. Renal response during acute unilateral ureteral obstruction in rats. *Neurourol Urodyn* 2001; 20:125–137

Chu MW, Wilson SR, Novick RJ, Stitt LW, Quantz MA. Does clopidogrel increase blood loss following coronary artery bypass surgery? *Ann Thorac Surg* 2004; 78(5):1536-1541

Ciapponi A, Pizarro R, Harrison J. Trimetazidine for stable angina. *Cochrane Database Syst Rev* 2005. 19CD003614

Cohen M, Demers C, Gurfinkel EP, Turpie AG, Fromell GJ, Goodman S, Langer A, Califf RM, Fox KA, Premmereur J, Bigonzi F. A comparison of low-molecular-weight heparin with unfractionated heparin for unstable coronary artery disease. Efficacy and Safety of Subcutaneous Enoxaparin in Non-Q-Wave Coronary Events Study Group. *N Engl J Med* 1997; 337: 447-452

Cohen ML. β_3-receptors mediate relaxation in stomach fundus whereas a fourth β receptor mediates tachycardia in atria from transgenic β_3-receptor knockout mice. *Receptors Channels* 2000; 7:17–23

Colantuoni A, Bertuglia S, Magistretti MJ, Donato L. Effects of *Vaccinium myrtillus* anthocyanosides on arterial vasomotion. *Arzneim Forsch/Drug Res* 1991; 41:905–909

Colin P, Ghaleh B, Monnet X, Su J, Hittinger L, Giudicelli JF, Berdeaux A.. Contributions of heart rate and contractility to myocardial oxygen balance during exercise. *Am J Physiol Heart Circ Physiol* 2003; 284:H676–H682

Collaborative overview of randomised trials of antiplatelet therapy--I: Prevention of death, myocardial infarction, and stroke by prolonged antiplatelet therapy in various categories of patients. Antiplatelet Trialists' Collaboration [published erratum appears in *BMJ* 1994; 308(6943):1540]. *BMJ* 1994; 308(6921):81-106

Collen D, Stassen JM, Yasuda T, Refino C, Paoni N, Keyt B, Roskams T, Guerrero JL, Lijnen HR, Gold HK. Comparative thrombolytic properties of tissue-type plasminogen activator inhibitor-1-resistant glycosylation variant, in a combined arterial and venous thrombosis model in the dog. *Thromb Haemost* 1994; 72: 98-104

Contro S, Haring OM, Goldstein W. Paradoxic action of amyl nitrite in coronary patients. *Circulation* 1952; 6:250–256

Cornett J. How Indians used desert plants. Nature Trails Press; 2000

Cow D. Some reactions of surviving arteries. *J Physiol* 1910; 42:125–143 de Lemos JA, Blazing MA, Wiviott SD, Lewis EF, Fox KA, White HD, Rouleau JL, Pedersen TR, Gardner LH, Mukherjee R, Ramsey KE, Palmisano J, Bilheimer DW, Pfeffer MA, Califf RM, Braunwald E. Early intensive vs a delayed conservative simvastatin strategy in patients with acute coronary syndromes: phase Z of the A to Z trial. *JAMA* 2004; 292:1307-1316

Degenring FH, Suter A, Weber M, Saller R. A randomised double blind placebo controlled clinical trial of a standardised extract of fresh Crataegus berries (Crataegisan) in the treatment of patients with congestive heart failure NYHA II. *Phytomedicine* 2003; 10:363–369

Demontis GC, Moroni A, Gravante B, Altomare C, Longoni B, Cervetto L, DiFrancesco D. Functional characterisation and subcellular localisation of HCN1 channels in rabbit retinal rod photoreceptors. *J Physiol* 2002; 542: 89–97

Di Napoli P, Taccardi A, Barsotti A. Long term cardioprotective action of trimetazidine and potential effect on the inflammatory process in patients with ischaemic dilated cardiomyopathy. *Heart* 2005; 91: 161–165

DiFrancesco D, Camm JA. Heart rate lowering by specific and selective I_f current inhibition with ivabradine: a new therapeutic perspective in cardiovascular disease. *Drugs* 2004; 64:1757–1765

Dong YL, Gangula PR, Fang L, Wimalawansa SJ, Yallampalli C. Uterine relaxation responses to calcitonin gene-related peptide and calcitonin gene-related peptide receptors decreased during labor in rats. *Am J Obstet Gynecol* 1998; 179:497–506

Dwivedi S, Aggarwal A, Agarwal MP, Rajpal S. Role of Terminalia arjuna in ischaemic mitral regurgitation. *Int J Cardiol* 2005; 100:507-508

Dyerberg J., Bang H. O., Hjorne N. Fatty acid composition of the plasma lipids in Greenland Eskimos. *Am J Clin Nutr* 1975; 28:958–966

Eikelboom JW, Mehta SR, Anand SS, Xie C, Fox KA, Yusuf S. Adverse impact of bleeding on prognosis in patients with acute coronary syndromes. Circulation 2006; 114:774-782

Elkayam A, Mirelman O, Peleg E, Wilchek M, Miron T, Rabinkov A, Oron-Herman M, Rosenthal T. The effects of allicin on weight in fructose-induced hyperinsulinemic, hyperlipidemic, hypertensive rats. *Am J Hypertension* 2003; 16: 1053–1056

Facchinetti F, Neri I, Genazzani AR. L-arginine infusion reduces preterm uterine contractions. *J Perinat Med* 1996; 24:283–285

Ferguson JJ, Califf RM, Antman EM, Cohen M, Grines CL, Goodman S, Kereiakes DJ, Langer A, Mahaffey KW, Nessel CC, Armstrong PW, Avezum A, Aylward P, Becker RC, Biasucci L, Borzak S, Col J, Frey MJ, Fry E, Gulba DC, Guneri S, Gurfinkel E, Harrington R, Hochman JS, Kleiman NS, Leon MB, Lopez-Sendon JL, Pepine CJ, Ruzyllo W, Steinhubl SR, Teirstein PS, Toro-Figueroa L, White H; SYNERGY Trial Investigators. Enoxaparin vs unfractionated heparin in high-risk patients with non-ST-segment elevation acute coronary syndromes managed with an intended early invasive strategy: primary results of the SYNERGY randomized trial. *JAMA* 2004; 292:45-54

Francois-Frank CA. Effect vasodilatateur du nitrite d'amyle sur les vaisseaux de l'corce crebrale et sur les vaisseaux du myocarde. *Compt Rend Soc Biol* 1903; 55:1448

Frere C, Cuisset T, Morange PE, Quilici J, Camoin-Jau L, Saut N, Saut N, Faille D, Lambert M, Juhan-Vague I, Bonnet JL, Alessi MC. Effect of cytochrome p450 polymorphisms on platelet reactivity after treatment with clopidogrel in acute coronary syndrome. *Am J Cardiol* 2008; 10:1088-1093

Frishman WH, Pepine CJ, Weiss RJ, Baiker WM. Addition of zatebradine, a direct sinus node inhibitor, provides no greater exercise tolerance benefit in patients with angina taking extended-release nifedipine: results of a multicenter, randomized, double-blind, placebo-controlled, parallel-group study. *J Am Coll Cardiol* 1995; 26: 305–312

Frishman WH, Retter A, Misailidis J, Ganem A, Sekhon J, Mohandas R, Khaski D, Sheikh F, Orlic D, Anversa P. Innovative pharmacologic approaches to treatment of myocardial ischemia. In: Frishman WH, Sonnenblick EH, Sica DA, editors. *Cardiovascular Pharmacotherapies.* 2nd edition. New York, NY, USA: McGraw-Hill; 2003. pp. 655–690

Garjani A, Nazemiyeh H, Maleki N, Valizadeh H. Effects of extracts from flowering tops of Crataegus meyeri A. Pojark. on ischaemic arrhythmias in anaesthetized rats. *Phytother Res* 2000; 14: 428–431

Giugliano RP, White JA, Bode C, Armstrong PW, Montalescot G, Lewis BS, van 't Hof A, Berdan LG, Lee KL, Strony JT, Hildemann S, Veltri E, Van de Werf F, Braunwald E, Harrington RA, Califf RM, Newby LK; EARLY ACS Investigators. Early versus delayed, provisional eptifibatide in acute coronary syndromes. *N Engl J Med* 2009; 360:2176-2190

Goldstein RE, Boccuzzi SJ, Cruess D, Nattel S. Diltiazem increases late-onset congestive heart failure in postinfarction patients with early reduction in ejection fraction. The Adverse Experience Committee; and the Multicenter Diltiazem Postinfarction Research Group. *Circulation* 1991; 83:52–60

Gradinak S, Coleman GM, Taegtmeyer H, Sweeney MS, Frazier OH. Improved cardiac function with glucose-insulin-potassium after coronary bypass surgery. *Ann Thorac Surg* 1989; 48:484–489

Hankey GJ, Eikelboom JW. Aspirin resistance. *Lancet* 2006; 367(9510):606-617.

Hanspal IS, Magid KS, Webb DJ, Megson IL. The effect of oxidative stress on endothelium-dependent and nitric oxide donor-induced relaxation: implications for nitrate tolerance. *Nitric Oxide* 2002; 6:263–270.

Herrera E, Barbas C. Vitamin E: action, metabolism and perspectives. *J Physiol Biochem* 2001; 57:43–56

Ho PM, Maddox TM, Wang L, Fihn SD, Jesse RL, Peterson ED, Rumsfeld JS. Risk of adverse outcomes associated with concomitant use of clopidogrel and proton pump inhibitors following acute coronary syndrome. *JAMA* 2009; 301:937-944

Hoffman BB. Adrenoceptor antagonist drugs. In: Katzung BG, editor. *Basic and Clinical Pharmacology.* 10th ed. New York: McGraw-Hill; 2007. pp. 141–58

Horowitz JD, Button IK, Wing L. Is perhexiline essential for the optimal management of angina pectoris? *Aust NZ J Med* 1995; 25:111–113

Horowitz JD, Pia STB, Macdonald PS, Goble AJ, Louis WJ. Perhexiline maleate treatment for severe angina pectoris - correlations with pharmacokinetics. *Int J Cardiol* 1986; 13: 219–229

Iliceto S, Scrutinio D, Bruzzi P, D'Ambrosio G, Boni L, Di Biase M, Biasco G, Hugenholtz PG, Rizzon P.. Effects of L-carnitine administration on left ventricular remodeling after acute anterior myocardial infarction: The L-Carnitine Ecocardiografia Digitalzzata Infarto Miocardico (CEDIM) trial. *J Am Coll Cardiol* 1995; 26:380–387

Inhibition of platelet glycoprotein IIb/IIIa with eptif ibatide in patients with acute coronary syndromes. The PURSUIT Trial Investigators. Platelet Glycoprotein IIb/IIIa in Unstable Angina: Receptor Suppression Using Integrilin Therapy. *N Engl J Med* 1998; 339:436-443

Inhibition of the platelet glycoprotein IIb/IIIa receptor with tirofiban in unstable angina and non-Q-wave myocardial infarction. Platelet Receptor Inhibition in Ischemic Syndrome Management in Patients Limited by Unstable Signs and Symptoms (PRISM-PLUS) Study Investigators [published erratum appears in *N Engl J Med* 1998; 339:415. *N Engl J Med* 1998; 338:1488-1497

IONA Study Group. Effect of nicorandil on coronary events in patients with stable angina: the impact of nicorandil in angina (IONA) randomised trial. *Lancet* 2002; 359: 1269–1275

Iyer RN, Khan AA, Gupta A, Vajifdar BU, Lokhandwala YY. L-carnitine moderatelyimproves the exercise tolerance in chronic stable angina. *J Assoc Physicians India* 2000; 48:1050–1052

Jayalakshmi R, Devaraj NS. Cardioprotective effect of tincture of Crataegus on isoproterenol-induced myocardial infarction in rats. *J Pharm Pharmacol* 2004; 56:921-926

Jayalakshmi R, Thirupurasundari CJ, Devaraj SN. Pretreatment with alcoholic extract of Crataegus oxycantha (AEC) activates mitochondrial protection during isoproterenol - induced myocardial infarction in rats. *Mol Cell Biochem* 2006; 292:59-67

Jula A, Marniemi J, Huupponen R, Virtanen A, Rastas M, Ronnemaa T. Effects of diet and simvastatin on serum lipids, insulin and antioxidants in hypercholesterolemic men: a randomized controlled trial. *JAMA* 2002; 287:598–605

Juurlink DN, Gomes T, Ko DT, Szmitko PE, Austin PC, Tu JV, Henry DA, Kopp A, Mamdani MM.. A population-based study of the drug interaction between proton pump inhibitors and clopidogrel. *CMAJ* 2009; 180:713-718

Kaumann AJ, Molenaar P. Modulation of human cardiac function through 4 β-adrenoceptor populations. *Naunyn. Schmiedebergs Arch Pharmacol* 1997; 355: 667–681

Kay MA. Healing with plants in the American and Mexican west. The University of Arizona Press; 1996

Kennedy JA, Unger SA, Horowitz JD. Inhibition of carnitine palmitoyltranferase-1 in rat heart and liver by perhexiline and amiodarone. *Biochem Pharmacol* 1996; 52:273-280

Keyt BA, Paoni NF, Refino CJ, L Berleau, H Nguyen, A Chow, J Lai, L Peña, C Pater, J Ogez. A faster-acting more potent form of tissue plasminogen activator. *Proc Natl Acad Sci USA* 1994; 91:3670-3674

Kim DH, Sabour S, Sagar UN, Adams S, Whellan DJ. Prevalence of hypovitaminosis D in cardiovascular diseases (from the National Health and Nutrition Examination Survey 2001 to 2004) *Am J Cardiol* 2008; 102:1540–1544

Klein L, O'Connor CM, Gattis WA, Zampino M, de Luca L, Vitarelli A, Fedele F, Gheorghiade M. Pharmacologic therapy for patients with chronic heart failure and reduced systolic function: review of trials and practical considerations. *Am J Cardiol* 2003; 91(9A): 18F–40F

Knishinsky R. Prickly pear cactus medicine. Healing Arts Press, Rochester, Vermont; 1971.

Kones R. After cardiac surgery, how does nutrition fit in with risk factors? *J Parent Enteral Nutr* 2010; 34:163-167

Kromhout D. The inverse relation between fish consumption and 20 years mortality from coronary disease. *N Engl J Med* 1985; 312:1205-1209

Kwon MJ, Song YS, Choi MS, Park SJ, Jeong KS, Song YO. Cholesteryl ester transfer protein activity and atherogenic parameters in rabbits supplemented with cholesterol and garlic powder. *Life Sci* 2003; 72:2953–2964

Lavie C. J., Milani R. V. Fish oils. In: Messerli F. H., editor. *Cardiovascular Drug Therapy.* Philadelphia: W.B. Saunders Company; 1996. pp. 1608–1613

Lavie C. J., Squires R. W., Gau G. T. Preventive cardiology: what is the role of fish and fish oils in primary and secondary prevention. *J Cardiopulm Rehabil* 1987; 7:526–533

Lee J. H., O'Keefe J. H., Lavie C. J., Marchioli R., Harris W. S. Omega-3 for cardioprotection. *Mayo Clin Proc* 2008; 83:324–332

Li XQ, Andersson TB, Ahlstrom M, Weidolf L. Comparison of inhibitory effects of the proton pump-inhibiting drugs omeprazole, esomeprazole, lansoprazole, pantoprazole, and rabeprazole on human cytochrome P450 activities. *Drug Metab Dispos* 2004; 32(8):821-827

Lietti A, Cristoni A, Picci M. Studies on Vaccinium myrtillus anthocyanosides. *Arzneim Forsch/Drug Res* 1976;26:829–32

Lincoff AM, Bittl JA, Harrington RA, Feit F, Kleiman NS, Jackman JD, Sarembock IJ, Cohen DJ, Spriggs D, Ebrahimi R, Keren G, Carr J, Cohen EA, Betriu A, Desmet W, Kereiakes DJ, Rutsch W, Wilcox RG, de Feyter PJ, Vahanian A, Topol EJ; REPLACE-2 Investigators. Bivalirudin and provisional glycoprotein IIb/IIIa blockade compared with heparin and planned glycoprotein IIb/IIIa blockade during percutaneous coronary intervention. *JAMA* 2003; 289:853-863

Lincoff AM, Kleiman NS, Kottke-Marchant K, Maierson ES, Maresh K, Wolski KE, Topol EJ. Bivalirudin with planned or provisional abciximab versus low-dose heparin and abciximab during percutaneous coronary revascularization: results of the Comparison of Abciximab Complications with Hirulog for Ischemic Events Trial (CACHET). *Am Heart J* 2002;143: 847-853

Liu Q, Docherty JC, Rendell J, Clanachan AS, Lopaschuk GD. High levels of fatty acids decrease the rate of recovery of intracellular pH in isolated rat hearts reperfused after ischemia. *Circulation* 1999; 100(I):1811

Liu Q, Docherty JC, Rendell JC, Clanachan AS, Lopaschuk GD. High levels of fatty acids delay the recovery of intracellular pH and cardiac efficiency in post-ischemic hearts by inhibiting glucose oxidation. *J Am Coll Cardiol* 2002; 39: 718–725

Lonn E, Bosch J, Yusuf S, Sheridan P, Pogue J, Arnold JM, Ross C, Arnold A, Sleight P, Probstfield J, Dagenais GR. Effects of long-term vitamin E supplementation on cardiovascular events and cancer: a randomized controlled trial. *JAMA* 2005; 293:1338–1347

Love BB, Biller J, Gent M. Adverse haematological effects of ticlopidine. Prevention, recognition and management. *Drug Saf* 1998;19:89-98.

Maragos CM, Morley D, Wink DA, Dunams TM, Saavedra JE, Hoffman A, Bove AA, Isaac L, Hrabie JA, Keefer LK. Complexes of ·NO with nucleophiles as agents for the controlled biological release of nitric oxide. Vasorelaxant effects. *J Med Chem* 1991; 34:3242–3247

Markham A, Plosker GL, Goa KL. Nicorandil—an updated review of its use in ischaemic heart disease with emphasis on its cardioprotective effects. Drugs 2000; 60:955–74

Maroko PR, Libby P, Sobel BE, Bloor CM, Sybers HD, Shell WE, Covell JW, Braunwald E. Effect of glucose-insulin-potassium infusion on myocardial infarction following experimental coronary artery occlusion. *Circulation* 1972; 45:1160–1175

McMahon FG, Vargas R. Can garlic lower blood pressure? A pilot study. *Pharmacotherapy* 1993;13: 406–407

Mehta RH, Roe MT, Mulgund J, Ohman EM, Cannon CP, Gibler WB, Pollack CV Jr, Smith SC Jr, Ferguson TB, Peterson ED.. Acute clopidogrel use and outcomes in patients with non-ST-segment elevation acute coronary syndromes undergoing coronary artery bypass surgery. *J Am Coll Cardiol* 2006; 48:281-286

Michel M.C. Tissue functions mediated by β_3-adrenoceptors - findings and challenges. *Naunyn Schmiedebergs Arch Pharmacol* 2010; 382:103–108

Michelangelo Oasis 5 Steering Committee, Mehta SR, Yusuf S, Granger CB, Wallentin L, Peters RJ, Bassand JP, Budaj A, Joyner C, Chrolavicius S, Fox KA. Design and rationale of the MICHELANGELO Organization to Assess Strategies in Acute Ischemic Syndromes (OASIS)-5 trial program evaluating fondaparinux, a synthetic factor Xa inhibitor, in patients with non-ST-segment elevation acute coronary syndromes. *Am Heart J* 2005; 150:1107

Michelson AD, Cattaneo M, Eikelboom JW, Gurbel P, Kottke-Marchant K, Kunicki TJ, et al. Aspirin resistance: po-sition paper of the Working Group on Aspirin Resistance. *J Thromb Haemost* 2005; 3:1309-1311.

Mills S, Bone K. Principles and practice of phytotherapy: modern herbal medicine. Edinburgh: Churchill Livingstone; 2000

Mills S, Bone K. The essential guide to herbal safety. Edinburgh: Churchill Livingstone; 2005.

Mohri M, Shimokawa H, Hirakawa Y, Masumoto A, Takeshita A. Rho-kinase inhibition with intracoronary fasudil prevents myocardial ischemia in patients with coronary microvascular spasm. *J Am Coll cardiol* 2003; 41: 15-19

Molenaar P. The 'state' of β-adrenoceptors. *Br J Pharmacol* 2003; 140:1–2

Murphy SA, Antman EM, Wiviott SD, Weerakkody G, Morocutti G, Huber K, Lopez-Sendon J, McCabe CH, Braunwald E; TRITON-TIMI 38 Investigators.. Reduction in recurrent cardiovascular events with prasugrel compared with clopidogrel in patients with acute coronary syndromes from the TRITON-TIMI 38 trial. *Eur Heart J* 2008; 29(20):2473-247

Murphy SA, Gibson CM, Morrow DA, Van de Werf F, Menown IB, Goodman SG, Mahaffey KW, Cohen M, McCabe CH, Antman EM, Braunwald E.. Efficacy and safety of the low-molecular weight heparin enoxaparin compared with unfractionated heparin across the acute coronary syndrome spectrum: a meta-analysis. *Eur Heart J* 2007; 28:2077-2086

Murrell W. Nitro-Glycerine in angina pectoris. *Lancet* 1879; 1:80–81

Nordt TK, Moser M, Kohler B, Ruef J, Peter K, Kübler W, Bode C. Augmented platelet aggregation as predictor of reocclusion after thrombolysis in acute myocardial infarction. *Thromb Haemost* 1998; 80:881-886

Occhiuto F, Circosta C, Briguglio F, Tommasini A, de Pasquale A (a). Comparative study of the cardiovascular activity of shoots, leaves and flowers of Crataegus oxyacantha: 1. Electrical activity and arterial pressure in the rat. *Plantes medicinales et phytotherapie* 1986; 20:37–51

Occhiuto F, Circosta C, Costa R, Briguglio F, Tommasini A (b). Comparative study of the cardiovascular activity of shoots, leaves and flowers of Crataegus oxyacantha: 2. Action of extracts and isolated pure active principles on the isolated rabbit heart. *Plantes medicinales et phytotherapie* 1986; 20:52–63

Ogiwara Y, Furukawa Y, Akahane K, Haniuda M, Chiba S. Bradycardic effects of AQ-A 39 (Falipamil) in situ and in isolated, blood-perfused dog hearts. Comparison with alinidine and verapamil. *Japanese Heart Journal* 1988; 29:849–861

Okin PM, Devereux RB, Jern S, Kjeldsen SE, Julius S, Nieminen MS, Snapinn S, Harris KE, Aurup P, Edelman JM, Dahlof B; Losartan Intervention for Endpoint reduction in hypertension Study Investigations Regression of electrocardiographic left ventricular hypertrophy by losartan versus atenolol: the Losartan Intervention for Endpoint reduction in Hypertension (LIFE) Study. *Circulation* 2003; 108:684-690

Oler A, Whooley MA, Oler J, Grady D. Adding heparin to aspirin reduces the incidence of myocardial infarction and death in patients with unstable angina. A meta-analysis. *JAMA* 1996; 276:811-815

Opie LH, Owen P. Effect of glucose-insulin-potassium infusions on arteriovenous difference of glucose and of free fatty acids and on tissue metabolic changes in dogs with developing myocardial infarction. *Am J Cardiol* 1976; 38:310–321

Opie LH. Calcium antagonists. *Lancet* 1980; i:806–809

O'queli E, Hiscock M, Dick R. Clopidogrel resistance. *Heart Lung Circ* 2007;16 Suppl 3:S17-28.

Ostadal P, Alan D, Vejvoda J, Kukacka J, Macek M, Hajek P, Mates M, Kvapil M, Kettner J, Wiendl M, Aschermann O, Slaby J, Holm F, Telekes P, Horak D, Blasko P, Zemanek D, Veselka J, Cepova J. Fluvastatin in the first-line therapy of acute coronary syndrome: results of the multicenter, randomized, double-blind, placebo-controlled trial (the FACS-trial). *Trials* 2010; 11: 61

Pache J, Kastrati A, Mehilli J, Bollwein H, Ndrepepa G, Schuhlen H, Martinoff S, Seyfarth M, Nekolla S, Dirschinger J, Schwaiger M, Schomig A. A randomized evaluation of the effects of glucose-insulin-potassium infusion on myocardial salvage in patients with acute myocardial infarction treated with reperfusion therapy. *Am Heart J* 2004; 148: e3

Packer M, O'Connor CM, Ghali JK, Pressler ML, Carson PE, Belkin RN, Miller AB, Neuberg GW, Frid D, Wertheimer JH, Cropp AB, DeMets DL. Effect of amlodipine on morbidity and mortality in severe chronic heart failure. Prospective Randomized Amlodipine Survival Evaluation Study Group. *N Engl J Med* 1996; 335:1107–1114

Patel DJ, Purcell HJ, Fox KM. Cardioprotection by opening of the KATP channel in unstable angina: Is this a clinical manifestation of myocardial preconditioning? Results of a randomized study with nicorandil. *Eur Heart J* 1999; 20:51–57

Patrono C. Aspirin resistance: definition, mechanisms and clinical read-outs. *J Thromb Haemost* 2003; 1:1710-1713

Pepine CJ, Handberg EM, Cooper-DeHoff RM, Marks RG, Kowey P, Messerli FH, Mancia G, Cangiano JL, Garcia-Barreto D, Keltai M, Erdine S, Bristol HA, Kolb HR, Bakris GL, Cohen JD, Parmley WW; INVEST Investigators. A calcium antagonist vs a non-calcium antagonist hypertension treatment strategy for patients with coronary artery disease. The International Verapamil-Trandolapril Study (INVEST): a randomized controlled trial. *JAMA* 2003; 290:2805–2816

Perez-Severiano F, Rodriguez-Perez M, Pedraza-Chaverri J, Maldonado PD, Medina-Campos ON, Ortíz-Plata A, Sánchez-García A, Villeda-Hernández J, Galván-Arzate S, Aguilera P, Santamaría A. S-Allylcysteine, a garlic-derived antioxidant, ameliorates quinolinic acid-induced neurotoxicity and oxidative damage in rats. *Neurochem Int* 2004; 45:1175–1183

Petesern JL, Mahaffey KW, Hasselblad V, Antman EM, Cohen M, Goodman SG, Langer A, Blazing MA, Le-Moigne-Amrani A, de Lemos JA, Nessel CC, Harrington RA, Ferguson JJ, Braunwald E, Califf RM. Efficacy and bleeding complications among patients randomized to enoxaparin or unfractionated heparin for antithrombin therapy in non-ST-segment elevation acute coronary syndromes: a systematic overview. *JAMA* 2004; 292:89-96

Pfeffer MA. Left ventricular remodelling after acute myocardial infarction *Annu Rev Med* 1995; 46:455-466

Pilcher J, Cooper DH, Turnell DC, Matenga J, Paul R, Lockhart JDF. Investigations of long-term treatment with perhexiline maleate using therapeutic monitoring and electromyography. *Ther Drug Monit* 1985; 7:54-60

Pittler MH, Schmidt K, Ernst E. Hawthorn extract for treating chronic heart failure: meta-analysis of randomized trials. *Am J Med* 2003; 114: 665–674

Pliml W, Von Arnim T, Stablein K, Hofmann H, Zimmer HG, Erdmann E. Effects of ribose on exercise-induced ischemia in stable coronary artery disease. *Lancet* 1992; 340:507–510

Poole-Wilson PA, Lubsen J, Kirwan BA, van Dalen FJ, Wagener G, Danchin N, Just H, Fox KA, Pocock SJ, Clayton TC, Motro M, Parker JD, Bourassa MG, Dart AM, Hildebrandt P, Hjalmarson A, Kragten JA, Molhoek GP, Otterstad JE, Seabra-Gomes R, Soler-Soler J, Weber S; Coronary disease Trial Investigating Outcome with Nifedipine gastrointestinal therapeutic system investigators.. Effect of long-acting nifedipine on mortality and cardiovascular morbidity in patients with stable angina requiring treatment (ACTION trial): randomised controlled trial. *Lancet* 2004; 364: 849–857

Randomised placebo-controlled trial of abciximab before and during coronary intervention in refractory unstable angina: the CAPTURE Study [published erratum appears in *Lancet* 1997;350(9079):744, *Lancet* 1997; 349(9063): 1429-1435

Rao SV, Jollis JG, Harrington RA, Granger CB, Newby LK, Armstrong PW, Moliterno DJ, Lindblad L, Pieper K, Topol EJ, Stamler JS, Califf RM. Relationship of blood transfusion and clinical outcomes in patients with acute coronary syndromes. *JAMA* 2004; 292:1555-1562

Rich JD, Cannon CP, Murphy SA, JQin J, Giugliano RP, Braunwald E. Prior aspirin use and outcomes in acute coronary syndromes. *J Am Coll Cardiol* 2010; 56:1376-1385

Richardson BW. Report on the physiological action of nitrite of amyl. *Rep Br Assoc Adv Sci* 1864; 34:120

Rosenfeldt FL, Haas SJ, Krum H, Hadj A, Ng K, Leong JY, Watts GF. Coenzyme Q10 in the treatment of hypertension: a meta-analysis of the clinical trials. J Hum Hypertens 2007; 21:297–306

Rupp H, Schulze W, Vetter R.Dietary medium-chain triglycerides can prevent changes in myosin and SR due to CPT-1 inhibition by etomoxir. *Am J Physiol* 1995; 269(3 Pt 2):R630-640

Ruzyllo W, Tendera M, Ford I, Fox KM. Antianginal efficacy and safety of ivabradine compared with amlodipine in patients with stable effort angina pectoris: a 3-month randomised, double-blind, multicentre, noninferiority trial. *Drugs* 2007; 67:393–405

Santopinto J, Gurfinkel EP, Torres V, Marcos E, Bozovich GE, Mautner B, McCabe CH, Antman EM. Prior aspirin users with acute non-ST-elevation coronary syndromes are at increased risk of cardiac events and benefit from enoxaparin *Am Heart J* 2001; 141:566–572

Savelieva I, Camm JA. Novel I_f current inhibitor ivabradine: safety considerations Camm J, Tendera M, editors. *Heart rate slowing by I_f current inhibition* Basel: Karger; 2006, 79–96 (*Advances in Cardiology, vol 43*)

Schloss K. Uber die XWirkung der Nitrite auf die Durchblutung des Herzens (Versuche am Herzen in situ) *Deutsches Arch Klin Med* 1913; 111: 310

Schmitt L, Fouillot JP, Nicolet G, Midol A.Opuntia ficus indica's effect on heart-rate variability in high-level athletes. *Int J Sport Nutr Exerc Metab* 2008; 18: 169-178

Schnabel P. Binding properties of β-blockers at recombinant β1-β2-, and β3-adrenoceptors. *J Cardiovasc Pharmacol* 2000; 36:466–471

Schofield RS, Hill JA. Role of metabolically active drugs in the management of ischemic heart disease. *Am J Cardiovascr Drugs* 2001; 1: 23-35

Schussler M, Holzl J, Fricke U. Myocardial effects of flavonoids from Crataegus species. *Arzneimittelforschung* 1995; 45:842–845

Serebruany VL, Steinhubl SR, Berger PB, Malinin AI, Bhatt DL, Topol EJ. Variability in platelet responsiveness to clopidogrel among 544 individuals. *J Am Coll Cardiol* 2005; 45: 246-251

Shimokawa H, Hiramori K, Iinuma H, Hosoda S, Kishida H, Osada H, Katagiri T, Yamauchi K, Yui Y, Minamino T, Nakashima M, Kato K. Anti-anginal effect of fasudil, a Rho-kinase inhibitor, in patients with stable effort anginaa multicenter study. *J Cardiovasc Pharmacol* 2002; 40:751-761

Siddiqui M A, Keam S J. Ranolazine: a review of its use in chronic stable angina pectoris. *Drugs* 2006; 66: 693–710

Sierra C, Coca A.The ACTION study: nifedipine in patients with symptomatic stable angina and hypertension. *Expert Rev Cardiovasc Ther* 2008; 6:1055–1062

Simoons ML; GUSTO IV-ACS Investigators. Effect of glyco-protein IIb/IIIa receptor blocker abciximab on outcome in patients with acute coronary syndromes without early coronary revascularisation: the GUSTO IV-ACS randomised trial. *Lance*t 2001;357(9272):1915-1924

Simpson D, Wellington K. Nicorandil: a review of its use in the management of stable angina pectoris, including high-risk patients. *Drugs* 2004; 64:1941–1955

Sinclair HM. The diet of Canadian Indians and Eskimos. *Proc Nutr Soc* 1953; 12:69–82

Singh RB, Niaz MA, Agarwal P, Beegum R, Rastogi SS, Sachan DS. A randomized, double-blind, placebo-controlled trial of L-carnitine in suspected myocardial infarction. *Postgrad Med J* 1996; 72:45–50

Sodi-Pallares D, Bisteni A, Medrano GA, Testelli MR, DeMicheli A. The polarizing treatment of acute myocardial infarction. *Dis Chest* 1963; 43:424–432

Sodi-Pallares D, Testelli MR, Fishleder BL, Bisteni A, Medrano GA, Friedland C, DeMicheli A. Effects of an intravenous infusion of a potassium-glucose-insulin solution on the electrocardiographic signs of myocardial infarction. *Am J Cardiol* 1962; 9: 166–181

Stacpoole PW, Henderson GN, Yan Z, Cornett R, James MO. Pharmacokinetics, metabolism and toxicology of dichloroacetate. *Drug Metab Rev* 1998; 30:499–539

Stewart S, Voss DW, Northey DL, Horowitz JD. Relationship between plasma perhexiline concentration and symptomatic status during short-term perhexiline therapy. *Ther Drug Monit* 1996; 18:635–639

Stone GW, McLaurin BT, Cox DA, Bertrand ME, Lincoff AM, Moses JW, White HD, Pocock SJ, Ware JH, Feit F, Colombo A, Aylward PE, Cequier AR, Darius H, Desmet W, Ebrahimi R, Hamon M, Rasmussen LH, Rupprecht HJ, Hoekstra J, Mehran R, Ohman EM; ACUITY Investigators. Bivalirudin for patients with acute coronary syndromes: the ACUITY trial. *N Engl J Med* 2006; 355: 2203-2216

Sugiyama S, Kitazawa M, Ozawa T, Suzuki K, Izawa Y. Anti-oxidative effect of coenzyme Q10. *Experentia* 1980; 36:1002–1003

Svedstrom U, Vuorela H, Kostiainen R, Huovinen K, Laakso I, Hiltunen R. High-performance liquid chromatographic determination of oligomeric procyanidins from dimers up to the hexamer in hawthorn. *J Chromatogr A* 2002; 968:53–60

Swahn E, Wallentin L. Low-molecular-weight heparin (Fragmin) during instability in coronary artery disease (FRISC). FRISC Study Group. *Am J Cardiol* 1997; 80(5A): 25E-29E

Swaminath G. Probing the β_2-adrenoceptor binding site with catechol reveals differences in binding and activation by agonists and partial agonists. *J Biol Chem* 2005; 280:22165–22171

Swaminathan JK, Khan M, Mohan IK, Selvendiran K, Devaraj SN, Rivera BK, Kuppusamy P. Cardioprotective properties of Crataegus oxycantha extract against ischemia-reperfusion injury. *Phytomedicine* 2010; 17:744-752

Taddei S, Virdis A, Ghiadoni L, Magagna A, Salvetti A. Vitamin C improves endothelium-dependent vasodilation by restoring nitric oxide activity in essential hypertension. *Circulation* 1998; 97: 2222–2229

Tankanow R, Tamer HR, Streetman DS, Smith SG, Welton JL, Annesley T, Aaronson KD, Bleske BE. Interaction study between digoxin and a preparation of hawthorn (Crataegus oxyacantha) *J Clin Pharmacol* 2003; 43: 637–642

Tardif JC, Ford I, Tendera M, Bourassa MG, Fox K., INITIATIVE Investigators Efficacy of ivabradine, a new selective I(f) inhibitor, compared with atenolol in patients with chronic stable angina. *Eur Heart J* 2005; 26:2529–2536

Tesoriere L, Butera D, Pintaudi M, Allegra M, Livrea MA. Supplementation with cactus pear (Opuntia ficus-indica) fruit decreases oxidative stress in healthy humans: a comparative study with Vit C. *Am J Clin Nutr* 2004; 80:391–395

Thadani U, Rodgers T. Side effects of using nitrates to treat angina. *Expert Opin Drug Saf* 2006; 5:667–674

The EURopean trial On reduction of cardiac events with Perindopril in stable coronary Artery disease Investigators Efficacy of perindopril in reduction of cardiovascular events among patients with stable coronary artery disease: randomised, double-blind, placebo-controlled, multicentre trial (the EUROPA study) *Lancet* 2003;362:782-788

The IONA Study Group. Trial to show the impact of nicorandil in angina (IONA): design, methodology, and management. *Heart.*2001; 85:e9

Theroux P, Ouimet H, McCans J, Latour JG, Joly P, Levy G, Pelletier E, Juneau M, Stasiak J, deGuise P. Aspirin, heparin, or both to treat acute unstable angina. *N Engl J Med* 1988; 319:1105-1111

Thollon C, Cambarrat C, Vian J, Prost J-F, Peglion JL, Vilaine JP. Electrophysiological effects of S 16257 a novel sino-atrial node modulator, on rabbit and guinea-pig cardiac preparations: comparison with UL-FS 49. *Br J Pharmacol* 1994; 112: 37–42

Tune JD, Gorman MW, Feigl EO. Matching coronary blood flow to myocardial oxygen consumption. *J Appl Physiol* 2004; 97:404–415

Tyrrell H. Ischemic heat disease and wine or garlic. *Lancet* 1979; 1: 1294

Urban P, Macaya C, Rupprecht HJ, Kiemeneij F, Emanuelsson H, Fontanelli A, Pieper M, Wesseling T, Sagnard L. Randomized evaluation of anticoagulation versus antiplatelet therapy after coronary stent implantation in high-risk patients: the multicenter aspirin and ticlopidine trial after intracoronary stenting (MATTIS). *Circulation* 1998; 98:2126-2132

Use of a monoclonal antibody directed against the platelet glycoprotein IIb/IIIa receptor in high-risk coronary angioplasty. The EPIC Investigation. *N Engl J Med* 1994; 330:956-956

Walker AF, Marakis G, Morris AP, Robinson PA. Promising hypotensive effect of hawthorn extract: a randomized double-blind pilot study of mild, essential hypertension. *Phytother Res* 2002; 16:48–54

Wang C, Harris WS, Chung M, Lichtenstein AH, Balk EM, Kupelnick B, Jordan HS, Lau J. n-3 fatty acids from fish or fish-oil supplements, but not alpha-linoleic acid, benefit cardiovascular disease outcomes in primary- and secondary-prevention studies: a systematic review. *Am J Clin Nutr* 2006; 84: 5-17

Wang PZ. Chinese Medicine Surgery. Ancient Chinese Medicine Press; 1988. pp. 164–183

Weerakkody GJ, Jakubowski JA, Brandt JT, et al (a) Comparison of speed of onset of platelet inhibition after loading doses of clopidogrel versus prasugrel in healthy volunteers and correlation with responder status. *Am J Cardiol* 2007; 100: 331–336

Weerakkody GJ, Jakubowski JA, Brandt JT, Payne CD, Naganuma H, Winters KJ (b). Greater inhibition of platelet aggregation and reduced response variability with prasugrel versus clopidogrel: an integrated analysis. *J Cardiovasr Pharmacol Ther* 2007; 12:205-212

Weihmayr T, Ernst E. Therapeutic effectiveness of Crataegus. *Fortschr Med* 1996; 114:27–29

Weitz JI. Low-molecular-weight heparins. *N Engl J Med* 1997; 337:688-698

Wisneski JA, Stanley WC, Neese RA, Gertz EW. Effects of acute hyperglycemia on myocardial glycolytic activity in humans. *J Clin Invest* 1990; 85:1648–1656

Wiviott SD, Braunwald E, McCabe CH, Horvath I, Keltai M, Herrman JP, Van de Werf F, Downey WE, Scirica BM, Murphy SA, Antman EM; TRITON-TIMI 38 Investigators. Intensive oral antiplatelet therapy for reduction of ischaemic events including stent thrombosis in patients with acute coronary syndromes treated with percu-taneous coronary intervention and stenting in the TRITON-TIMI 38 trial: a subanalysis of a randomised trial. *Lancet* 2008; 371(9621):1353-1563.

Wiviott SD, Braunwald E, McCabe CH, Montalescot G, Ruzyllo W, Gottlieb S, Neumann FJ, Ardissino D, De Servi S, Murphy SA, Riesmeyer J, Weerakkody G, Gibson CM, Antman EM; TRITON-TIMI 38 Investigators. Prasugrel versus clopidogrel in patients with acute coronary syndromes. *N Engl J Med* 2007; 357:2001-2015.

Yallampalli C, Garfield RE, Byam-Smith M. Nitric oxide inhibits uterine contractility during pregnancy but not during delivery. *Endocrinology* 1993; 133: 1899–1902

Yamagami T, Shibata N. Bioenergetics in clinical medicine: studies on coenzyme Q10 and essential hypertension. *Res Commun Chem Pathol Pharmacol* 1975; 11:273–88

Yasuda T, Hashimura K, Matsu-ura Y, Kato Y, Ueda T, Mori I, Kijima Y. Nicorandil, a hybrid between nitrate and ATP-sensitive potassium channel opener, preconditions human heart to ischemia during percutaneous transluminal coronary angioplasty. *Jpn Circ J* 2001; 65:526–530

Yusuf S, Mehta SR, Xie C, Ahmed RJ, Xavier D, Pais P, Zhu J, Liu L. Effects of reviparin, a low-molecular-weight heparin, on mortality, reinfarction, and strokes in patients with acute myocardial infarction presenting with ST-segment elevation. *JAMA* 2005; 293: 427-435

Zaza A, Rocchetti M. Regulation of the sinoatrial pacemaker: selective If inhibition by ivabradine. In: Fox K, Ferrari R, editors. *Heart rate management in stable angina.* Abingdon: Taylor & Francis; 2005. pp. 51–67

Žiberna l, Lunder M, Može Š, Vanzo A, Drevenšek G. Cardioprotective effects of bilberry extract on ischemia-reperfusion-induced injury in isolated rat heart. *BMC Pharmacol* 2009; 9(Suppl 2): A55

10

Coronary Arterial Drug-Eluting Stent: From Structure to Clinical

Tim Wu and Stephen McCarthy
Biomedical Engineering and Biotechnology,
University of Massachusetts Lowell, MA,
USA

1. Introduction

1.1 Cardiovascular diseases and Percutaneous Coronary Intervention (PCI)

Coronary Artery Disease (CAD) is the chronic blocking or narrowing of the coronary arteries caused by neointimal hyperplasia of the arterial wall. It has been the number one killer in the United States since 1900 and remains a common cause of death in the Western world despite therapeutic advances. Approximately 14 million Americans have CAD, 500,000 people die from acute myocardial infarction, and one million more survive but with a 1.5 to 15 times greater risk of mortality or morbidity than the rest of the population each year. The annual health care cost of the disease is in excess of $112 billion [1]. The current levels of predictors of heart disease risk, such as obesity, diabetes, and smoking, suggests that this will continue to be a significant public health problem for the foreseeable future [2].

The options for CAD treatments include medications, percutaneous coronary arterial interventions (PCI, including angioplasty and stenting), or coronary artery bypass graft surgery (CABG). In general, patients with coronary narrowing that does not limit coronary artery blood flow receive medications and lifestyle modification to help prevent progression. If a patient has coronary atherosclerosis that limits blood flow in the coronary arteries, balloon angioplasty and stenting can be offered. In patients with multiple areas of coronary artery narrowing or blockage, CABG is generally recommended.

1.1.1 Coronary Artery Bypass Graft Surgery (CABG)

Of those patients with coronary artery disease, about 10% undergo CABG surgery. Patients with severe narrowing or blockage of the left main coronary artery or those with disease involving two or three coronary arteries are generally considered for bypass surgery. In a CABG, the surgeon uses a portion of a healthy vessel (either an artery or vein) from the leg, chest, or arm to create a detour or bypass around the blocked portion of the coronary artery. Depending on how many coronary arteries (and main branches) are blocked, patients typically receive 1 to 5 bypasses. The most commonly used bypass vessels are the saphenous vein from the leg, the internal mammary artery from the chest, and the radial artery from the arm. During a CABG, a heart-lung machine artificially maintains circulation while the surgeon operates on the heart. CABG operations require general anesthesia and typically 4 to 7 days in the hospital. It may take up to 3 months to fully recover from the surgery.

1.1.2 Percutaneous Interventions (PCIs)

Percutaneous Interventions (PCIs), which include percutaneous transluminal coronary artery angioplasty (PTCA) and coronary artery stenting (CAS) are the major therapies for CAD treatment. PTCA involves insertion of an expandable balloon catheter against a primary atherosclerotic plaque or secondary restenotic lesion to increase vessel patency and blood flow. Clinical stenting was introduced in 1986 with the Wallstent to repair abrupt closure after PTCA and has revolutionized interventional cardiology [3]. In CAS, the stent (a tiny metal scaffolding) functions to brace the vessel wall and reduce the risk of restenosis following angioplasty. CAS reduces the rate of angiographic and clinical restenosis compared to PTCA alone. This results in a significant reduction in the frequency of major adverse cardiac events (MACE) after PCI driven mainly by a reduction in target vessel revascularization (TVR). CAS not only increases procedural success rates, but also increases the safety of procedures by decreasing the need for emergency CABG surgery. As a result, stents are currently utilized in over 85% of the two million PCIs in US and the total direct cost for those life-saving procedures is over $5 billion annually.

1.2 Problems in current DESs

Since the introduction of the stent, there exist two serious complications: namely, thrombosis (subacute and late-stage) and in-stent restenosis (ISR). While subacute thrombosis has been controlled with the use of dual anti-platelet therapy, late-stage thrombosis occurring in drug-eluting stents (DESs) has been a big concern recently. Restenosis remains among the most challenging problems in interventional cardiology. The recent development of DESs is a major breakthrough as a potential solution for the restenosis problem.

1.2.1 In-stent Restenosis (ISR)

Restenosis, the re-narrowing of an opened artery after stenting or PTCA procedure, is due to a proliferative response of the intima, a layer of cells that lines the lumen of the vessel composed of connective tissue and smooth muscle cells (SMC). In restenosis, vascular neointimal hyperplasia results in complete blockage of the original artery and insufficient oxygenation of cardiac tissue, leading to cardiac arrhythmia or cardiac arrest. Restenosis has been the biggest problem in PCI until the recent successful development of DESs. Initially, the restenosis rate in PTCA procedures was over 50% within six months post balloon dilation. Stenting lowers this rate to 20-30%. Both Sirolimus (Cypher®, Cordis Inc, Fla) and Paclitaxel (Taxus®, Boston Scientific Inc, Natick, MA) coated DESs can significantly reduce the rate of restenosis to <10%[4-6]. However, restenosis in patients with high risk such as small vessels, diabetes, and long diffusion diseased arteries still remains unacceptably high (30%-60% in bare metal stents [BMSs] and 6%-18% in DESs)[7-9] despite DES implantation.

ISR formation is a multi-factorial, sequential process. Although the detailed mechanism of the arterial tissue response to an implanted stent is still under investigation, it is generally believed that three stages are involved in the process. 1) Thrombotic Phase (day 0-3): this phase is the initial response of the artery tissue to stent implantation characterized with rapid activation, adhesion, aggregation and deposition of platelets and neutrophils to form a thrombus at the injured site. 2) Recruitment Phase: this phase occurs between days 3 to 8 and is characterized by an intensive inflammatory cell infiltration. In this phase, inflammatory cells are activated and infiltrate into the injured vessel wall. Subsequently, the recruited inflammation cells provide the key stimulus for subsequent smooth muscle cell (SMC) proliferation and migration. 3) Proliferate Phase: This phase lasts 1 to 3 months depending on the thickness of the residual thrombus and the rate of growth. At this stage, inflammation cells colonize the residual thrombus, forming a "cap" across the mural thrombus. The cells progressively proliferate, resorbing residual thrombus until all thrombus is gone and is replaced by the neointima tissue [10-12].

The process of neointimal growth, which consists of SMCs, extracellular matrix, and macrophages recruited over a period of several weeks, is similar to the process of tumor tissue growth [13]. This pathologic similarity between tumor cell growth and benign neointimal formation has led to the discovery of anti-tumor drugs such as Paclitaxel as effective agents for the treatment of ISR [12, 13].

1.2.2 Stent thrombosis

In spite of restenosis remaining a clinical problem in approximately 10% of patients with DES implantation, it can often be successfully treated with repeat implantation. The greatest concern, however, has been for stent thrombosis which is associated with a high rate of myocardial infarction and death. The rate of early stent thrombosis (less than 30 days following implantation) appears similar in both BMSs and DESs (Cypher® and Taxus®) [14]. However, late stent thrombosis has been increasingly reported beyond 12 months following DES implantation with the greatest risk occurring as a result of premature discontinuation of anti-platelet therapy [15-19]. Although the precise mechanism of late stage stent thrombosis is unknown, it is generally believed that the combination of delayed endothelialization due to anti-proliferative therapy and persistence of the nonerodable polymer contribute to a hypersensitivity reaction, possibly with some residual active drug that may not be eluted [20, 21].

2. The structure and components of a drug eluting stent

Drug eluting stents are comprised of three major parts: 1) drug delivery platform (metal stent) to hold the drug and provide supporting forces for the collapsed artery; 2) drug coating polymer to attach the drug on the stent surface; 3) anti restenosis drugs released from the stent to inhibit restenosis formation after stent implantation. We review each component systemically in order to have an anatomic understanding of drug eluting stent.

2.1 Stent platforms

2.1.1 Stent materials

2.1.1.1 Non degradable material

316L stainless steel: 316L stainless steel (316L SS) is the most commonly used metal material in stents due to its excellent mechanical properties and corrosion resistance and is used in the first generation DESs, Cypher (sirolimus-eluting stent, Cordis, Warren, NJ) and Taxus (paclitaxel-eluting stent, Boston Scientific, Natick, MA). However, its ferromagnetic nature and low density make it a non-MRI compatible and poorly visible fluoroscopic material. Furthermore, the release of nickel, chromate and molybdenum ions is likely to provoke immune reactions and inflammatory responses, which may result in ISR[22]. Therefore, a number of materials have been used as coatings to improve its visibility and biocompatibility.

Co-Cr: Co-Cr alloy exhibits superior radial strength and improved radiopacity compared to 316L SS. It allows for thinner stent struts, which is a significant advantage because the thickness of stent struts is a important factor on the reduction of restenosis in BMSs[23, 24]. At the same time, it reduces device profile and consequently improves its deliverability to the target lesion. Co-Cr platforms are employed in the second generation DES, Xience V (everolimus-eluting stent, Abott Vascular, CA) and Endeavor (zotarolimus-eluting stent, Medtronic Vascular, Santa Rosa, CA).

Ta: The highly stable surface oxide layer, preventing electron exchange between the metal and the absorbed biological species[25, 26], make Ta an excellent corrosion resistant material. Ta has been coated on 316L SS to improve corrosion properties and biocompatibility of 316L SS[27]. Its high density and non-ferromagnetic properties[28,29] make Ta an excellent fluoroscopically visible and MRI compatible material. However, its poor mechanical properties make Ta stents have higher rates of recoil compared to 316L SS based stents and result in enhanced neointimal formation[30]. Although no Ta based stents have been approved by FDA for general use to date, a bare Ta stent has been used by Cordis® (Johnson & Johnson, USA) in clinical trials and released commercially in Japan, Canada and Europe[31].

Ti: Although Ti has excellent biocompatibility and corrosion resistance, pure Ti is not commonly used for making stents due to its low tensile strength and ductility. However, Ti alloys might be optimum for stents. Ti-nitride-oxide coating on 316L SS was biologically inert, reducing platelet and fibrinogen deposition, and neointimal hyperplasia[32]. Promising results were reported in clinical trials by the Titan stent (Hexacath, France) using this coating[33,34]. Moreover, Ti-based Ta and niobium alloys showed excellent haemocompatibility[35], indicating they have potential applications for stents. An extensively used Ti alloys in stents is Ni-Ti.

Ni-Ti: Ni-Ti alloy is also a common material for stents which has good biocompatibility, radial force and shape memory. However, the release of nickel ions and their toxic effects on tissues have been reported[36, 37]. In addition, it is suspected of producing mild inflammation when contacting monocytes[38]. In order to solve these problems, the surface of Ni-Ti is passivated to increase the Ti oxide concentration and decrease the Ni concentration[39, 40], and it is coated by some materials such as polyurethane[41], Ti nitride[42] and polycrystalline oxides[43] to improve the corrosion resistance. Another problem is that the Ni-Ti alloy does not have adequate visibility under fluoroscopy[44] though it can be visualized by MRI[45]. Ni-Ti is used by ACT-One™ (Progressive Angioplasty Systems, USA)[46], Paragon (Progressive Angioplasty Systems, USA)[47], and Radius (Scimed, USA)[48] in clinical trials.

Pt-Ir: The bare stents made from Pt-Ir alloy of 90% platinum and 10% iridium have been implanted in animal models, showing excellent radiopacity and a reduction in both thrombosis and neointimal proliferation with less inflammatory reactions. However, their recoiling percentage was much higher (16%) than the 316L SS stents (5%)[49, 50]. Though Pt-Ir alloy stents have been proved safe and effective in a human clinical trial[51], the biocompatibility and haemocompatibility of Pt-Ir alloys needs be further investigated.

2.1.1.2 Biodegradable metallic materials

Besides the aforementioned non-degradable metallic stents, a new concept is biodegradable metallic stent. The recently used biodegradable metallic materials are pure Fe[52] and Mg alloys[53].

Pure Fe: The degradation of Fe was completed through the oxidation of Fe into ferrous and ferric irons which were dissolved into biological media[54]. It is reported that ferrous ions could reduce the proliferation rate of vascular smooth muscle cell *in vitro* by influencing growth-related gene expression and therefore may antagonize restenosis *in vivo*[54]. The pure Fe (more than 99.5%) stents with strut thickness varied from 100 to 120μm have been implanted successfully in rabbit and porcine and endothelialization was observed[52, 55]. However, further investigation is needed on the modification of the composition and design of the stent to expedite the degradation process[55].

Mg alloys: Mg and its alloys has been used as orthopedic materials[56], but it is a new principle to apply these materials to coronary stents[53]. Unlike pure Fe, pure Mg is not suitable for making stents due to mechanical and corrosion properties. There are two Mg alloys, AE21[53] and WE43[57], used for making stents. These materials are radiolucent and thus cannot be imaged by X-rays. However, they can be visualized by intravascular ultrasound and MRI[58]. The Lekton Magic stent (Biotronik, Switzerland) is made from WE43, which is safe and can provide sufficient support to the collapsed arteries within its degradation time (2-3 months)[59,60]. It has been implanted in porcine models, and the preliminary clinical data showed promising results that after one-month implantation of magic stents, 18 out of 20 patients had normal flow while 30%-40% restenosis occurred in the other 2 patients[57]. However, mixed results were found in a human study using a Biotronik's Mg absorbable metal stents[61,62], indicating further evaluation is needed.

2.1.2 Stent geometric design

Self-expanding vs. balloon-expandable: Basically, there are two stent types: the self-expanding and the balloon-expandable stents. The self-expanding stent is made of a coil, mesh or zigzag configuration that is constrained with an outer sheath. The stent elastically springs open to a predetermine size after the sheath is removed. The balloon-expandable stent is crimped and premounted on a balloon, and expanded by the inflation of the balloon whose diameter determines the size of expanded stent. Though the self-expanding stent will expand to a calculated size automatically, it is not recommended and seldom used at present because it continues to expand in the weeks after deployment and thus leads to the stent migration to the adventia and the stent cross-sectional area increasing accompanied by medial compression[63, 64].

Coil vs. Tube: Generally, the balloon-expandable stent is classified into two groups: the tube and the coil design. The tubular stent is cut from a steel tube or a flat sheet of metal which is then rolled and welded to form a tube. The coil design is composed of a continuously wound wire or a series of flat sheet coils, which has a greater strut width with gaps and fewer or no connections between struts compared with the tubular stent[65]. These characteristics make coil stents more flexible but have poor radial strength and the wide gap allows tissue prolapse[66]. As a result, coil design is being replaced by the tube design gradually.

Slotted tube vs. Modular: Tubular balloon-expandable stents also can be divided into two types: slotted tube and modular design. Both of them are cut from a tube of metal. A clinical study showed slotted tube stents resisted restenosis more than the modular stents (22.1% vs 25.2%)[67]. The slotted tube stent also has two kinds: one is closed cell design, and the other one is open cell design. The former one is loser to the original concept of slotted tubes, while the latter is more like the modular stent. In a clinical study, less platelet activation was found in the implantation of closed cell stents than the open cell stents, which may have resulted from a greater degree of tissue prolapsed with the open cell stents[68].

Long vs. Short: It has been proven that stent length is associated with restenosis rate and clinical events (mainly target lesion revascularization): 20 mm length stent resulted in 22.6% angiographic restenosis rate; 27 mm length stent led to 36% angiographic restenosis rate; and 43 mm length stent produced 67.5% angiographic restenosis rate[69]. Similar results were found in another clinical study that showed the angiographic restenosis rates were 20.8% and 37.3%, respectively, in the implantation of 16 mm and ≥ 32 mm BMSs, and the angiographic restenosis rates were 7.2% and 10.3% for the implantation of the same length of DESs[70]. Therefore, stent length is still a problem in DESs. On the one hand, the DESs can reduce restesnosis in both long and short lesions compared with BMSs, but a long stent is expected to cover all the diseased area. On the other hand, a long DES may increase the occurrence of restenosis.

Wide vs. Narrow: As with stent length, the stent width is another problem in both BMSs and DESs. The same study mentioned above showed the angiographic rates were 40.8% in the 2.5 mm diameter vs. 12.9% in the 3.5 mm diameter BMSs, and 8.8% vs. 5.5% in the same diameter DESs[70]. Although the study suggested that the wide diameter stent is more favorable than the narrow one, the width is still a problem which has not been eliminated by DESs.

More struts vs. less: An animal study, of stainless steel stents with different configurations implanted in rabbit iliac arteries, indicated that the stents with 12 struts per cross section had 50% to 60% less mural thrombus and 2-fold less neointimal area than those of identical stents with only 8 struts per cross section[71]. However, another animal study showed the neointimal growth is not related to the number of struts, but associated with the stretching of arteries and the injury depth caused by the implantation of stents[72]. Therefore, further research is needed to evaluate the impact of the number of struts in a stent on thrombosis and restenosis.

Thick vs. thin struts: As discussed above, the injury depth and the stretching of the coronary arteries have a great impact upon neointimal growth[72], and the two parameters are vary inversely with the thickness of the stent struts. Thinner struts slice into tissue more easily and hence induce more deep injury to the coronary arteries, but unlike thicker struts, they cause less angulations and stretching of the arterial wall. The effect of strut thickness on restenosis incidence was evaluated in both ISAR-STEREO and ISAR-STEREO 2 trials[23, 24]. In the ISAR-STEREO trial, 326 patients were implanted with thin-strut stents (strut thickness is 50 μm) while in the other 325 patients were assigned to receive thick-strut stents (strut thickness is 140 μm) randomly. The results showed the incidence of angiographic restenosis was 15.0% in the thin-strut group vs. 25.8% in the thick-strut group (P=0.003), clinical restenosis was also significantly reduced, with a reintervention rate of 8.6% among thin-strut patients vs 13.8% among thick-strut patients (relative risk, 0.62; 95% CI, 0.39 to 0.99; P=0.03), and no difference was observed in the combined 1-year rate of death and myocardial infarction (MI)[23]. In the ISAR-STEREO 2 trial, a total of 611 patients with symptomatic coronary artery disease were randomly assigned to receive two different kind of stents in both design and strut thickness: the thin-strut ACS RX Multilink stent with interconnected ring design (Guidant, Advanced Cardiovascular Systems, Santa Clara, California) (strut thickness 50μm) were implanted into 309 patients while the thick-strut BX Velocity stent with closed cell design (Cordis Corp., Miami, Florida) (strut thickness 140μm) were implanted into 302 patients. The results showed the incidence of angiographic restenosis was 17.9% in the thin-strut group vs. 31.4% in the thick-strut group ($p < 0.001$), a target-vessel revascularization (TVR) due to restenosis was required in 12.3% of the thin-strut group vs. 21.9% of the thick-strut group ($p = 0.002$), and no significant difference was observed in the combined incidence of death and MI at one year[24]. Therefore, the stents with thinner struts is preferred for the design of new stents as they can reduce angiographic and clinical restenosis more than those with thicker struts.

Square vs. round strut cross-section: Another note worthy stent geometry is the shape of the strut cross-section. An *in vitro* study showed the migration distance of human aortic endothelial cells along the surface of the flat pieces of 316L stainless steel with the sharpest edge angles of the bottom surfaces (35°) was significantly greater than with larger angles (70°, 90°, and 140°, $P < 0.05$) under static and flow conditions, indicating the edge angle of stent struts does influence the rate of endothelialization. The stents with smaller edge angles and slopes facilitate endothelialization as compared with the larger angles[73]. In addition, when compared to those with smaller edge angles, the stents with larger angels have sharper edges in the direction of blood flow, which may interfere with blood by slicing the blood cells. Therefore, the square strut cross-section is not recommended and the round strut cross-section without corners or sharp edges is popular at present.

Rough vs. smooth surface: The stent surface topography is thought to play an important role in stent performance. Though some studies showed a smooth, polished surface reduced thrombus adhesion and neointimal growth[74], it does not mean extremely smooth surfaces are optimal for re-endothelialization. Recently, an *in vitro* study suggested that a stent surface with a microscopic pattern of parallel grooves disposed in the direction of blood flow leads to a faster re-endothelialization process than the stent with smooth surface[75]. In addition, in a recent animal study, a similar result was observed a stent with a microscopic parallel grooves accelerated the endothelialization rate significantly 1 week after implantation in porcine carotid arteries compared to smooth stents[76, 77]. In order to determine the relationship between the stent surface topography and outcome in patients undergoing implantation of stents with rough and smooth surfaces, a clinical trial of 200 patients with significant stenosis in native coronary vessels were randomly assigned in a double-blind study to receive either a rough or a smooth-surface stent. The study indicated rough stent surface does not increase late lumen loss after stent implantation as compared with a conventional smooth stent surface, and the angiographic restenosis rates were 25% with rough-surface stents vs 35% with smooth surface stents (P=0.19)[78]. Therefore, a relatively rough surface is better for stent performance than a smooth one.

Symmetry of Deployment: Previous studies suggested that the degree of restenosis is related to the symmetry of stent expansion and increased neointimal thickening was found in the unevenly deployed stents[71, 79]. In the presence of calcified lesions, the stents usually were expanded asymmetrically[80, 81]. It is believed that the symmetry of stent deployment might be influenced by the balloon folding patterns[82]. Currently, trefoil or tetrafoil folding is common, which prevents excessive expansion of one side of the stent[83].

2.2 Drug delivery vehicles – Coating polymer

Polymers are large molecule compounds consisting of repeating structural units typically connected by covalent chemical bonds, which can be broadly classified into nonbiodegradable and biodegradable polymers when used as drug carriers in DESs.

2.2.1 Non biodegradable polymers

Both the first and the second generation of DESs are using nonbiodegradable polymers to control the drug-elution profile. In the first generation of DES, Cypher (sirolimus-eluting stent, Cordis, Warren, NJ) used polyethylene-co-vinyl acetate (PEVA)/poly-n-butyl methacrylate (PBMA) to delivery sirolimus, while Taxus (paclitaxel-eluting stent, Boston Scientific, Natick, MA) used polystyrene-b-isobutylene-b-styrene (SIBS) to delivery paclitaxel. Both stents can reduce restenosis significantly compared to BMSs[70,84-86], however, an increase in the rate of MI and mortality was reported in patients following 18 months to 3 years after the implantation of Cypher or Taxus[87-90]. In the second generation of DES, Xience V (everolimus-eluting stent, Abott Vascular, CA) employed a fluoropolymer to carry everolimus, while Endeavor (zotarolimus-eluting stent, Medtronic Vascular, Santa Rosa, CA) employed phosphorylcholine (PC) to carry zotarolimus. Compared with the respective BMS, the target vessel revascularization (TVR) was reduced significantly by both Endeavor and Xience V stents[91,92]. Xience V stents reduced angiographic late loss without an increase of stent thrombosis compared with Taxus stents in the SPIRIT III study[93], whereas Endeavor stents showed a higher incidence of restenosis compared with Cypher stents in the ENDEAVOR III trial[94]. However, both Endeavor and Taxus stents had an equivalent target lesion revascularization rate in a later trial[95]. In addition, there were no cases of very late stent thrombosis in earlier ENDEAVOR trials over 4 years indicating Endeavor stents are safe in the long-term[96].

2.2.2 Biodegradable polymers

As nonbiodegradable polymers may lead to inflammatory response[97], the biodegradable polymers applied for stent coatings to delivery drugs are being investigated. The most commonly used polymers now are polylactic acid (PLA), polyglycolic acid (PGA) and their copolymer, polylactic-co-glycolic acid (PLGA)[98, 99], which are fully metabolized to water and carbon dioxide and excreted via the respiratory system. Despite a series of promising preliminary data that was reported[100-103], the development of biodegradable polymers in DES is still challenging. On the one hand, the degradation of polymers are affected by a variety of factors[104] such as the pH, the polymer's size, molecular weight and crystallinity, etc, making the drug release control difficult. On the other hand, the accumulated acidic products from polymer degradation may result in significant inflammatory response of the vessel wall and therefore lead to restenosis.

2.2.3 Other materials and methods

Other stents that do not use a polymer at all are still under development. For example, a titanium–nitric oxide alloy has been applied to stainless steel stents with encouraging results, including decreased platelet adhesion and neointimal hyperplasia compared with BMS[34]. A microporous stainless steel stent (Yukon, Translumina, Germany) allows for dose-adjustable, multiple drugs, and on-site coating[105] [63]. The system is therapeutically effective with rapamycin[106]. A nanoporous hydroxyapetite (a biocompatible crystalline derivative of calcium phosphate) coating, which can be impregnated with anti-restenotic drugs, is currently under development[107]. A stainless steel stent coated with nanoporous aluminium oxide and tacrolimus showed disappointing results, however, with evidence of particle debris shed from the coating contributing to increased neointimal hyperplasia[108]. An interesting drug delivery system developed recently is composed of magnetic nanoparticles (MNPs) loaded with endothelial cells and a 304 grade stainless steel[109]. The endothelial cells were loaded on polylactide modified MNPs and then moved by a magnetic field gradient towards the stent surface after injection, which enabled artificial endothelialization and repeated dosing, showing promising future. However, further evaluation in animal studies and clinical trials is required.

2.3 Therapeutic agents

2.3.1 Sirolimus and its analogues

Sirolimus: Sirolimus (rapamycin), a macrocyclic lactone used in the Cypher stents, binds to FK-binding protein 12 and subsequently inhibits the mammalian target of rapamycin (mTOR). The mTOR prevents the degradation of p27kip1, a cyclin-dependgdent kinase inhibitor, thereby inhibits the migration and proliferation of SMCs[110, 111]. However, the mTOR is also a downstream target of the phosphatidylinositol-3 kinase pathway, which inhibits the tissue factor in endothelial cells and monocytes[112-114]. Therefore, the inhibition of mTOR by sirolimus leads to increasing expression and activity of tissue factor in endothelial cells[112].

Zotarolimus: The former name of zotarolimus is ABT-578, which is one of the sirolimus analogues developed by Abbott laboratories. The extremely lipophilic property and low water solubility[115] make zotarolimus a better candidate for DES than sirolimus. It has been employed in Medtronic's Endeavor stents which was approved by FDA in 2008 and showed better endothelialization than Cypher at 14 days post implantation[116]. It is also used in Zomaxx stents developed by Abbott laboratories[117].

Everolimus: Everolimus is another sirolimus analogue, which is also used as an immunosuppressive agent [118]. As with sirolimus, it inhibits smooth muscle cell proliferation and in-stent neointimal growth[119, 120]. However, compared to sirolimus, everolimus has a better pharmacokinetic profile and bioavailability when used in organ transplant[121]. When it is used in intracoronary elution, everolimus absorbs to local tissue more rapidly and has a longer celluar residence time and activity[122]. It has been used in another FDA approved stent, Xience V, which also showed better endothelialization than Cypher at 14 days post implantation of stents[116].

Biolimus A9: Biolimus A9 has similar immunosuppressive potency to sirolimus, but it is absorbed by vessel walls more readily and enters cells more rapidly[123, 124]. It has been investigated in two PLA coated stainless steel stents, Biomatrix (Biosensors International, Singapore) and Nobori (Terumo, Japan) [124-126]. The biolimus-eluting stent has been proven to be safe and effective in reducing neointimal proliferation when compared to BMSs and Taxus in the Nobori 1 trial[126].

2.3.2 Paclitaxel and its analogues

Paclitaxel: Paclitaxel, a lipophilic diterpenoid, binds to β-subunit of the tubulin heterodimer, promoting tubulin polymerization and cell cycle arrest, thus inhibiting the migration and proliferation of SMCs[127, 128]. Notwithstanding, an important regulator of endothelial and monocytic tissue factor induction[113, 114], c-Jun NH2-terminal kinase, is also activated by paclitaxel[129, 130], and, consequently, enhances the activity of tissue factor in endothelial cells [130].

Coroxane: To improve the solubility of paclitaxel and reduce non-drug-related toxicties[131], a protein-engineered nanoparticle albumin bound paclitaxel (nab-paclitaxel) named Coroxane was developed by Abraxis Bioscience Inc.. The phase 1 study has been conducted showing 10-30 mg/m^2 doses of the drug are safe for humans[132]. The phase II study is ongoing.

Docetaxel: Docetaxel is a semi-synthetic analogue of paclitaxel used for the treatment of ovarian, breast and non-small cell lung cancer[133]. Compared to paclitaxel, docetaxel has better anti-proliferative properties[134], however, it has dose-dependent cytotoxicity[135].

2.3.3 Others

Tacrolimus: Tacrolimus (FK-506 or Fujimycin or Prograf), a hydrophobic macrolide immunosuppressant drug, is a T cell inhibitor resulting in cell apoptosis by holding cells in the G0 phase of the cell cycle and has a different mechanism from that of sirolimus[136, 137]. Moreover, unlike the mTOR inhibitors and paclitaxel, tacrolimus does not increase expression of tissue factor since it has a preferential effect on SMCs as suppressed endothelial cells[112, 130, 138, 139]. Although some studies showed that tacrolimus-eluting stents can significantly reduce neointimal proliferation[108, 140], a study on Janus, a new design of tacrolimus-eluting stent (Sorin Biomedica Cardio, Italy), indicated the performance of Janus was no better than a BMS[141]. Other tacrolimus-eluting stents and their long term outcomes are still under investigation[142].

Pimecrolimus: Pimecrolimus (SDZ ASM 981), an analogue of ascomycin, has similar effects and mechanism of tacrolimus. It has received substantial interest for its significant anti-inflammatory activity, immunomodulatory capabilities and low systemic immunosuppressive potential[143].

Curcumin: Curcumin, a component of turmeric, exhibits a variety of biological activities such as anti-proliferative activity, anti-inflammatory, anti-oxidant activity, wound healing ability, and anti-microbial activity[144-146]. Thus, curcumin is an excellent candidate in the application of coronary stents to inhibit the proliferation of SMCs and prevent inflammatory response, and hence prevent the occurrence of restenosis.

Resveratrol: Resveratrol (3, 5, 4'- trihydroxystilbene), is a phytoalexin found in various plants, such as grapes, berries, peanuts and wines, and has many biological activities including anti-fungal, anti-bacterial, anti-viral, anti-oxidant, and anti-inflammatory activity[147, 148]. It is most important, however, that resveratrol has the potential to be used as a therapeutic agent in DES to inhibit thrombosis and restenosis because of its ability to block the aggregation of human platelets and prevent the proliferation of vascular smooth muscle cells[149-152].

CD 34 antibody: Contrary to SMC inhibition, a novel prohealing technology is used in the Genous™ stent (Orbus Neich, Fort Lauderdale, Florida), which is a stainless steel stent coated with murine monoclonal antihuman CD34 antibodies that attracts endothelial progenitor cell to enhance re-endothelialization. The reported results indicate that the Genous™ stent is effective and promising[153-156].

Anti-VEGF: Another similar concept is the bevacizumab-eluting stent (Biocompatibles Ltd., London, UK)[157]. Bevacizumab, a specific anibody of vascular endothelial growth factor (VEGF), was coated on the surface of BiodivYsio stent to inhibit the development of the vaso vasorum and thereby promote atheromatous plaque stability. Further investigation is in progress.

Drug Combinations: Besides developing new individual drugs to inhibit thrombosis and restenosis, combining the known effective drugs together on the stents is a novel method. For example, pimecrolimus and paclitaxel were loaded together on Symbio stents; heparin and sirolimus were coated on Synchronnium stents; genistein were combined with sirolimus[158].

3. Current commercially available and investigational DESs

Currently, four drug-eluting stents have been approved by the FDA for the U.S. market including: Sirolimus coated Cypher® stent (Cordis, Inc.), Paclitaxel coated Taxus® stent (Boston Scientific, Inc.), Zotarolimus coated Endeavour® stent(Medtronic, Minneapolis, MN) and Everolimus coated Xience® Stent (Abbott, Redwood city, California). Cook, MIV Therapeutics, Inc. and a few others including MicroMedical Group, Inc. have been working hard to enter the stent market as well. The table below provides a summary of currently available and investigational DESs and their status.

Among currently available nonbiodegradable DESs, both Cypher® and Taxus® stents have been well- accepted by clinical cardiologists and patients. The incidences of in-stent restenosis in both stents are effectively confined to less than 10%. However, the common problem faced with both stents is late-stage thrombosis which occurs at approximately 0.4% after one year of implantation. Endeavour® and Xience® are relatively new to the market, and therefore their long-term clinical safety and efficacy need to be further investigated.

Cypher® and Taxus® stents, the first generation of DESs, are constructed from 316L stainless steel, while recently approved Endeavour® and Xience® stents are made from

Cobalt chrome. All four approved DESs are coated with nonbiodegradable polymers. Nonbiodegradable polymers were used rather than biodegradable polymers primarily due to the bio-incompatibility issues of existing biodegradable polymers.

Generations	Brand Name	Drugs	Platforms			Polymers		Manufacturers	Current Status	
			Platforms	Strut thickness	Materials	Nondegrad.	Biodegrad.		FDA	CE Mark
First	Taxus®	Paclitaxel	Nir®	132	316LSS	SIBS		BSC	Approved	
	Cypher®	Sirolimus	BxVelocity	140	316LSS	PEVA/PBMA		Cordis, J&J	Approved	
Second	Endeavour®	Zotarolimus	Driver	91	Cobalt	PC		Medtronic	Approved	
	Xience ®	Everolimus	ML-VISION®	81	Cobalt	Fluropolymer		Abbott	Approved	
New Generation and Pipeline	BioMatrix	Biolimus A9	S stent	N/A	316LSS		PLA	Biosensor Int		yes
	Nobori	Biolimus A9	Nobori Stent	112	316lss		PLA	TERUMO		yes
	Xtent	Biolimus A9	NX™ DES	Cobalt--adjustable length			PLA	Xtent		inv.
	BioFreedom	Biolimus A9		112	316LL	No polymer-Texture		Biosensor Int		inv.
	Janus	Tacrolimus		110	316ll	No polymer--Rreservoir		Sorin		yes
	Yukon	Sirolimus		87	316ll	No polymer--microporous		Yukon		yes
	Genous	Anti-CD 34 antibody		100	316ll	No Polymer		OrbusNeich		yes
	JACTax Stent	Paclitaxol	JACTax Stent		316L	PLA with microdroplet		Labcoat		inv.
	MIV	Siroliumus	Miv	87	Cobalt	Hap		MIV therapeutics		

PEVA: Poly(ethylene-co-vinyl acetate; PBMA: polybutyl methacrylate; PC: Phosphorylcholine; PLA: Poly(acitic acid); PTFE: Polyetrafluoroethylene; SIBS: styrene-b-isobutylene-b-styrene; PLGA: Poly(Lactide-co-Glycolide); ACP: amorphous calcium phosphate; N/A: Not available, BVS: bioabsorable everolimus-eluting stent, Inv.: Investigation

Table 1. The current commercially available and investigational DESs and their status

3.1 Cypher® stent

Cypher® stent has 8-33 mm in length and is offered in 2.5-3.5 mm diameters. Its coating matrix is composed of three nonbiodegradable polymers: Parylene C coated primer layer for improving adhesion of polymer to the metal surface, followed by a layer of polyethylene-co-vinyl acetate (PEVA)/poly n-butyl methacrylate (PBMA) copolymer containing the active agent of Sirolimus. The top layer is a drug-free coating of PBMA to control drug release and to prevent a burst effect. The Cypher® stent releases 50% of its Sirolimus content during the first week after implantation and 85% of the drug over 30 days. All of the Sirolimus is eluted over 90 days.

3.2 Taxus® stent

Taxus® stent comes in lengths of 8-28mm and diameters of 2.5-3.75mm. The stent is coated with non-biodegradable poly (styrene-b-isobutylene-b-styrene), known as TransLute polymer. The stent provides a burst release of Paclitaxel during the initial 48 hours followed by slow release over the next 10 days and no further release after 30 days.

3.3 Endeavour® DES

Endeavour® stent is a cobalt chrome stent with strut thickness of 91 μm (originally S660 stent). The stent was coated with 4.3 μm of phosphorylcholine polymer and the immunosuppressive drug: Zotarolimusan an analog of Sirolimus.

3.4 Xience® DES

Xience® *stent* is the most recently FDA approved DES. The stent is made by using Abbott's cobalt chrome Multilink® Vision stent as a platform, coated with 7.6um of nonbiodegradable fluropolymer and another Sirolimus analogue drug, Everolimus.

4. Fully Biodegradable Drug Eluting Stent (BDES)

Despite a tremendous amount of capital invested in developing fully biodegradable stents to overcome the drawbacks existing in current nonbiodegradable stents, only five fully biodegradable stents have been investigated in humans so far:

1. The Igaki-Tamai bioabsorbable stent (Igaki Medical Planning Company, Kyoto, Japan)
2. Biodegradable everolimus eluting XIENCE V stent (BVS, Abbott Vascular, Santa Clara, CA, USA).
3. Tyrosine polycarbonate biodegradable stent (Reva Medical Inc, San Diego, CA)
4. Salicylate-based polyanhydride ester biodegradable sirolimus-eluting stent (Ideal™ Bioabsorbable Therapeutics Inc., CA, USA), and
5. Biodegradable magnesium alloy stent (Biotronik AG, Berlin, German)

Table 2 below summarizes the physical, chemical and structural characteristics of these five stents (159).

4.1 The Igaki-Tamai Bioabsorbable Stent

Igaki-Tamai Bioabsorbable Stent is the first absorbable stent that was implanted in humans. It is constructed from poly-L-lactic acid (PLLA). The stent is designed in a zig-zag helical coil structure with a 170um strut thickness. The stent is delivered by a balloon-mounted self-expanding sheathed system with warmed contrast medium. As PLLA is radiolucent, gold markers at each end provide radio-opacity for stent identification. The stent does not release any antiproliferative drug. In the preliminary, first-in-man prospective, nonrandomized clinical trial that enrolled 50 patients, a 4-year follow-up of all the patients (100%) revealed a low complication rate with 1 in-hospital stent thrombosis causing a Q-wave MI, 1 non cardiac death, and 18% repeat PCI and no surgical revascularization. Although there have been no further human coronary implants and the focus is now on a peripheral application, this stent is important in the history of PCI with absorbable stents.

4.2 Biodegradable everolimus-eluting XIENCE V stent

XIENCE Stent has a backbone of circumferential hoops of crystalline PLA, with a strut thickness of 150μm, linked directly together or held by straight bridges achieving a radial strength similar to the Multi-link Vision metal stent. At both ends of the stent, two adjacent radio-opaque metal markers facilitate correct fluoroscopic positioning. The stent was coated with everolimus(8.2 μg/mm) and amorphous PLA matrix in the ratio of 1:1. Eighty percent of the coated drug is released in 30 days, which is similar to the release patterns of the Xience V™ and Cypher® DESs. The stent has been evaluated in an observational first-in-man study of 30 patients with single *de novo* coronary artery lesions. At the 2-year follow-up, the device has been shown to be safe with no cardiac deaths, target lesion revascularizations, nor stent thromboses and only one non-Q wave MI. In-stent late loss amounted to 0.43 ± 0.44 mm at 6 months and 0.48 ± 0.28 mm at 2 years. Binary restenosis was observed in 7.7% of patients (2/26) at 6 months and in 0% of patients at 2 years (0/19). One third of stent struts had resolved after 2 years as assessed by optical coherence tomography. Although these data are encouraging, the small number of patients enrolled in the trial and the simplicity of the lesions treated means that a great deal of work remains to be done before the device can be considered for routine use in clinical practice. The stent is currently commercially available in Europe.

4.3 Tyrosine polycarbonate biodegradable REVA stent

The REVA stent is made from monomeric units of the common amino acid *L*-tyrosine, chemically modified to incorporate iodine molecules so as to make this stent radiopaque. This polymer degrades to carbon dioxide and water in a similar fashion to PLA. The stent struts were designed with a "slide and lock'" feature that enables strut thickness to be reduced without compromising radial integrity. The RESORB first-in-man trial showed unfavorable outcomes between 4 and 6 months post-implantation with a higher-than-anticipated target lesion revascularization rate driven mainly by reduced stent diameter

4.4 Polyanhydride ester (PAE) polymeric stent

The PAE stent is made by incorporating salicylic acid into the backbone of a PAE polymer. The stent surface is coated with Sirolimus with complete elution of the drug by 30 days. The stent offers the advantages of being absorbable and providing anti-inflammatory and antiproliferative properties. In the first-in-man Whisper trial, a stent with strut thickness of 200um and a crossing profile of 2.0 mm with a stent-to-artery coverage of 65% was implanted in 8 patients. Because of the higher-than-expected intimal hyperplasia in this FIM study, a subsequent design with thinner struts, a higher dose of Sirolimus, and a lower percent wall coverage is currently under investigation.

4.5 Absorbable magnesium stent

The AMS stent is composed of 93% magnesium and 7% rare-earth metals. It degrades within the body over a 2-to-3-month time frame, forming inorganic salts containing calcium, chloride, oxide, sulfates and phosphates. The AMS stent has been evaluated in an observational study (PROGRESS) of 71 patients with an angiographic and IVUS assessment at 4 months and clinical follow-up at 1 year. The relatively high in-stent late loss of 1.08 ± 0.49 mm at 4 months translated into a TLR rate of 48.4% at 1 year. The main contributors to restenosis, as detected by IVUS at 4 months, were a decrease of external elastic membrane volume and neointimal hyperplasia, but only small remnants of the stent material were observed at 4 months.

5. Future Development of DES

Ideal DES, from a clinical aspect, should possess the following characteristics: a remarkable ease of use, unparalleled efficacy, impeccable safety, and restoration of conduit vessel physiology. However, from an engineering point of view, it is impossible to incorporate all parameters to make an "apple-pie" DES. Therefore the next generation of DES will be continuously developed by optimizing these three components through a variety ways including the new material selection, new platform design, and new drug incorporation, etc.

Stents	Strut Material	Coating Material	Design	Absorption Products	Drug Elution	Stent Radiopacity	Depolyment	Strut Thickness (um)	Crossing Profile (mm)	Stent-to-Artery Ratio(%)	Duration Radial Support	Absorption Time
Igaki-Tamai	PLLA	Nil	Zig-Zag helical coils with straight bridge	Lactic acid, CO_2, and H_2O	Nil	Gold marker	Self Expanding & heated balloon	170	?	24	6 mo	2y
Bioabsorable Magnesium Alloy	Metal Magnesium Alloy	Nil	Sinusoidal in-phase hoop linked by straight bridge	Not applicable	Nil	Nil	Balloon	165	1.2	10	Days or weeks	< 4mo
BVS 1.0	PLLA	PDLA	out-of-phase hoop with straight & direct link	Lactic acid, CO_2 and H_2O	Everolimus	Platinum marker	Balloon	156	1.4	25	weeks	2y
BVS 1.1	PLLA	PDLA	In-phase hoop with straight and direct link	lactic acid, CO_2, and H_2O	Everolimus	Platinum marker	Balloon	156	1.4	25	3 mo	2y
REVA	Tyrosine-Derived Polycarbonate	Nil	Side and lock	Amino acids ethanol and CO_2	Nil	Idodine impregnated	Balloon	200	1.7	55	3-6 mo	2y
BTI Bioabsorable Therapeutics Incoporated	Salicylate linker	Salicylate different linker	Tuber with laser cut void	Salicylate, CO_2, and H_2O	Sirolimus & Salicylate	Nil	Balloon	200	2	65	3 mo	6 mo

Table 2. Comparison of the Preoterties Among 5 Absorable Stents

The challenges faced by emerging technologies are to reduce restenosis in high-risk lesions, without compromising healing, in order to avoid late thrombotic complications and to improve system deliverability to allow treatment of more complex patients. Currently, a number of strategies are being utilized to achieve these goals through the development of novel stent platforms, coating with biodegradable polymers or moving away from polymers, and with new generations and/or combinations of biological agents that both inhibit proliferation and promote endothelialization. With the recent positive data from Abbott's ABSORB trial, *clinical consensus is building that fully bioabsorbable stents (BDS) represent the next generation in DES.* Table 3 summarizes the potential benefits for the biodegradable DES.

May limit late-stent thrombosis
Allows late favorable positive remodeling
May reduce long-term dual antiplatelet therapy
Has Larger drug-loading capacity
Addresses patient's concerns about permanent implants
Faciltates noninvasive diagnosis imaging(MR/CT)
Surgical option not restricted
Easier repeat revascularization

Table 3. Potential Benefits of Biodegradable Stent.

6. References

[1] Cardiovascular disease statistics. *American Heart Association*. 1988: ICD/9, 390-459.

[2] Stamler J. Epidemiology, established major risk factors, and the primary prevention of coronary heart disease. *Cardiology*. 1991;2

[3] Sigwart U, Puel J, Mirkovitch V, Joffre F, Kappenberger L. Intravascular stents to prevent occlusion and re-stenosis after transluminal angioplasty. *New England Journal of Medicine*. 1987;316:701-706

[4] Sousa JE, Costa MA, Abizaid A, Sousa AGMR, Feres F, Mattos LA, Centemero M, Maldonado G, Abizaid AS, Pinto I. Sirolimus-eluting stent for the treatment of in-stent restenosis: A quantitative coronary angiography and three-dimensional intravascular ultrasound study. *Circulation*. 2003;107:24

[5] Grube E, Silber S, Hauptmann KE, Mueller R, Buellesfeld L, Gerckens U, Russell ME. Taxus i. *Circulation*. 2003;107:38-42

[6] Babapulle MN, Eisenberg MJ. Coated stents for the prevention of restenosis: Part i. *Circulation*. 2002;106:2734-2740

[7] Iijima R, Ikari Y, Miyazawa A, Nakajima H, Hara K. Predictors of restenosis after implantation of 2.5 mm stents in small coronary arteries. *Circulation Journal*. 2004;68:236-240

[8] Schofer J, Schlüter M, Gershlick AH, Wijns W, García E, Schampaert E, Breithardt G. Sirolimus-eluting stents for treatment of patients with long atherosclerotic lesions in small coronary arteries: Double-blind, randomised controlled trial (e-sirius). *Lancet*. 2003;362:1093-1099

[9] Muramatsu T, Tsukahara R, Ho M, Ito Y, Ishimori H, Hirano K, Nakano M, Matsushita M, Leung W. Clinical outcome of stent implantation in small coronary arteries using different type of coronary stents. *J Invasive Cardiol.* 2001;13:634-639

[10] Welt FGP, Rogers C. Inflammation and restenosis in the stent era. *Arterioscler. Thromb. Vasc. Biol.* 2002;22:1769-1776

[11] Shah PK. Inflammation, neointimal hyperplasia, and restenosis: As the leukocytes roll, the arteries thicken. *Circulation.* 2003;107:2175-2177

[12] Bennett MR. In-stent stenosis: Pathology and implications for the development of drug eluting stents. *Heart* 2003;89:218-224

[13] Cotran RS, Kumar V, Collins T, Robbins SL. *Robbins pathologic basis of disease.* 6th Ed. Philadelphia: WB Saunders; 1999.

[14] Ong ATL, Hoye A, Aoki J, Van Mieghem CAG, Rodriguez Granillo GA, Sonnenschein K, Regar E, McFadden EP, Sianos G, Van Der Giessen WJ, De Jaegere PPT, De Feyter P, Van Domburg RT, Serruys PW. Thirty-day incidence and six-month clinical outcome of thrombotic stent occlusion after bare-metal, sirolimus, or paclitaxel stent implantation. *J Am Coll Cardiol.* 2005;45:947-953

[15] Iakovou I, Schmidt T, Bonizzoni E, Ge L, Sangiorgi GM, Stankovic G, Airoldi F, Chieffo A, Montorfano M, Carlino M, Michev I, Corvaja N, Briguori C, Gerckens U, Grube E, Colombo A. Incidence, predictors, and outcome of thrombosis after successful implantation of drug-eluting stents. *JAMA.* 2005;293:2126-2130

[16] Ong ATL, McFadden EP, Regar E, De Jaegere PPT, Van Domburg RT, Serruys PW. Late angiographic stent thrombosis (last) events with drug-eluting stents. *J Am Coll Cardiol.* 2005;45:2088-2092

[17] Wang F, Stouffer GA, Waxman S, Uretsky BF. Late coronary stent thrombosis: Early vs. Late stent. *Catheterization and Cardiovascular Interventions.* 2002;55:142-147

[18] Wenaweser P, Rey C, Eberli FR, Togni M, Tuller D, Locher S, Remondino A, Seiler C, Hess OM, Meier B. Stent thrombosis following bare-metal stent implantation: Success of emergency percutaneous coronary intervention and predictors of adverse outcome. *European Heart Journal.* 2005;26:1180-1187

[19] McFadden EP, Stabile E, Regar E, Cheneau E, Ong ATL, Kinnaird T, Suddath WO, Weissman NJ, Torguson R, Kent KM. Late thrombosis in drug-eluting coronary stents after discontinuation of antiplatelet therapy. *Lancet.* 2004; 364:1519-1521

[20] Virmani R, Guagliumi G, Farb A, Musumeci G, Grieco N, Motta T, Mihalcsik L, Tespili M, Valsecchi O, Kolodgie FD. Localized hypersensitivity and late coronary thrombosis secondary to a sirolimus-eluting stent should we be cautious? *Circulation.* 2004;109:701-705

[21] Joner M, Finn AV, Farb A, Mont EK, Kolodgie FD, Ladich E, Kutys R, Skorija K, Gold HK, Virmani R. Pathology of drug-eluting stents in humans:: Delayed healing and late thrombotic risk. *Journal of the American College of Cardiology.* 2006;48:193-202

[22] Köster R, Vieluf D, Kiehn M, Sommerauer M, Kähler J, Baldus S, Meinertz T, Hamm CW. Nickel and molybdenum contact allergies in patients with coronary in-stent restenosis. *Lancet.* 2000;356:1895-1897

[23] Kastrati A, Mehilli J, Dirschinger J, Dotzer F, Schühlen H, Neumann F-J, Fleckenstein M, Pfafferott C, Seyfarth M, Schömig A. Intracoronary stenting and angiographic results : Strut thickness effect on restenosis outcome (isar-stereo) trial. *Circulation*. 2001;103:2816-2821

[24] Pache J, Kastrati A, Mehilli J, Schühlen H, Dotzer F, Hausleiter J, Fleckenstein M, Neumann F-J, Sattelberger U, Schmitt C, Müller M, Dirschinger J, Schömig A. Intracoronary stenting and angiographic results: Strut thickness effect on restenosis outcome (isar-stereo-2) trial. *Journal of the American College of Cardiology*. 2003;41:1283-1288

[25] Zitter H, Plenk Jr H. The electrochemical behavior of metallic implant materials as an indicator of their biocompatibility. *Journal of Biomedical Materials Research*. 1987;21:881-896

[26] Johnson PF, Bernstein JJ, Hunter G, Dawson WW, Hench LL. An in vitro and in vivo analysis of anodized tantalum capacitive electrodes: Corrosion response, physiology, and histology. *Journal of Biomedical Materials Research*. 1977;11:637-656

[27] Macionczyk F, Gerold B, Thull R. Repassivating tantalum/tantalum oxide surface modification on stainless steel implants. *Surface & Coatings Technology*. 2001;142:1084-1087

[28] Teitelbaum GP, Raney M, Carvlin MJ, Matsumoto AH, Barth KH. Evaluation of ferromagnetism and magnetic resonance imaging artifacts of the strecker tantalum vascular stent. *CardioVascular and Interventional Radiology*. 1989;12:125-127

[29] Matsumoto AH, Teitelbaum GP, Barth KH, Carvlin MJ, Savin MA, Strecker EP. Tantalum vascular stents: In vivo evaluation with mr imaging. *Radiology*. 1989;170:753-755

[30] Barth KH, Virmani R, Froelich J, Takeda T, Lossef SV, Newsome J, Jones R, Lindisch D. Paired comparison of vascular wall reactions to palmaz stents, strecker tantalum stents, and wallstents in canine iliac and femoral arteries. *Circulation*. 1996;93:2161-2169

[31] Ozaki Y, Keane D, Nobuyoshi M, Hamasaki N, Popma JJ, Serruys PW. Coronary lumen at six-month follow-up of a new radiopaque cordis tantalum stent using quantitative angiography and intracoronary ultrasound. *The American Journal of Cardiology*. 1995;76:1135-1142

[32] Windecker S, Mayer I, De Pasquale G, Maier W, Dirsch O, De Groot P, Wu Y-P, Noll G, Leskosek B, Meier B, Hess OM. Stent coating with titanium-nitride-oxide for reduction of neointimal hyperplasia. *Circulation*. 2001;104:928-933

[33] Mosseri M, Tamari I, Plich M, Hasin Y, Brizines M, Frimerman A, Miller H, Jafari J, Guetta V, Solomon M. Short-and long-term outcomes of the titanium-no stent registry. *Cardiovascular Revascularization Medicine*. 2005;6:2-6

[34] Windecker S, Simon R, Lins M, Klauss V, Eberli FR, Roffi M, Pedrazzini G, Moccetti T, Wenaweser P, Togni M, Tuller D, Zbinden R, Seiler C, Mehilli J, Kastrati A, Meier B, Hess OM. Randomized comparison of a titanium-nitride-oxide-coated stent with a stainless steel stent for coronary revascularization: The tinox trial. *Circulation*. 2005;111:2617-2622

[35] Biehl V, Wack T, Winter S, Seyfert UT, Breme J. Evaluation of the haemocompatibility of titanium based biomaterials. *Biomolecular Engineering*. 2002;19:97-101

[36] Heintz C, Riepe G, Birken L, Kaiser E, Chakf N, Morlock M, Delling G, Imig H. Corroded nitinol wires in explanted aortic endografts: An important mechanism of failure? *Journal of Endovascular Therapy*. 2001;8:248-253

[37] Berger-Gorbet M, Broxup B, Rivard C, Yahia LH. Biocompatibility testing of niti screws using immunohistochemistry on sections containing metallic implants. *Journal of Biomedical Materials Research*. 1996;32:243 - 248

[38] Wataha JC, Lockwood PE, Marek M, Ghazi M. Ability of ni-containing biomedical alloys to activate monocytes and endothelial cells in vitro. *Mater Res*. 1999;45:251-257

[39] Shabalovskaya SA. On the nature of the biocompatibility and on medical applications of niti shape memory and superelastic alloys. *Biomedical materials and engineering*. 1996;6:267-289

[40] Maitz MF, Shevchenko N. Plasma-immersion ion-implanted nitinol surface with depressed nickel concentration for implants in blood. *Journal of Biomedical Materials Research Part A*. 2006;76:356–365

[41] Mazumder MM, De S, Trigwell S, Ali N, Mazumder MK, Mehta JL. Corrosion resistance of polyurethane-coated nitinol cardiovascular stents. *Journal of Biomaterials Science, Polymer Edition*. 2003;14:1351-1362

[42] Starosvetsky D, Gotman I. Corrosion behavior of titanium nitride coated ni-ti shape memory surgical alloy. *Biomaterials*. 2001;22:1853-1859

[43] Shih CC, Lin SJ, Chung KH, Chen YL, Su YY. Increased corrosion resistance of stent materials by converting current surface film of polycrystalline oxide into amorphous oxide. *Journal of Biomedical Materials Research*. 2000;52:323-332

[44] Schürmann K, Vorwerk D, Kulisch A, Stroehmer-Kulisch E, Biesterfeld S, Stopinski T, Günther RW. Experimental arterial stent placement: Comparison of a new nitinol stent and wallstent. *Investigative radiology*. 1995;30:412-420

[45] Adams GJ, Baltazar U, Karmonik C, Bordelon C, Lin PH, Bush RL, Lumsden AB, Morrisett JD. Comparison of 15 different stents in superficial femoral arteries by high resolution mri ex vivo and in vivo. *Journal of Magnetic Resonance Imaging*. 2005;22:125-135

[46] Nakamura S, Degawa T, Nishida T, Anzai H, Mitsuo K, Sakatani H, Tsunoda T, Ui K, Yabuki S, Yamaguchi T. Preliminary experience of act-one^{tm} coronary stent implantation. *J. Am. Coll. Cardiol*. 1996;27:53

[47] Holmes DR, Lansky A, Kuntz R, Bell MR, Buchbinder M, Fortuna R, O'Shaughnessy CD, Popma J. The paragon stent study: A randomized trial of a new martensiti nitinol stent versus the palmaz-schatz stent for treatment of complex native coronary arterial lesions. *The American Journal of Cardiology*. 2000;86:1073-1079

[48] Isshiki T, Eto K, Ochini M, Milani H, Kondo K, Takoshita S, Sato T. Nitinol radius stent induces less platelet aggregation than stainless steel palmaz-schatz/glanturco-rubin ii stents. *JACC*. 1998;31:312

[49] Hijazi ZM, Homoud M, Aronovitz MJ, Smith JJ, Faller GT. A new platinum balloon-expandable stent (angiostent) mounted on a high pressure balloon: Acute and late results in an atherogenic swine model. *The Journal of invasive cardiology*. 1995;7:127-134

[50] Bhargava B, Scheerder ID, Ping QB, Yanming H, Chan R, Kim HS, Kollum M, Cottin Y, Leon MB. A novel platinum-iridium, potentially gamma radioactive stent: Evaluation in a porcine model. *Catheterization and Cardiovascular Interventions*. 2000;51:364-368

[51] Foti R, Tamburino C, Galassi AR, Russo G, Nicosia A, Grassi R, Monaco A, Azzarelli S, Mammana C, Calvi V. Safety, feasibility and efficacy of a new single-wire stent in the treatment of complex coronary lesions: The angiostent. *Cardiologia*. 1998;43:725-730

[52] Peuster M, Wohlsein P, Brugmann M, Ehlerding M, Seidler K, Fink C, Brauer H, Fischer A, Hausdorf G. A novel approach to temporary stenting: Degradable cardiovascular stents produced from corrodible metal-results 6-18 months after implantation into new zealand white rabbits. *Heart*. 2001;86:563-569

[53] Heublein B, Rohde R, Kaese V, Niemeyer M, Hartung W, Haverich A. Biocorrosion of magnesium alloys: A new principle in cardiovascular implant technology? *Heart* 2003;89:651-656

[54] Mueller PP, May T, Perz A, Hauser H, Peuster M. Control of smooth muscle cell proliferation by ferrous iron. *Biomaterials*. 2006;27:2193-2200

[55] Peuster M, Hesse C, Schloo T, Fink C, Beerbaum P, von Schnakenburg C. Long-term biocompatibility of a corrodible peripheral iron stent in the porcine descending aorta. *Biomaterials*. 2006;27:4955-4962

[56] Staiger MP, Pietak AM, Huadmai J, Dias G. Magnesium and its alloys as orthopedic biomaterials: A review. *Biomaterials*. 2006;27:1728-1734

[57] Di Mario C, Griffiths H, Goktekin O, Peeters N, Verbist JAN, Bosiers M, Deloose K, Heublein B, Rohde R, Kasese V. Drug-eluting bioabsorbable magnesium stent. *Journal of Interventional Cardiology*. 2004;17:391-395

[58] Eggebrecht H, Rodermann J, Hunold P, Schmermund A, Bose D, Haude M, Erbel R. Novel magnetic resonance-compatible coronary stent: The absorbable magnesium-alloy stent. *Circulation*. 2005;112:e303-304

[59] Sharkawi T, Cornhill F, Lafont A, Sabaria P, Vert M. Intravascular bioresorbable polymeric stents: A potential alternative to current drug eluting metal stents. *Journal of Pharmaceutical Sciences*. 2007;96:2829 - 2837

[60] Bosiers M, Deloose K, Verbist J, Peeters P. Will absorbable metal stent technology change our practice? *Journal of cardiovascular surgery*. 2006;47:393-397

[61] Zartner P, Cesnjevar R, Singer H, Weyand M. First successful implantation of a biodegradable metal stent into the left pulmonary artery of a preterm baby. *Catheterization and Cardiovascular Interventions*. 2005;66:590-594

[62] Schranz D, Zartner P, Michel-Behnke I, Akinturk H. Bioabsorbable metal stents for percutaneous treatment of critical recoarctation of the aorta in a newborn. *Catheterization and Cardiovascular Interventions*. 2006;67:671-673

[63] Waale WHE, Van Der Veen FH, Leeuwen C, Lankveld M, Havenith M, Bar FW, Oppen J, Wellens HJJ. Modulation of healthy pig coronary arteries by self-expanding stents. *Journal of Interventional Cardiology*. 1996;9:45-52

[64] Bramwell O, Leon MB. Acute and chronic effects of self-expanding nitinol stents in porcine coronary arteries. *Coronary Artery Disease*. 1997;8:45-46

[65] Mosseri M, Rozenman Y, Mereuta A, Hasin Y, Gotsman MS. New indicator for stent covering area. *Catheterization and cardiovascular diagnosis*. 1998;44:188 - 192
[66] Leon MB, Popma JJ, O'haughnessy C, Dean LS, Lansky AJ, Fry ETA, Curran MJ. Quantitative angiographic outcomes after gianturco-roubin stent implantation in complex lesion subsets. *Circulation*. 1997;96: I-593
[67] Heuser R, Lopez A, Kuntz R, Reduto L, Badger R, Coleman P, Whitlow P, Iannone LA, Safian R, Yeung A. Smart: The microstent's ability to limit restenosis trial. *Catheterization and Cardiovascular Interventions*. 2001;52:269 - 277
[68] Gurbel PA, Callahan KP, Malinin AI, Serebruany VL, Gillis J. Could stent design affect platelet activation? Results of the platelet activation in stenting (past) study. *Journal of Invasive Cardiology*. 2002;14:584-589
[69] Foley DP, Pieper M, Wijns W, Suryapranata H, Grollier G, Legrand V, de Scheerder I, Hanet C, Puel J, Mudra H. The influence of stent length on clinical and angiographic outcome in patients undergoing elective stenting for native coronary artery lesions; final results of the magic 5l study. *European Heart Journal*. 2001;22:1585-1593
[70] Stone GW, Ellis SG, Cox DA, Hermiller J, O'Shaughnessy C, Mann JT, Turco M, Caputo R, Bergin P, Greenberg J. A polymer-based, paclitaxel-eluting stent in patients with coronary artery disease. *N. Engl. J. Med.* 2004;350:221-231
[71] Garasic JM, Edelman ER, Squire JC, Seifert P, Williams MS, Rogers C. Stent and artery geometry determine intimal thickening independent of arterial injury. *Circulation*. 2000;101:812-818
[72] Gunn J, Arnold N, Chan KH, Shepherd L, Cumberland DC, Crossman DC. Coronary artery stretch versus deep injury in the development of in-stent neointima. *Heart*. 2002;88:401-405
[73] Hamuro M, Palmaz JC, Sprague EA, Fuss C, Luo J. Influence of stent edge angle on endothelialization in an in vitro model. *Journal of Vascular and Interventional Radiology*. 2001;12:607-611
[74] De Scheerder I, Verbeken E, Van Humbeeck J. Metallic surface modification. *Seminars in interventional cardiology* 1998;3:139-144
[75] Palmaz JC, Benson A, Sprague EA. Influence of surface topography on endothelialization of intravascular metallic material. *Journal of Vascular and Interventional Radiology*. 1999;10:439-444
[76] Fuss C, Sprague EA, Bailey SR, Palmaz JC. Surface micro grooves (mg) improve endothelialization rate in vitro and in vivo. *Am J Cardiol*. 2001;37:70A
[77] Palmaz JC, Bailey S, Marton D, Sprague E. Influence of stent design and material composition on procedure outcome. *Journal of Vascular Surgery*. 2002;36:1031-1039
[78] Dibra A, Kastrati A, Mehilli J, Pache J, von Oepen R, Dirschinger J, Schomig A. Influence of stent surface topography on the outcomes of patients undergoing coronary stenting: A randomized double-blind controlled trial. *Catheterization and Cardiovascular Interventions*. 2005;65:374 - 380
[79] Rogers C, Edelman ER. Endovascular stent design dictates experimental restenosis and thrombosis. *Circulation*. 1995;91:2995-3001

[80] Albrecht D, Kaspers S, Fussl R, Hopp HW, Sechtem U. Coronary plaque morphology affects stent deployment: Assessment by intracoronary ultrasound. *Catheterization and cardiovascular diagnosis*. 1996;38:229 - 235

[81] Henneke KH, Regar E, Konig A, Werner F, Klauss V, Metz J, Theisen K, Mudra H. Impact of target lesion calcification on coronary stent expansion after rotational atherectomy. *American Heart Journal*. 1999;137:93-99

[82] Narracott AJ, Lawford PV, Gunn JPG, Hose DR. Balloon folding affects the symmetry of stent deployment: Experimental and computational evidence. *Engineering in Medicine and Biology Society, 2007. EMBS 2007. 29th Annual International Conference of the IEEE*. 2007:3069-3073

[83] Narracott AJ, Hose DR, Lawford PV, Gunn J. Measurement of the symmetry of in vitro stent expansion: A stereo-photogrammetric approach. *Journal of medical engineering & technology*. 2003;27:59-70

[84] Morice MC, Serruys PW, Sousa JE, Fajadet J, Ban Hayashi E, Perin M, Colombo A, Schuler G, Barragan P, Guagliumi G. A randomized comparison of a sirolimus-eluting stent with a standard stent for coronary revascularization. *N. Engl. J. Med.* 2002;346:1773-1780

[85] Moses JW, Leon MB, Popma JJ, Fitzgerald PJ, Holmes DR, O'Shaughnessy C, Caputo RP, Kereiakes DJ, Williams DO, Teirstein PS. Sirolimus-eluting stents versus standard stents in patients with stenosis in a native coronary artery. *N. Engl. J. Med.* 2003;349:1315-1323

[86] Stone GW, Ellis SG, Cannon L, Mann JT, Greenberg JD, Spriggs D, O'Shaughnessy CD, DeMaio S, Hall P, Popma JJ, Koglin J, Russell ME, for the TVI. Comparison of a polymer-based paclitaxel-eluting stent with a bare metal stent in patients with complex coronary artery disease: A randomized controlled trial. *JAMA*. 2005;294:1215-1223

[87] Aziz S, Morris JL, Perry RA. Late stent thrombosis associated with coronary aneurysm formation after sirolimus-eluting stent implantation. *J. Invasive. Cardiol.* 2007;19:E96-98

[88] Camenzind E. Treatment of in-stent restenosis--back to the future? *N. Engl. J. Med.* 2006;355:2149-2151

[89] Camenzind E, Steg PG, Wijns W. Stent thrombosis late after implantation of first-generation drug-eluting stents: A cause for concern. *Circulation*. 2007;115:1440-1455

[90] Pfisterer ME. The basket-late-study. Basel stent cost-effectiveness trial--late thrombotic events trial. *Herz*. 2006;31:259

[91] Tsuchida K, Piek JJ, Neumann FJ, Van Der Giessen WJ, Wienler M, Zeiher AM, Grube E, Haase J, Thuesen L, Hamm CW. One-year results of a durable polymer everolimus-eluting stent in fife novo coronary narrowings(the spirit first trial). *EuroIntervention*. 2005;1:266-272

[92] Fajadet J, Wijns W, Laarman GJ, Kuck KH, Ormiston J, Munzel T, Popma JJ, Fitzgerald PJ, Bonan R, Kuntz RE. Randomized, double-blind, multicenter study of the endeavor zotarolimus-eluting phosphorylcholine-encapsulated stent for treatment of native coronary artery lesions: Clinical and angiographic results of the endeavor ii trial. *Circulation*. 2006;114:798-806

[93] Stone GW, Midei M, Newman W, Sanz M, Hermiller JB, Williams J, Farhat N, Mahaffey KW, Cutlip DE, Fitzgerald PJ, Sood P, Su X, Lansky AJ, for the SIIII. Comparison of an everolimus-eluting stent and a paclitaxel-eluting stent in patients with coronary artery disease: A randomized trial. *JAMA*. 2008;299:1903-1913

[94] Kandzari DE, Leon MB, Popma JJ, Fitzgerald PJ, O'Shaughnessy C, Ball MW, Turco M, Applegate RJ, Gurbel PA, Midei MG. Comparison of zotarolimus-eluting and sirolimus-eluting stents in patients with native coronary artery disease a randomized controlled trial. *J. Am. Coll. Cardiol.* 2006;48:2440-2447

[95] Slottow TLP, Steinberg DH, Waksman R. Overview of the 2007 food and drug administration circulatory system devices panel meeting on patent foramen ovale closure devices. *Circulation*. 2007;116:677-682

[96] Meredith IT, Ormiston J, Whitbourn R, Kay IP, Muller D, Popma JJ, Cutlip DE, Fitzgerald PJ. Four-year clinical follow-up after implantation of the endeavor zotarolimus-eluting stent: Endeavor i, the first-in-human study. *Am. J. Cardiol.* 2007;100:56-61

[97] Finn AV, Nakazawa G, Joner M, Kolodgie FD, Mont EK, Gold HK, Virmani R. Vascular responses to drug eluting stents: Importance of delayed healing. *Arterioscler. Thromb. Vasc. Biol.* 2007;27:1500-1510

[98] Hollinger JO. Preliminary report on the osteogenic potential of a biodegradable copolymer of polyactide (pla) and polyglycolide (pga). *J. Biomed. Mater. Res.* 1983;17:71-82

[99] Gunatillake PA, Adhikari R. Biodegradable synthetic polymers for tissue engineering. *Eur Cells Mat*. 2003;5:1-16

[100] Ge J, Qian J, Wang X, Wang Q, Yan W, Yan Y, Fan B, Ge L, Liu X. Effectiveness and safety of the sirolimus-eluting stents coated with bioabsorbable polymer coating in human coronary arteries. *Catheter Cardiovasc Interv*. 2007;69:198 - 202

[101] Lee CH, Lim J, Low A, Zhang XL, Kyaing TT, Chan MY, Wong HB, Lim YT, Tan HC. Sirolimus-eluting, bioabsorbable polymer-coated constant stent (cura[tm]) in acute st-elevation myocardial infarction: A clinical and angiographic study (curami registry). *J Invasive Cardiol*. 2007;19:182-185

[102] Aoki JO, Andrew T. L., Abizaid A, Tien HP, Bonnier H, Mcclean DR, Verheye S, Belardi J, Condado JA, Pieper M, Sousa JE, Bressers M, Symons J, Litvack F, Sianos G, Serruys PW. One-year clinical outcome of various doses and pharmacokinetic release formulations of paclitaxel eluted from an erodable polymer—insight in the paclitaxel in-stent controlled elution study (pisces). *EuroIntervention*. 2005;1:165-172

[103] Serruys PW, Sianos G, Abizaid A, Aoki J, den Heijer P, Bonnier H, Smits P, McClean D, Verheye S, Belardi J, Condado J, Pieper M, Gambone L, Bressers M, Symons J, Sousa E, Litvack F. The effect of variable dose and release kinetics on neointimal hyperplasia using a novel paclitaxel-eluting stent platform: The paclitaxel in-stent controlled elution study (pisces). *J. Am. Coll. Cardiol.* 2005;46:253-260

[104] Middleton JC, Tipton AJ. Synthetic biodegradable polymers as orthopedic devices. *Biomaterials*. 2000;21:2335-2346

[105] Wessely R, Hausleiter J, Michaelis C, Jaschke B, Vogeser M, Milz S, Behnisch B, Schratzenstaller T, Renke-Gluszko M, Stöver M, Wintermantel E, Kastrati A, Schömig A. Inhibition of neointima formation by a novel drug-eluting stent system that allows for dose-adjustable, multiple, and on-site stent coating *Arteriosclerosis, Thrombosis, and Vascular Biology*. 2005;25:748-753

[106] Mehilli J, Kastrati A, Wessely R, Dibra A, Hausleiter J, Jaschke B, Dirschinger J, Schömig A. Randomized trial of a nonpolymer-based rapamycin-eluting stent versus a polymer-based paclitaxel-eluting stent for the reduction of late lumen loss *Circulation*. 2006;113:273-279

[107] Rajtar A, Kaluza GL, Yang Q, Hakimi D, Liu D, Tsui M, Lien M, Smith D, Clubb FJ, Troczynski T. Hydroxyapatite-coated cardiovascular stents. *EuroIntervention*. 2006;2:113-115

[108] Kollum M, Farb A, Schreiber R, Terfera K, Arab A, Geist A, Haberstroh J, Wnendt S, Virmani R, Hehrlein C. Particle debris from a nanoporous stent coating obscures potential antiproliferative effects of tacrolimus-eluting stents in a porcine model of restenosis. *Catheter Cardiovasc Interv*. 2005;64:85-90

[109] Polyak B, Fishbein I, Chorny M, Alferiev I, Williams D, Yellen B, Friedman G, Levy RJ. High field gradient targeting of magnetic nanoparticle-loaded endothelial cells to the surfaces of steel stents. *Proc. Natl. Acad. Sci. U.S.A.* 2008;105:698-703

[110] Sun J, Marx SO, Chen HJ, Poon M, Marks AR, Rabbani LRE. Role for p27kip1 in vascular smooth muscle cell migration. *Circulation*. 2001;103:2967-2972

[111] Tanner FC, Boehm M, Akyurek LM, San H, Yang ZY, Tashiro J, Nabel GJ, Nabel EG. Differential effects of the cyclin-dependent kinase inhibitors p27kip1, p21cip1, and p16ink4 on vascular smooth muscle cell proliferation. *Circulation*. 2000;101:2022-2025

[112] Steffel J, Latini RA, Akhmedov A, Zimmermann D, Zimmerling P, Luscher TF, Tanner FC. Rapamycin, but not fk-506, increases endothelial tissue factor expression implications for drug-eluting stent design. *Circulation*. 2005;112:2002-2011

[113] Steffel J, Luscher TF, Tanner FC. Tissue factor in cardiovascular diseases molecular mechanisms and clinical implications. *Circulation*. 2006;113:722-731

[114] Guha M, Mackman N. The phosphatidylinositol 3-kinase-akt pathway limits lipopolysaccharide activation of signaling pathways and expression of inflammatory mediators in human monocytic cells. *Journal of Biological Chemistry*. 2002;277:32124-32132

[115] Seabra-Gomes R. Percutaneous coronary interventions with drug eluting stents for diabetic patients. *Heart*. 2006;92:410 – 419

[116] Joner M, Nakazawa G, Finn AV, Quee SC, Coleman L, Acampado E, Wilson PS, Skorija K, Cheng Q, Xu X, Gold HK, Kolodgie FD, Virmani R. Endothelial cell recovery between comparator polymer-based drug-eluting stents. *Journal of the American College of Cardiology*. 2008;52:333-342

[117] Lasave LI, Costa JdR, Abizaid AA, Feres F, Tanajura LF, Staico R, Abizaid AA, Beraldo P, Sousa AMR, Sousa JEMR. A three-dimensional intravascular ultrasound comparison between the new zotarolimus-eluting stent (zomaxx™) and the non-drug-eluting trimaxx™ stent. *Journal of Invasive Cardiology*. 2007;19:303-308

[118] Dunn C, Croom KF. Everolimus: A review of its use in renal and cardiac transplantation. *Drugs*. 2006;66:547-570

[119] Farb A, John M, Acampado E, Kolodgie FD, Prescott MF, Virmani R. Oral everolimus inhibits in-stent neointimal growth. *Circulation*. 2002;106:2379-2384

[120] Waksman R, Pakala R, Baffour R, Hellinga D, Seabron R, Kolodgie F, Virmani R. Optimal dosing and duration of oral everolimus to inhibit in-stent neointimal growth in rabbit iliac arteries. *Cardiovascular Revascularization Medicine*. 2006;7:179-184

[121] Patel JK, Kobashigawa JA. Everolimus: An immunosuppressive agent in transplantation. *Expert opinion on pharmacotherapy*. 2006;7:1347-1355

[122] Grube E, Buellesfeld L. Everolimus for stent-based intracoronary applications. *Reviews in cardiovascular medicine*. 2004;5:S3-S8

[123] Grube E, Buellesfeld L. Biomatrix biolimus a9-eluting coronary stent: A next-generation drug-eluting stent for coronary artery disease. *Expert Review of Medical Devices*. 2006;3:731-741

[124] Costa RA, Lansky AJ, Abizaid A, Müeller R, Tsuchiya Y, Mori K, Cristea E, Leon MB, Eduardo Sousa J, Schmidt T. Angiographic results of the first human experience with the biolimus a 9 drug-eluting stent for de novo coronary lesions. *American Journal of Cardiology*. 2006;98:443-446

[125] Grube E, Hauptmann KE, Buellesfeld L, Lim V, Abizaid A. Six-month results of a randomized study to evaluate safety and efficacy of a biolimus a 9 eluting stent with a biodegradable polymer coating. *EuroIntervention*. 2005;1:53-57

[126] Chevalier B, Serruys PW, Silber S, Garcia E, Suryapranata H, Hauptmann K, Wijns W, Schuler G, Fath-Ordoubadi F, Worthley SG, Thuesen L, Meredith IT, Bressers M, Nagai H, Paunovic D. Randomised comparison of nobori™, biolimus a9-eluting coronary stent with ataxus®, paclitaxel-eluting coronary stent in patients with stenosis in native coronary arteries: The nobori 1 trial. *EuroIntervention*. 2007;2:426-434

[127] Sollott SJ, Cheng L, Pauly RR, Jenkins GM, Monticone RE, Kuzuya M, Froehlich JP, Crow MT, Lakatta EG, Rowinsky EK. Taxol inhibits neointimal smooth muscle cell accumulation after angioplasty in the rat. *Journal of Clinical Investigation*. 1995;95:1869-1876

[128] Abal M, Andreu JM, Barasoain I. Taxanes: Microtubule and centrosome targets, and cell cycle dependent mechanisms of action. *Current Cancer Drug Targets*. 2003;3:193-203

[129] Wang TH, Wang HS, Ichijo H, Giannakakou P, Foster JS, Fojo T, Wimalasena J. Microtubule-interfering agents activate c-jun n-terminal kinase/stress-activated protein kinase through both ras and apoptosis signal-regulating kinase pathways. *Journal of Biological Chemistry*. 1998;273:4928-4936

[130] Stahli BE, Camici GG, Steffel J, Akhmedov A, Shojaati K, Graber M, Luscher TF, Tanner FC. Paclitaxel enhances thrombin-induced endothelial tissue factor expression via c-jun terminal nh2 kinase activation. *Circulation Research*. 2006; 99:149-155

[131] Green MR, Manikhas GM, Orlov S, Afanasyev B, Makhson AM, Bhar P, Hawkins MJ. Abraxane®, a novel cremophor®-free, albumin-bound particle form of paclitaxel for the treatment of advanced non-small-cell lung cancer. *Annals of Oncology.* 2006;17:1263-1268

[132] Margolis J, McDonald J, Heuser R, Klinke P, Waksman R, Virmani R, Desai N, Hilton D. Systemic nanoparticle paclitaxel (nab-paclitaxel) for in-stent restenosis i (snapist-i): A first-in-human safety and dose-finding study. *Clin. Cardiol.* 2007;30:165-170

[133] Clarke SJ, Rivory LP. Clinical pharmacokinetics of docetaxel. *Clinical Pharmacokinetics.* 1999;36:99-114

[134] Yasuda S, Noguchi T, Gohda M, Arai T, Tsutsui N, Nakayama Y, Matsuda T, Nonogi H. Local delivery of low-dose docetaxel, a novel microtubule polymerizing agent, reduces neointimal hyperplasia in a balloon-injured rabbit iliac artery model. *Cardiovascular Research.* 2002;53:481-486

[135] Silvestrini R, Zaffaroni N, Orlandi L, Oriana S. In vitro cytotoxic activity of taxol and taxotere on primary cultures and established cell lines of human ovarian cancer. *Stem Cells.* 1993;11:528-535

[136] Gottschalk AR, Quintans J. Apoptosis in b lymphocytes: The wehi-231 perspective. *Immunology and Cell Biology.* 1995;73:8-16

[137] Halloran PF. Immunosuppressive drugs for kidney transplantation. *New England Journal of Medicine.* 2004;351:2715-2729

[138] Mohacsi PJ, Tuller D, Hulliger B, Wijngaard PL. Different inhibitory effects of immunosuppressive drugs on human and rat aortic smooth muscle and endothelial cell proliferation stimulated by platelet-derived growth factor or endothelial cell growth factor. *Journal of Heart and Lung Transplantation.* 1997;16:484-492

[139] Matter CM, Rozenberg I, Jaschko A, Greutert H, Kurz DJ, Wnendt S, Kuttler B, Joch H, Grünenfelder J, Zünd G, Tanner FC, Lüscher T. Effects of tacrolimus or sirolimus on proliferation of vascular smooth muscle and endothelial cells. *Journal of Cardiovascular Pharmacology.* 2006;48:286-292

[140] Grube E, Buellesfeld L. Rapamycin analogs for stent-based local drug delivery. Everolimus- and tacrolimus-eluting stents. *Herz.* 2004;29:162-166

[141] Morice MC, Bestehorn HP, Carrie D, Macaya C, Aengevaeren W, Wijns W, Dubois C, De Winter R, Verheye S, Hoffmann S. Direct stenting of de novo coronary stenoses with tacrolimus-eluting versus carbon-coated carbostents. The randomized jupiter ii trial. *EuroIntervention.* 2006;2:45-52

[142] Tanimoto S, W vdG, H vB, Sorop O, Kukreja N, Fukaya K, Nishide T, Nakano R, Maeda H, Serruys PW. Mahoroba™: Tacrolimus eluting coronary stent. *EuroIntervention.* 2007;3:149-153

[143] Gupta AK, Chow M. Pimecrolimus: A review. *Journal of the European Academy of Dermatology & Venereology.* 2003;17:493-503

[144] Dorai T, Aggarwal BB. Role of chemopreventive agents in cancer therapy. *Cancer letters.* 2004;215:129-140

[145] Gupta KK, Bharne SS, Rathinasamy K, Naik NR, Panda D. Dietary antioxidant curcumin inhibits microtubule assembly through tubulin binding. *FEBS Journal.* 2006;273:5320-5332

[146] Ruby AJ, Kuttan G, Babu KD, Rajasekharan KN, Kuttan R. Anti-tumour and antioxidant activity of natural curcuminoids. *Cancer letters*. 1995;94:79-83

[147] Docherty JJ, Fu MM, Tsai M. Resveratrol selectively inhibits neisseria gonorrhoeae and neisseria meningitidis. *Journal of Antimicrobial Chemotherapy*. 2001;47:243-244

[148] de la Lastra C, Villegas I. Resveratrol as an antioxidant and pro-oxidant agent: Mechanisms and clinical implications. *Biochemical Society Transactions*. 2007;35:1156-1160

[149] Mnjoyan ZH, Fujise K. Profound negative regulatory effects by resveratrol on vascular smooth muscle cells: A role of p53–p21$^{waf1/cip1}$ pathway *Biochemical and Biophysical Research Communications*. 2003;311:546-552

[150] Olas B, Wachowicz B. Resveratrol, a phenolic antioxidant with effects on blood platelet functions. *Platelets*. 2005;16:251-260

[151] Poussier B, Cordova AC, Becquemin JP, Sumpio BE. Resveratrol inhibits vascular smooth muscle cell proliferation and induces apoptosis. *Journal of Vascular Surgery*. 2005;42:1190-1197

[152] Pace-Asciak CR, Hahn S, Diamandis EP, Soleas G, Goldberg DM. The red wine phenolics trans-resveratrol and quercetin block human platelet aggregation and eicosanoid synthesis: Implications for protection against coronary heart disease. *Clinica Chimica Acta*. 1995;235:207-219

[153] Aoki J, Serruys PW, van Beusekom H, Ong ATL, McFadden EP, Sianos G, van der Giessen WJ, Regar E, de Feyter PJ, Davis HR. Endothelial progenitor cell capture by stents coated with antibody against cd34 the healing-fim (healthy endothelial accelerated lining inhibits neointimal growth-first in man) registry. *Journal of the American College of Cardiology*. 2005;45:1574-1579

[154] Duckers HJ, Silber S, De Winter R, Heijer PD, Rensing B, Rau M, Mudra H, Benit E, Verheye S, Wijns W. Circulating endothelial progenitor cells predict angiographic and intravascular ultrasound outcome following percutaneous coronary interventions in the healing-ii trial: Evaluation of an endothelial progenitor cell capturing stent. *EuroIntervention*. 2007;3:67-75

[155] Duckers HJ, Soullie T, Peter DH, Rensing B, Robbert DW, Rau M, Mudra H, Silber S, Benit E, Velheye S, Wiins W, Serruys PW. Accelerated vascular repair following percutaneous coronary intervention by capture of endothelial progenitor cells promotes regression of neointimal growth at long term follow-up : Final results of the healing ii trial using an endothelial progenitor cell capturing stent (genous r stent)™. *EuroIntervention*. 2007;3:350-358

[156] Co M, Tay E, Lee CH, Poh KK, Low A, Lim J, Lim IH, Lim YT, Tan HC. Use of endothelial progenitor cell capture stent (genous bio-engineered r stent) during primary percutaneous coronary intervention in acute myocardial infarction: Intermediate-to long-term clinical follow-up. *American Heart Journal*. 2008;155:128-132

[157] Stefanadis C, Toutouzas K, Stefanadi E, Kolodgie F, Virmani R, Kipshidze N. First experimental application of bevacizumab-eluting pc coated stent for inhibition of vasa vasorum of atherosclerotic plaque: Angiographic results in a rabbit atheromatic model. *Hellenic Journal of Cardiology*. 2006;47:7-10

[158] Kukreja N, Onuma Y, Daemen J, Serruys PW. The future of drug-eluting stents. *Pharmacological Research.* 2008;57:171-180

[159] Yosinobu Onuma and Patrick W. Serruys. Bioresorbable Scaffold : The Advent of a New Era in Percutaneous Coronary and Peripheral Revascularization? *Circulation* 2011, 123:779-797

11

Pursuing Candidate Stem Cells for Optimal Cardiac Regeneration in Patients Suffered from Acute Coronary Syndrome

Mohaddeseh Behjati
Isfahan University of Medical Sciences
Iran

1. Introduction

It has been estimated that cardiovascular diseases will increase to 23.3 million in 2030 [Mathers & Loncar, 2006]. Acute myocardial infarction (AMI) typically occurs as a result of death of millions of myocytes, replaced by non-contractile scar tissue, which imposes a great load burden on surviving myocytes [Segers & Lee, 2010]. Despite of the fundamental progress in the treatment of cardiovascular diseases, a substantial limitation is still present. Current reperfusion strategies afford a great myocardial salvage but limited regenerative capacity of the human heart is a barrier for complete myocardial recovery after necrotic events. Thus, the heart responds to injury by scar formation and persistence muscle damage. Massive cell death and replacement of fibrotic tissue lead to cavitary dilatation and negative left ventricular (LV) remodeling [Ren et al., 2005]. The aftermath event is contractile dysfunction and terminal failure. Thus, regenerating the infracted heart should be adjunct to the therapeutic strategies capable to restore the blood supply to the territory of the infarct related artery. These needs can be met using a cluster of cells with self-renewal capacity, clonal expansion and ability to differentiate into multiple cell lineages. Pluripotent embryonic stem cells (ESCs) or multipotent adult stem cells (ASCs) showed remarkable capacity in heart regeneration. But it needs to be emphasized that heart is not just a pump and orchestrated temporospatial activities consisting sequential electrical stimulation and mechanical contraction are highly demanded. By now, our knowledge about the genetic bases and natural underlying events of cardiovascular disease precede the advancement of therapeutic strategies. A candidate therapeutic strategy should improve cardiac remodeling and function through formation of new blood vessels and inducing reconstitution of functional myocardium. Thus, the aim of this chapter is to focus on the different aspects of stem cell therapy as a growing field for cell-based strategies.

2. Stem cells

Human ESCs (hESCs) isolated from the inner cell mass of the blastocyst stage of human embryo [Ding et al., 2011]. These cells have a unique ability to differentiate into various derivatives of three germ layers and construct ~ 220 diverse cell types of adult human body [Mingxia et al., 2011, Ding et al., 2011]. Application of clinically unsuitable or developmentally arrested embryos can overcome the ethical problems related to embryo manipulation. Obtaining cells from single blastomeres of human embryo hampers the need for embryo destruction. Induced pluripotent stem cells (iPSCs) using cellular reprogramming via forced expression of certain stimulating factors essential for maintenance of stemness, brought the ultimate solution without the need to human embryo [David et al., 2011]. By transferring the nuclear materials of somatic cells into the oocytes conferred pluripotency or totipotency of somatic cells became possible [Gurdon & Wilmut, 2011]. Despite of some epigenetic variations between iPSCs (mainly factor-free) and ESCs, these cells are similar in terms of proliferation, morphology, differentiation potential, imprinting, chromatin profiles and global gene/protein expression signature [Nordin et al., 2011]. This technology bypasses the need for the embryo or the desired tissue as heart. Thus, it is ethically accepted for both therapeutic applications and diagnostic measures like patient's disease modeling in vitro in order to find a treatment. Disease-specific iPS cells are also of paramount importance for achievement of this goal. In this way, tissue matching for organ transplantation is not a matter more. These goals are achievable using exogenous expression of two pluripotency transcription factors (e.g. Nanong, Oct4 and Sox2) and two proto-oncogenes (e.g. c-Myc and Klf4) [Nordin et al., 2011]. Induction of these programming factors is possible through application of retroviral and lentiviral vectors. Both of these vectors act for a period of time and then get silenced state once the endogenous genes had taken over the management of pluripotency [Stadtfeld & Hochedlinger, 2010]. The larger insert capacity of defective lentiviral vectors let them to deliver all of the programming factors without the need for separate individual vectors [Sinn et al., 2005]. In contrast with retroviruses, lentiviral vectors potently infect both dividing and non-dividing cells [Škalamera et al., 2011]. Viral vectors without integration into the genomic material of the target cells, like Adenovirus, have been used but their extremely low efficiency has faded their wide application [Okita & Yamanaka, 2011, Stadtfeld et al., 2008]. In addition to genetic manipulation, cell preconditioning and reprogramming could be performed thorough chemical and pharmacological cell manipulation. The advent of virus-free induction methods seems a revolutionary step in stem cell biotechnology. Despite of their low efficiency, Transposons, protein and mRNA-based induction methods seem advantageous due to their transgene-free nature [Si-Tayeb, 2010]. Small molecules as chromatin-modifying agents like Valporic acid (VPA) are also promising options for transgene-free cell reprogramming with replacement of potentially oncogenic-reprogramming factors [Medvedev et al., 2011]. In addition to the induction methods, knowledge about the through interplay between reprogramming factors will help in identification of more powerful reprogramming strategies. In this context, the effect of c-Myc in augmentation of the Oct4, Sox2 and Klf4 has been consequently associated with enhanced proliferation and differentiation arrest [Takahashi. et al., 2007]. Fully programmed cells raised safety concerns due to induced tumorigenicity by applied preconditioning factors as c-Myc [Kooreman & Wu, 2010]. Recently it has been suggested that creation of iPSCs using L-Myc instead of c-Myc brings less tumorigenicity [Nakagawa et al., 2010]. iPSCs are characterized by the expression of the above mentioned transcription factors and cell surface molecules (e.g. SSEA-3/4, Tra-1-60 and Tra-1-81) [Swelstad & Kerr, 2009]. High alkaline phosphatase and telomerase activity, rapid proliferation, lack of contact inhibition and high nucleus to cytoplasmic ratio with prominent nuclear growing in flat colonies are also further confirmatory indices of successful iPSC achievement [Kooreman & Wu, 2010]. The major criterion for pluripotency is demonstration of the cell lineage's ability to reconstitute tissue composed of three layers by creating chimeras, tetraploid complementation or teratoma formation tests [Swelstad & Kerr, 2009]. Teratoma assay in immunodeficient SCID mice is currently used to test pluripotency in vivo for human iPSCs [Tan et al., 2008]. Teratoma formation (mature or immature) with differentiated ESC- or –iPSC-derived cells is attributed to the insufficient purity and remnant undifferentiated cell population within the transplanted cells [Kooreman & Wu, 2010]. Teratoma formation with injected mouse ESC (mESC)-derived beating embryoid bodies and undifferentiated mESCs is seen in experimental studies [Lin et al., 2010]. Transplantation of pure hESC-derived cardiomyocytes (82.6±6.6%) into immunodeficient rats was not associated with teratoma formation [Laflamme et al., 2007]. For ultimate translation of pluripotent stem cells into clinical benefits, highly purified cells and early detection of teratoma using novel non-invasive tracking strategies and advanced molecular imaging are warranted.

Despite of the substantial progresses made in the field of reprogramming, low reprogramming efficiencies (0.01-0.1% of input cells), slow kinetics of process, partial reprogramming and genetic instability of the manipulated cells hamper clinical application of iPSCs [Utikal et al., 2009, Kanawaty & Henderson, 2009, Stadtfeld et al., 2008]. The type of original somatic cell used for iPSCs, its cycle status and genetic/epigenetic background affect the functional/molecular characteristic of the derived cells [Polo et al., 2010]. These factors, in addition to the "epigenetic memory" of hiPSCs affect the total reprogramming efficiency [Polo et al., 2010]. Thus, alternative promising stem cell source with remarkable plasticity as easily extracted adult stem cells (ASCs), hematopoietic stem cells (HSCs), adipose-derived stem cells and derived MSCs seem useful surrogates [Lodi et al., 2011]. ASCs showed wide range of paracrine effects as cytoprotection, enhanced angiogenesis, recruitment of hematopoietic stem cells and activation of resident cardiac stem cells for endogenous repair [Gnecchi et al., 2008]. Umbilical cord blood (UCB) containing hematopoietic (UC-HS) and mesenchymal stem cells (UC-MS) with higher immunological tolerance are another cell source [Mihu et al., 2008]. Generally, UC-MS grafts are more beneficial than BM-MSCs [In 't Anker et al., 2010].

The activated vs. silenced pluripotency gene cluster is needed for proper programming. Mitotic errors, mutation occurrence and karyotypic changes have been observed in hESCs cultured over long passages [Kooreman & Wu, 2010]. Alterations in imprinted region on chromosome 12, location of pluripotency marker Nanog gene, have been proposed in the tumorigenicity of pluripotent cells [Draper et al., 2004]. Suppressed p53 signaling necessary for reprogramming brings tumorigenicity to the derived stem cells [Hong et al., 2009]. Tumorigenicity is an inherent property of pluripotent cells which is reduced upon differentiation. Thus, decreased tumorigenicity of the pluripotent cells means parallel decrease in their pluripotency and self-renewal potentials. Despite of the presence of intact spindle assembly checkpoints (SAC), mitotic failure-induced polyploidy has been observed in ESCs without occurrence of apoptosis [Kooreman & Wu, 2010]. In contrast with phenotypically resistant ESCs to DNA-damaging agents, embryoid bodies (EB) undergo caspase-3-induced apoptosis by these agents [Kooreman & Wu, 2010]. Human EB aggregates could be propagated from embryonic germ (EG) cells with multi-lineage differentiation potential and limited proliferation [Wobus & Löser, 2011]. It has been speculated that hEG cells might be an alternative to hESCs in future for therapeutic applications [Wobus & Löser, 2011]. Embryonic-like stem cells as Spermatogonial stem cells (SGSCs), parthenogenetic stem cells (PSCs) and male germline stem cells in pre-menopausal women can also give rise into fully active cardiomyocytes [Guan et al., 2007, Zimmermann, 2011].

3. Image platform

Molecular imaging for in vivo tracking the proliferating and viable stem cells made a substantial help in the field of bench to bedside application of stem cells. Pre-transplantation labeling through cell inoculation with nanoparticles or reporter gene is helpful [Kooreman & Wu, 2010]. Semiconductor quantum dots capable to emit different light wavelengths show photostable bright image signals but their aggregation inside the cytosol made the process of cell delivery difficult [Kooreman & Wu, 2010]. Non-specific binding is another issue. Mesenchymal stem cells have been tracked by MRI after labeling with Ferumoxides [Kraitchman et al., 2003, Amado et al., 2005, Arai et al., 2006]. MRI signals elicited by changes in T2 relaxation are induced due to the endocytosis of the iron oxide particles (SPIOs) or ultrasmall superparamagnetic iron oxide particles (USPIOs) [Kooreman & Wu, 2010]. MRI signals are detectable for a period between three weeks up to two months but these signals can already exist in the presence of dead stem cells due to engulfed iron particles in scavenging macrophages [Lee et al., 2009]. Alternatively, direct stem cell labeling applying radionucleotides has been used for circulating-progenitor cells successfully [Hofmann et al., 2005]. The radionucleotide-bound cells could be detected using SPECT, PET, gamma camera and cardiac magnetic resonance tracing [Kooreman & Wu. 2010]. Ultimately, the tracking duration of the radionucleotide-bound cells depends greatly on the individual half-lives of the applied radionucleotide [Kooreman & Wu, 2010]. The enhanced false-positive rate, attributed to the radionucleotide leakage into the non-target cells is still a remained limitation for this highly valuable labeling technique [Kooreman & Wu, 2010].

Reporter gene imagining using intracellular enzyme, cell surface receptor, transmembrane protein and intracellular storage protein probes can provoke detectable signals after interaction with the used exogenous reporters [Cao et al., 2006, MacLaren et al., 1999, Miyagawa et al., 2005, Liu et al., 2009]. Facilitated evaluation of survival and proliferation of the mother stem cells is possible through transferring stably integrated reporter genes [Kooreman & Wu, 2010]. However, concerns persist with regards to the altered cellular behaviors due to the inserted gene [Kooreman & Wu. 2010]. Assurance can be achieved using safer site-specific integration approaches [Keravala et al., 2009]. Double fusion construct containing firefly luciferase (Fluc) which interact with the reporter probe D-luciferin and enhanced green florescence protein (eGFP) can be used for cell tracking in small animals [van der Bogt et al., 2006]. Low-energy photons (2-3 ev) made by Fluc suitable for high-throughput bioluminescence imaging (BLI) and signals of eGFP can be detected using ultrasensitive CCD camera and postmortem histology experiments, respectively [Kooreman & Wu, 2010]. In vivo monitoring of survival, proliferation and migration of the injected intramyocardial mESCs were performed using triple-fusion construct composed of Fluc, monomeric red fluorescent protein (mRFP) and Herpes simplex virus truncated thymidine kinase (HSVttk) [Cao et al., 2006]. PET is preferred to BLI due to the greater anatomical details and applicability in humans [Yaghoubi et al., 2009]. Indeed, easily performed and sensitive imaging modalities like BLI are able to detect early stages of teratoma formation [van der Bogt et al., 2006, Lee et al., 2009]. Early detected teratomas can be ablated by its targeting using reporter-suicide gene construct [Cao et al., 2007]. But limited signal penetration in larger animals and lack of provided spatial three-dimensional data hurdles clinical application of BLI using Fluc reporter gene [Kooreman & Wu, 2010]. Higher spatial resolution of PET and MRI made them good candidate for clinical application but their substantial low detection threshold remained an obstacle [Kooreman & Wu, 2010]. Thus, combining image modalities is of crucial importance especially for clinical insights about identification of the safe limit of stem cell numbers without teratoma formation. Using BLI, Lee et al found safe limit of undifferentiated hESCs for cardiac transplantation into SCID mice to be 1×10^4 [Lee et al., 2009]. Progress in tracking strategies should be in parallel with identification of the appropriate markers for tracking of both stem cell homing and cardiac differentiation. Markers of undifferentiated cells as Oct4, hTert (human telomerase reverse transcriptase) and Dusp6 (dual specifity phosphatase 6) have been shown to be decreased during cardiac trans-differentiation [Wobus & Löser, 2011]. Thus, markers of mesoderm and early cardiogenesis as GATA-4 and Brachyury were found to be suitable for tracking cardiac differentiation [Wobus & Löser, 2011]. Precise imaging technologies should solve uncertainties real cardiomyocyte trans-differentiation vs. cell fusion. Cell fusion as an overlooked phenomenon occurs due to the autoflorescence problems regarding label transfer to neighboring cells or fusion of donor and recipient cells [Reinecke et al., 2008]. The former is avoidable using cell lineage markers as genetic materials [Reinecke et al., 2008]. This process gives rise to bi-nucleated, mono-nucleated cells with tetraploid synkaryon or cells with normal karyotype during division [Wang et al., 2003]. This phenomenon might be occurred after trans-differentiation into myocardium.

4. Culture conditions

The first ESC was cultured on mouse embryonic fibroblast- feeder layer cells (MEF-FL) [Wobus, 2010]. Growing of stem cells in suspension as aggregates or removing of feeder fibroblasts promotes differentiation of ESCs [Dambrot et al., 2011]. Derivatives of three germ layers like mesoderm (cardiomyocytes, blood and vascular endothelial cells) were derived by this method [Dambrot et al., 2011]. By advent of novel culture media stem cells could be kept in undifferentiated state even in the absence of feeder cells. Commercial culture media as mTeSR®1 and TeSR™2 (STEMCELL technologies) in combination with matrix containing a mixture of human collagen IV, fibronectin, vitronectin and laminin are beneficial in this context [Dambrot et al., 2011]. The goal of these culture conditions is to promote stem cell scale up while keeping karyotypic stability through successive enzymatic passages or suspension cultures. This field of stem cell technology needs to be promoted further.

5. Special considerations

Surveys to find the candidate stem cell should be parallel with search to find the candidate animal model. By now, mice are the most common used animal models due to the feasibility of the mutation induction and targeted deletion in them. Despite of these advantages, there are some fundamental differences between mouse and human heart. The predominantly expressed isoform of Myosin heavy chain (MHC) in fetal and adult mice are βMHC and αMHC, respectively [Dambrot et al., 2011]. The inverse pattern is seen in humans. The higher beating rate of mice (500 bpm) is surprisingly different from human heart (70 bpm)

[Dambrot et al., 2011]. Some inherent properties of mESCs and hESCs are noteworthy but their clinical significance is still unknown. mESCs and hESCs differ in expression of surface markers and culture requirements, mainly attributed to the more naïve state of mESCs [Dambrot et al., 2011]. Regarding culture requirements for maintenance of undifferentiated state, mESCs are leukemia inhibitory factor (LIF)-dependent but humans are dependent to basic fibroblast growth factor (bFGF) and Activin/Nodal-controlled signaling pathways [Tesar et al., 2007, Xu et al., 2008]. Indeed, mESCs express SSEA-1 surface molecule rather than SSEA-3/4 in hESCs [Wobus & Löser, 2011]. These basic differences make scientist to seek for a more comprehensively matched research model for regenerative purposes and diagnostic applications. In vitro drug screening, drug geneotoxicity/mutagenecity, chemical safety assessment, predictive toxicology and cardiac safety pharmacology are other avenues for beneficial application of stem cell technology. Due to species-specific pharmaco-toxicological effects, animal models are not representative for human beings. Indeed, high number of animals needed for in vitro compound screening and toxicology tests [Wobus & Löser, 2011]. In vitro human cellular tests overcame the limitations of inadequate standardized animal-based tests [Wobus & Löser, 2011]. These species specific toxicology tests using immortalized human cell cultures were not real representative of normal cell types and mortal primary human cells loose their tissue-specific functions in cultures [Wobus & Löser, 2011]. Thus, stem cells can provide a good source of cells without the need for immortalization measures; facilitate human-specific cardiac pharmaco-toxicology test systems. These stem-cell based compound screening, is of paramount importance for drugs synthesized for treatment of acute ischemic events. Stem cells can be potentially used for preimplantation genetic diagnosis (PGD) and –screening (PGS) of cases with genetic predisposition to cardiac ischemic events, but this aspect of stem cell technology needs to be wrought further: extended EST (Embryonic Stem Cell Test).

Creating predictive in vitro human models of acute coronary events may be possible using cardiac stem cells. Stem cell-based models might be helpful both diagnostically and therapeutically. In terms of diagnosis and treatment, induction of gain-of function (selective turn-on) and loss-of-function (selective turn-off) mutations allows selective genetic manipulation of stem cells serving as vehicles. In addition, these assays are complementary to understand the effects of constitutively expressed genes in cell function and during the differentiation process. Loss-of-function mutations will potentially serve in identifying the cardiac lethality and survival genes. Generally, non-homologous joint recombination, homologous recombination, site-specific double-strand breaks and transpositional recombination are used strategies for genomic manipulation of stem cells [Dambrot et al., 2011]. Direct stem cell reprogramming using three cardiac transcription factors, mouse fibroblasts can be differentiated into the cardiomyocytes [Ieda et al., 2010]. Examination of a cocktail of genes, introduced Gata4, Mef2c and Tbx5 as "master regulator genes" for rapid and stable direct reprogramming of fibroblasts into cardiomyocytes [Dambrot et al., 2011]. This method showed superior efficiency to iPSC technology by eliminating concerns regarding the presence of residual undifferentiated cells [Ieda et al., 2010]. Accelerated delivery of cells to the patients with lower costs is other benefit of this method [Dambrot et al., 2011]. But the inability of these emerged cardiomyocytes to expand in vitro is its major limitation [Dambrot et al., 2011]. Adipose-derived stem cells are also an attractive easily accessible source of stem cells for clinical application. These cells safely improve both angiogenesis and myogenesis in injured heart. Finally, it should be beer in mind that the goal of stem cell differentiation methods should be achievement of functional myocardium.

6. Cardiac differentiation

By depletion of differentiation-repressing factors or growing cells as EBs, hESCs are easily committed to the target lineage [Dambrot et al., 2011]. EB-based directed differentiation occurs on specific matrixes in the presence of multiple inducers as growth factors, differentiation repressors or small molecules [Mohr et al., 2010, Boheler et al., 2002, Zwi et al., 2009, Mummery et al., 2007, Passier et al., 2006]. This method showed more success with mESCs rather than hESCs [Huangfu et al., 2008]. Spin EBs created from exactly defined cell numbers and centrifugated in V-shaped wells enhanced directed differentiation down the cardiac lineage [Ng et al., 2005, Ng et al., 2008]. Its yield is comparable with cardiomyocyte achievement of less than 5% of all cells using "hanging drop" EBs [Yoon et al., 2006]. Spontaneously beating cardiac clusters in the EB-outgrowths, varying in number from 8 to 70%, will be stable for up to three months [He et al., 2003, Kehat et al., 2001, Xu et al., 2002]. Contracting EB depends on the applied growth factors, cell line used and size of EB [Burridge et al., 2007, Pal & Khanna, 2007, Mikkola et al., 2006, Niebruegge et al., 2009, Mohr et al., 2010]. Moreover, crucial additions of major regulators of cardiac development as fibroblast growth factor (FGF), transforming growth factor-β (TGF-β), bone morphogenic protein (BMP), activin, vascular endothelial growth factor (VEGF), stem cell factor (SCF), ascorbic acid and members of Wnt family added the yield of this technique [Dambrot et al., 2011]. Some inhibitors like Wnt-inhibitor DKK1 (added to culture media at late stages), mitogen-activated protein kinase inhibitor (p38 MAPK) and glycogen synthase kinase 3 (GSK3) inhibitor added more to this yield [Dambrot et al., 2011]. Co-cultures with visceral endoderm-like cell lines (END) in serum-free media supplanted with Insulin or their conditioned medium is an alternative approach [Passier et al., 2005, Freund et al., 2008]. This method, applies mechanical rather than enzymatic passage of undifferentiated cells [Dambrot et al., 2011]. Co-culture with END-2 cell line led a more homogenous ventricular cardiomyocyte population [Mummery et al., 2003]. Laflamme et al achieved cardiomyocytes more efficiently than EB-derived cells using high-density monolayer model in serum-free medium in the presence of BMP4 and activin A [Laflamme et al., 2007]. Achievement of homogenous mature cardiac cells as homogenous atrial, ventricular, conduction fibers or a mixture of them is the main goal of directed cardiomyocyte differentiation [Dambrot et al., 2011]. Currently applied technique yield a heterogeneous cell population with cardiomyocytes ranging from 1% to ~50% of the total cell mass [Dambrot et al., 2011]. Indeed, the premature phenotype of induced cells is an important issue which needs maturation induction using cell re-plating or END-2 co-culture methods followed by limited three-dimensional culturing [Otsuji et al., 2010]. Cyclic stretches or forcing alignments might enhance tissue maturity further. Gradient centrifugation method isolates largely-sized cardiomyocytes, physically [Xu et al., 2006]. Cardiomyocyte harvesting based on the cell surface receptors like protein fetal liver kinase 1 [Flk1; also known as VEGF-receptor or kinase insert domain-containing receptor (KDR)] has been demonstrated [Yang et al., 2008]. This method will provide a mixed population of cells like endothelial progenitor cells (EPCs), endothelial cells, smooth muscle cells and some other undifferentiated cells [Dambrot et al., 2011]. An easy and reversible method of isolation has been introduced using reversible mitochondria labeling by tetramethylrhodamine methyl ester perchlorate

(TMRM) in the mixed cell population [Hattori et al., 2010]. This labeling yields three cell fractions as follow: cardiomyocyte with high fluorescent fraction, intermediate fraction of non-cardiomyocyte viable cells and dead low fraction or blood cells [Hattori et al., 2010]. In this way, cardiomyocytes are maintained more than 50 days in cultures [Hattori et al., 2010]. Alternation in culturing protocols might insight to valuable information about alternative approaches for obtaining cardiomyocytes. A yield up to 50% cardiomyocytes was achieved using feeder-dependent enzymatic passage of hESCs in knockout serum replacement (KOSR) followed by spin EBs and addition of BMP4 and activin A with subsequent re-plating [Ng et al., 2008]. As a complication of acute coronary syndrome, conduction defects are notable which calls attention for the importance of nodal cell achievement besides cardiomyocytes. For this purpose, inhibition of neuregulin (NRG)-1β/ErbB pathway has been shown to enhance nodal-like cell achievement, in vitro [Zhu et al., 2010].

7. Resident cardiac stem cells

Mammalian cardiomyocytes are not totally terminally differentiated post-mitotic cells and cardiomyocyte turn-over has been observed in adult hearts [Walsh et al., 2010]. In aggregate, CSCs seem more efficient and natural for cardiogenesis than other non-heart origin stem cells. Resident CSCs restore the dead myocardium by proliferation and differentiation into newly mechanically effective myocardium [Dergilev et al., 2011]. These cells are tissue-specific, mostly pre-committed to cardiac lineage fate [Limana et al., 2011]. Thus, activation of the few resident cardiac stem cells (rCSCs) available in the heart via exogenous factors might exert beneficial effects [Leri et al., 2005]. But their insufficient numbers limit the benefits derived from their activation. Some resident cardiac progenitor cells are explained here.

Side-population (SP) cells are some resident which trans-differentiate into mature cardiomyocytes by co-culture with mature ventricular myocytes. SP cells express Abcg2 transporter and exporters of Hoechst dye [Balbuena et al., 2011]. The immediate replacement of SP cell by bone marrow cells after AMI suggests the presence of homing mechanism and phenotypic conversion [Guan & Hasenfuss, 2007]. This inspires the possibility of SP cell hunting from peripheral blood and avoiding their extraction by surgery and cardiac biopsy. Among SP cells the maximum potency for cardiac differentiation belongs to the Sca-1^{+}, CD31^{-} cells [Pfister et al., 2005]. Cardiac SP-derived Cardiospheres, self-adherent clusters derived from mild enzymatic digestion of cardiomyocytes, express both endothelial and stem cell markers [Chamuleau et al., 2009, Reinecke et al., 2008]. These cells belong to CSCs and contain firm cardiac stemness phenotypes [Guan & Hasenfuss, 2007]. Cardiosphere-derived stem cells as well as C-Kit^{+} cells are able to differentiate into the major cardiac vascular and muscular specialized cells [Guan & Hasenfuss, 2007].

Skeletal myoblasts were the first relevant cells used clinically [Guan & Hasenfuss, 2007]. Upon transplantation into the infracted myocardium, these cells were clonally expanded, propagated and differentiated into myotubes clustering in specific foci and improved cardiac contractility [Guan & Hasenfuss, 2007, Taylor et al., 1998, Scorsin et al., 2000]. However, there is some controversies regarding the arrhythmogenicity of these cells [Moreno et al., 2010]. Another cardiac stem cell capable to contribute to approximately all cellular elements of the cardiac interstitium and coronary vasculature is referred as epicardium-derived cell (EPDC) [Lie-Venema et al., 2007]. EPDCs transplanted into mouse heart, improved LV function and attenuated pathologic remodeling mostly through an indirect paracrine pathway [Winter et al., 2007]. The clinical efficacy of these cells for human application is not yet well clarified.

8. Stem cell-based therapies for ACS

Inadequate cardiac regeneration and cell death with subsequent progressive remodeling following acute ischemic insults make a vicious cycle toward further degeneration: degeneration begets degeneration. Measures should be performed to break this vicious cycle at earlier reversible stages. Despite of the potential role of stem cells in the regeneration of advanced stages of disease spectrum, it will bring battery of influential effects if used at the acute phase of ischemic event. Final goal should be replacement of the damaged and necrotic regions with alive and regenerative cells. Stem cell nomenclatures based on their function, phenotype, special characteristics and practical applications for heart regeneration seem helpful. Stem cell-based cardiac repair put forth new therapeutic paradigms for treatment of relentless progression of heart diseases after acute myocardial insults. But it is still in its infancy.

9. Pre-administration perquisites

Prior planning for stem cell-based therapies, issues regarding their safety and feasibility should be determined. Ethical considerations for stem cell-based therapies should be identified based on the district rules. The risks and benefits of the proposed procedure, the superiority of this procedure over other approaches and its probable durability and reproducibility should be reviewed with patient. Signed informed consents are perquisite for stem cell-based therapies. Pre-hospital issues to potentiate outcomes of the cases intended for this treatment modality are unknown. In clinically indicated cases, electrolyte abnormalities should be corrected before stem cell implantation. Patients should be evaluated for arrhythmogenic clinical grounds. It is not yet determined if patients at high risk for development of life-threatening arrhythmia are eligible for stem cell-based therapies. By virtue of the predisposition to arrhythmia in ischemic myocardium, the amplified arrhythmia risk might not be clinically favored. The benefits should be weighted in patients with currently under treatment of fatal arrhythmia or cases with remarkable past history respective to these arrhythmias.

After all, it is noteworthy that each stem cell-based therapy should be administrated in equipped hospitals. Isolated stem cells should be transferred to intervention room easily. Perhaps, the best condition is performance of stem cell-based therapies in hospitals equipped with stem cell laboratories. This minimizes troubles and cautions related to cell transferring. Moreover, time wasting would be minimized. For this purpose, standardized cell isolation protocols and scale-up procedures should be emerged before wide clinical applications. Expanded stem cells should be characterized prior to clinical application. Of note, pre-administration evaluation of cell sterility, quality and functionality both in vitro (migratory and colony forming abilities) and in vivo (ability to reperfuse blood flow to ischemic district) should be performed. Technical challenges must be met thoroughly before clinical stem cell application. The impact of quality of cell processing and purity of the final cell on the final outcomes has been previously clarified. In an equipped hospital, a trained assembled team composed of basic stem-cell researcher, cardiologist and nurses is necessary. Caring nurses must be able to recognize and deal with the challenges specified to stem cells recipients. Cardiac surgeon should also be attendant if surgical cell delivery is intended. Thus, those qualified centers should have on-site surgical back-up. Both team and hospital should have certificates for these operations by maintenance of good tissue practice (GTP) and GMP (good manufacturing practice). Periodic quality control should not be missed. Minimal stem-cell based procedures per year for the team and hospital need to be defined by experts. High-volume operation centers might offer less risk to the patient compared with low-volume ones. Poor clinical attainments might be reflection of technical failure. But, to date there is no absolute definition for primary and late procedural success and failure. Of course, clinical failure attributed to time delay to reperfusion and major adverse cardiac events due complications of angioplasty should be discriminated from pure cell-related outcomes.

10. Administration of regenerative agents

By now the maximized cell migration and adhesion through percutaneous delivery of stem cells is done with stop-flow balloon catheter to achieve total flow occlusion within three minutes followed by stem cell infusion and reflow through deflation [Nuri & Hafeez, 2011]. In the case of extensive MI and multi-vessel disease, the eligible vessel should be identified. The superiority of antegrade vs. retrograde and proximal vs. distal stem cell delivery is not yet elucidated. Inflamed necrotic myocardium makes a hot microenvironment for delivered stem cells. The impact of this even slightly higher temperature on the efficacy of stem cells should undergo exploration. If any, cooling devices assembled with mechanical cell delivery instruments seem attractive. Perhaps stem cell eluting stents containing stem cell seeding on stem cell-friendly biomaterials without the problem of much scaffolding become available in future. If so, combination of drug-release plus stem cell-eluting stents and other combination might become revolutionary. Cells delivered directly through intracoronary route, need migration out of the vessel walls into the adjacent myocardium. This method brings the risk of coronary artery obstruction due to the plagued stem cells and consequently leads to further myocardial damage [Grieve et al., 2010]. The diameter of the target vessel and number of delivered cells seem detrimental with respect to cell stasis and vessel obstruction. The inherent risk of embolic events "cell embolism" is another limitation for intracoronary administration of stem cells [Zhang et al., 2007]. The underperfused myocardium potentially makes an unfavored environment for stable graft survival.

Intravenous stem cell injection has been shown to be safe for allogenic MSCs [Vassalli & Moccetti, 2011]. By intravenous cell administration, the majority of infused cells were shown to be harbored in kings and this cell trapping consequently limit the efficacy of this approach [Wang. et al., 2011]. Poor cell survival and drastic safety outcomes due to the extensive cell redistribution throughout the body limits this delivery approach. Alternatively, direct intramyocardial cell delivery is possible through transendocardial (percutaneous) or transepicardial (surgical) cell injection into the LV walls [Nuri & Hafeez, 2011]. Percutaneous route or "interventional cardiomyoplasty" requires retrograde passage of specially designed injection catheters into the left ventricle via femoral or arterial access [Psaltis et al., 2010]. Direct cell injection into the scar tissue or hibernated myocardium can be performed during open heart surgery or minimally invasive thoracostomy. Traumatic myocardial perforation especially at the site of freshly infracted tissue is a major side effect of this method.

The goal of catheter based needle intramyocardial cell injection should be promoted cell dispersion with limited immediate cell washout. Since formation of cell clusters rather than cell dispersion is proposed as a mechanism of arrhythmia-induction following stem cell application, dispersed-delivery techniques should be sought. Strategies which enhance homogenous and aligned cell integration with host tissue are more desired. But the most important item is delivery of healthy cells, not crushed or squeezed cells.

Myocyte-specific strategies prevent tumor formation and growth in other tissues and allow safe systemic delivery bypassing complicated local delivery approaches. Factors specific for cardiomyocytes in the contracting walls bordering the infract zone should be identified. This strategy might be potentially with pronounced efficacy without imposing side effects like hypertrophy on remote resident cardiomyocytes. Implantation of tissue-engineered autologous myoblast sheets showed promising results in rat, canine and porcine ischemic models [Sawa et al., 2010]. Sheets would cover larger area with fewer arrhythmogenic potential. Since stem cell therapy is not just based on the administration of crude stem cells, approaches for delivery of other regenerative agents should also be discussed here.

Stem cell application might be possible through seeding of stem cells on appropriate scaffolds and cell delivery at the site of damage. A step further back, might be approaches based on the enhanced homing of stem cells via promoted endogenous or exogenous stimuli with high specifity for stem cells involved in cardiac regeneration. Providing an accommodation for stem cells released after acute ischemic insult into the circulation, will be another alternative. These approaches will minimize the untoward effects of the exogenously delivered stem cells. A combination of exogenous stem cell administration and activation of endogenous stem cells using endogenous or exogenous stimulating factors might be attractive. Last, integrated and multi-disciplinary stem cell therapy for ACS needs fusing basic and clinical researches to narrow the gaps. Moreover, identification of key proteins involved in cardiac regeneration and cell differentiation opened the field of "Protein therapeutics". Proteins should be modified in the way to limit immunogenicity and rapid degradation in plasma and tissues. Delivered proteins exert paracrine effects on neighboring myocardium. Regardless of the type of regenerative agent, each candidate method should elicit a durable effect in a significant number of myocytes.

Irrespective of the applied method for myocardial cell delivery, cells should be engrafted in suitable place. Viable myocardial segments are most desired sites for cell delivery. Patients who suffered from ACS might have chronic scar tissues rather than freshly made scar due to the acute event. Obviously, cell grafting at the sites of chronic scars would be of no benefit. In addition, most of the directly injected cells die off soon due to the lack of nutrient and blood supply from necrotic tissue without live myocyte syncytium. Cell loss during and after transplantation lowers the efficacy of stem cell therapy.

Targeting the ideal site of cell deployment is of paramount value. This site reflects the mentioned regenerative focus which can send out constructive signals. Thus, numerous 3-D intracardiac navigation systems as electromechanical mapping techniques have been developed for correct cell seeding [Banovic et al., 2011]. Interrogation using intracardiac echocardiography might yield more. Mapping catheters integrated with injection ports conjunct with manipulated guiding catheters might help in direct endomyocardial injection mapping for targeted cell delivery. Optimal imaging techniques should be applied to both guide characterization of the cell-delivery site and monitoring the functionality and efficacy of the transplanted cells. Stem cell scintigraphy, lineage tracing and intravital imaging protocols might be helpful. Since the heterogeneity of the grafted stem cells with native myocytes is the principal cause of arrhythmia induction, one potential application of imaging modalities might be detection of patients with greatest uncoupling between grafted and native cells. In this way, patents at high risk for development of arrhythmia presumably could be identified earlier. Patients at high risk of arrhythmogenicity can receive prophylactic measures before development of life-threatening arrhythmias. Whether if routine stem cell tracking after application of stem cell-based therapies is valuable or not should be determined clinically. Labeled grafts facilitate following of applied cells, but need advent of non-toxic and or timely degrades labels. Non-invasive objectifying of myogenic cell grafts and assessment of the fate and bio-distribution of applied cells might be valuable in certain patient populations at risk of early stem cell failure. If so, such at risk patients should be characterized by risk assessment algorithms. Indeed, the importance of early detection of residual ischemia in patients seems valuable. Residual ischemia might limit the potential benefits of applied stem cell-based therapies as soon as the time of application. All of the deteriorating underlying conditions like anemia and poor glycemic control, in recipients of stem-cell based therapies should be approached similar to the patients receiving standard medical cares.

11. Post-administration perquisites

Induction of malignant arrhythmia by transplanted stem cells has been demonstrated in several studies. This increased incidence has been attributed to the non-synchronized contraction and electromechanical non-incorporation of novel myocytes with background cells [Song et al., 2011]. Other mechanisms as Anisotropy, scar-implanted cell interaction and the presence of immature cardiomyocytes with intrinsic pacemaker activities are also speculated [Dambrot et al., 2011]. Recipients should be monitored in-hospital with more intense attention to electrocardiographic evidences of arrhythmia. Electrolyte abnormalities in favor of arrhythmogenicity should be identified and eliminated earlier. Routine electrolyte evaluation might be remarkable after stem cell implantation for reduction of the risk of arrhythmia. In the case of life-threatening arrhythmia, prophylactic and therapeutic anti-arrhythmic approaches should be provided for the patient. At least in-hospital monitoring interval before discharge should be determined. Indeed, the optimal hospitalization place for the recipient should also be evaluated. When the recipient should be sent to the step-down wards out of CCU? Certainly, the observation unit for the recipient should be equipped with central monitoring systems for the occurrence of fatal and non-fatal arrhythmias. Really, the interval with the greatest risk of arrhythmia induction should be determined. The impact of traditional risk factors and multiple comorbidities on either exogenous and mobilized endogenous stem cell outcomes or organ toxicities should be determined clearly. Irrelative to the type of applied therapies, ongoing risk factor modification and life-style modification should be started at early hospitalization in patients suffered from acute coronary syndrome. These strategies impact the general efficiency of applied therapies as stem cell-based treatments in the recipient patients. After stem cell transplantation, recipient should be followed-up for functional performance, clinical complications and mortality. Follow-up modalities and intervals should be determined. In this context, stem cell-specific comorbidity index (CI) charts derived from long-term patient follow-ups are helpful.

12. Clinical trials

The first clinical attempt of cell therapy was performed using BMC (bone-marrow derived cells). Rapid transfer of BMCs from bench to bedside without the need for ex-vivo expansion facilitates their clinical applications. BMCs showed modest and reproducible improvement in cardiac function by enhanced angiogenesis, augmented myocardial perfusion [Segers & Lee, 2008, Sun et al., 2009]. Reduced end-systolic volume by these cells reflects reduced negative remodeling [Orlic et al., 2001]. Un-fractionated BMCs encompass heterogeneous stem cell population including stromal cells, circulating progenitor cells (CPCs), EPC, MSC and HSC [Soejitno et al., 2010]. These cells release biologically active factors in favor of healing of the infracted myocardium [Henning, 2011]. Meta-analysis demonstrated a mean absolute increase 3-4% in ejection fraction by intracoronary infusion of patient's own reconstituted BMC aspirate [Rangappa et al., 2010]. Despite of the patient's pain relief and improved systolic and diastolic cardiac performance, the ultimate long-term effects were limited [Passier et al., 2008, Mummery et al., 2010, van Ramshorst et al., 2009]. Practically, there is no proved superiority between BMCs and CPCs in terms of clinical utilities and both are readily aspirated and administrated in contrary with difficult expansion of competent cardiac stem cells (CSCs) [Soejitno et al., 2010]. Ex-vivo expanded BMCs and unfractionated CPCs were infused post AMI via intracoronary rout in Transplantation of progenitor cells and regeneration enhancement in acute myocardial infarction (TOPCARE-AMI) trial [Schächinger et al., 2004]. It showed improved regional and global wall motion up to 9 and 1.2 percentage points from baseline during 4-month follow-up [Soejitno et al., 2010]. Significant enhancement was found in coronary blood flow reserve, cardiac geometry and myocardial viability [Schächinger et al., 2004]. EPCs augment tissue perfusion through pro-neovasculogenic functions and show very low efficient cardiac trans-differentiation in co-culture with mature cardiomyocytes [Kawamoto & Asahara, 2007, Badorff et al., 2003]. These cells increase perfusion of the ischemic tissue [Murohara et al., 2000, Kawamoto et al., 2001, Kalka et al., 2000]. In bone marrow transfer to enhance ST-elevation infarct regeneration (BOOST) trial, Mononucleated BMCs applied days after post-MI coronary intervention, increased regional and global cardiac performance during 6-month follow-up [Wollert et al., 2004]. Similar to TOPCARE-AMI trial, most improvement was seen in infarct border zone. But unexplained statistically insignificant decline in LVEF after 18 and 61 months later occurred in treatment arm [Meyer et al., 2006, Meyer et al., 2009]. Sustained improvements in LV function after 12-month of follow-up has been underlined through post-PCI BMC application in Reinfusion of Enriched Progenitor cells And Infarct Remodeling in Acute Myocardial Infarction (REPAIR-AMI) trial [Schächinger et al., 2006]. There are some discouraging data from Autologous Stem Cell Transplantation in Acute Myocardial Infarction trial (ASTAMI) and Multicenter, randomized trial of intracoronary infusion of autologous mononuclear bone marrow cells or peripheral mononuclear blood cells after primary PCI (HEBE) trial which failed to demonstrate clinical benefits of intracoronary transfusion of BMC and BMC or CPC, respectively [van der Laan et al., 2008, Lunde et al., 2006]. Similar negative results with BMC were achieved by Leuven AMI trial with intracoronary application of BMCs 24 hrs after reperfusion in AMI cases [Janssens et al., 2006]. These patients showed improvement in regional function of only infracted segment [Janssens et al., 2006]. The same, Regeneration by Intracoronary Infusion of Selected Population of Stem Cells in Acute Myocardial Infarction (REGENT) trail failed to show promising outcomes of intracoronary infusion of bone marrow-derived selected $CD34^{+}CXCR4^{+}$ cells and non-selected mononuclear cells on LVEF or volumes [Tendera et al., 2009]. However, a trend in favor of cell therapy was found in patients with severely depressed LVEF [Schaefer et al., 2010]. In TOPCARE-AMI study, the potential role of BMCs in the pathogenesis of In-Stent restenosis and thrombosis has been advocated [Assmus et al., 2002, Schächinger et al., 2004]. These concerns are based on the advocates respective to enhanced restenosis due to progenitor cell-mediated plaque angiogenesis or inflammation [Assmus et al., 2006]. Increased restenosis rate seen with $CD133^{+}$cells arose these questions, but evidences support the risk related to the local inflammation due to applied mouse antibody for cell isolation [Assmus et al., 2006]. Contrary, mobilized BM-derived putative EPCs designated to decrease complications of iatrogenic vascular injury [Kawamoto & Asahara, 2007]. In this regard, REPAIR-AMI trial showed a substantial decreased necessity for revascularization procedures in patients with engrafted BMCs [Schächinger et al., 2006]. FINCELL study has declared that there is no globally increased risk of restenosis attributable to BMCs [Huikuri et al., 2008]. The increased risk of intramyocardial calcification in rats received BMCs have been found with no similar finding in related human cases [Kang. et al., 2004, Yoon. et al., 2004]. The clinical safety of BMCs regarding to adverse events and induction of malignant arrhythmia has been shown in BOOST and FINnish study of autologous bone marrow-derived stem CELLs in acute myocardial infarction (FINCELL) trials [Wollert et al., 2004, Huikuri et al., 2008]. SWiss multicenter Intracoronary Stem cells Study in Acute Myocardial Infarction. SWISS-AMI trial using autologous bone marrow mononucleated cells (BM-MNCs) is currently underway [Sürder et al., 2010].

The limited efficacy of BMCs led scientists for alternative stem cell source. MSCs are potentially differentiated into functional beating cardiomyocytes, especially by exposure to certain DNA-methylation inhibitors [Lu et al., 2010]. MSCs improved contractility by prevention of remodeling in the vicinity of non-infracted myocardium [Soejitno et al., 2010]. MSCs, easily isolated and expanded in vitro, are effective in restriction of ischemic wave propagation in the area adjacent to infarction by accelerating inflammation, angiogenesis activation, prevention of apoptosis and reducing the scar size and volume [Sokolova & Pavlichenko, 2010]. Unsurprisingly, efficacy of these cells proved clinically without adequate clues of remuscularization [Soejitno et al., 2010].Very low degree of cardiogenesis and donor cell incorporation (just seven MSC-derived cardiomyocytes per heart) was also seen [Soejitno et al., 2010]. These data inspire the presence of an indirect paracrine mechanism of actions [Mangi et al., 2003, Noiseux et al., 2006, Gnecchi et al, 2005, Gnecchi et al., 2006]. These paracrine effects also impact on the extent of scar and fibrotic tissue by exertion of anti-inflammatory, anti-apoptosis and anti-remodeling properties [Gnecchi et al., 2008, Burdon. et al., 2011]. Immunomodulatory actions and low immunogenicity of MSCs allow their safe application for allogenic transplantation [Pittenger & Martin, 20004, Aggarwal & Pittenger, 2005]. Another examined stem cell source for cardiac regeneration is hESCs. hESCs, cultured reliably and differentiated robustly into cardiomyocytes regenerate myocardium in infracted hearts, attenuate heart remodeling and contribute to LV systolic force development [Henning. 2011]. Despite their unambiguous cardiogenesis, limited data are available regarding their advanced maturation and seamless myocardial integration in vivo. To overcome obstacles regarding the risk of teratocarcinoma formation by hESCs, application of differentiated hESCs toward cardiac progenitor cells prior to transplantation into the hearts seems beneficial. The large pool of generated hESCs cardiac progenitor cells needed for this purpose is a limitation for this proposition. Ultimately, prevention of immune rejection and enhanced graft survival over long term are necessary to improve myocardial performance. There are some few studies with CD34 or CD133 positive cells, CD34 and CXCR4 double positive cells, hESC-CMs (cardiomyocytes) and hESC-CPCs (cardiac progenitor cells). A quiescent progeny of epiblast-derived progenitor stem cells, BM-derived very small embryonic-like cells (VSELs), enhanced LV contractility more efficient than that of HSCs in experimental MI models [Wojakowski et al., 2011]. But studies are limited for proper conclusions regarding clinical readiness and utilities of these cells.

13. Experiments on stem cell homing after ACS

Granulocyte-Colony stimulating factor (G-CSF) is the only safe exogenous factor has been investigated widely for the treatment of acute ischemic phase. Despite of the low myogenic differentiation potential of the homed hematopoietic stem cells by G-CSF, its angiogenic and anti-apoptotic effects on cardiomyocytes assumed to be beneficial [Segers & Lee, 2008, Harada et al., 2005]. It also accelerates infarct healing through facilitated infiltration of macrophages into the necrotic tissue and activation of matrix metalloproteinases (MMPs) [Minatoguchi et al., 2004]. G-CSF used within the early 37 hours after MI, showed modest but tangible effects on cardiac performance without any significant impact on mortality rate or vessel stenosis [Abdel-Latif et al., 2008]. G-CSF enriches and mobilizes a specific $CD34^{+}CD133^{+}$ sub-fraction of hematopoietic cells from whole blood [Powell et al., 2005]. Some contradictory results seen with application of G-CSF are attributed to its inhibitory effects on CXCR4 activity with consequent decrease in migration and homing of progenitor cells into the infarct tissue [Dimmeler, 2010]. Application of G-CSG mobilized cells in AMI showed more benefits rather than application of G-CSF alone [Kang et al., 2007]. Regarding stem cells homing, Hepatocyte-growth factor (HGF) has been demonstrated to decrease infarct size by improving angiogenesis and exerting anti-apoptosis properties on the damaged myocardium [Urbanek et al., 2005, Wang et al., 2004, Nakamura et al., 2000]. HGF has chemotactic effects on putative cardiac stem cells [Segers & Lee.2010]. Alternatively, Delivered protease resistant Stroma-derived factor (SDF-1 S4V) using self-assembled peptide nanofibers enhanced both vascular density and cardiac function in rats with AMI [Segers et al., 2007].

Stimulating Factor in Acute Myocardial Infarction (SITAGR-AMI) trial with administration of CD26/dipeptidyl peptidase 4 inhibitor in AMI, which augments SDF concentration, is currently underway [Theiss et al., 2010]. SDF potentially recruits endothelial progenitor cells (EPCs) [Segers & Lee.2010]. EPCs and BM-derived putative progenitor cells are potentially homed into infarcted heart tissue after by Erythropoietin (EPO) [Westenbrink et al., 2007]. Due to le discrepancies between preclinical and clinical results, large randomized placebo-controlled clinical trials are underway to scrutinize therapeutic benefits of EPO treatment for acute coronary syndromes. After all, the efficacy of each promising homing factor depends on the presence of relatively intact stem cell pool.

AMI is not just a fault with cardiac myocyte and defects in large vessels and microvasculature compose one tail of the spectrum. Although angiogenic factors as VEGF and FGF seem hypothetically beneficial, they failed to meet the primary endpoints in clinical trials [Segers & Lee, 2008]. This unsuccessful application has been attributed to the formation of tortuous, aberrant and leaky vessel walls [Carmeliet, 2005, Lee et al., 2000]. Formation of non-leaky vessels need orchestrated action of various proteins at different time intervals beyond mere VEGF and FGF. Thus, a comprehensive approach would be application of functional proteins at various time points but it is yet impossible. The tumorgenecity of angiogenic factors is also a great concern [Segers & Lee, 2008].

There are some limited experiments regarding the beneficial role of proteins capable to induce cell cycle reentry of cardiomyocytes for regeneration purposes. Some are explained here. Extracellular matrix play a fundamental role in remodeling is prevention of ventricular rupture after AMI [Matsumur et al., 2005]. Periostin delivered into the infracted rat myocardium through a patch of Gelfoam, induced cell cycle reentry of adult myocytes in the border zone of MI and stimulated mitosis of surviving myocytes [Kühn et al., 2007]. Although controversial, it improved cardiac function with decreased scar formation and remodeling of non-infarcted myocardium [Segers & Lee, 2010]. Another protein able to establish myocyte reentry is neuregulin, a member of epidermal growth factor family involved in proliferation and differentiation of cardiomyocytes [Lemmens et al., 2007]. Increased cardiac function and decreased infarct size were seen with daily intraperitoneal administration of neuregulin [Bersell et al., 2009]. This improvement was attributed to the proliferation of existing myocytes rather than prohibition of apoptosis or differentiation of progenitor cells [Bersell et al., 2009].

14. Limitations and clinical pearls

Ladder diagrams, evidence-based guidelines and evidence-based therapies for the use of stem cells in the cases afflicted with ACS should be prepared. The witnessed "Go with Guidelines" in the treatment of acute coronary syndrome should be extended to the field of cardiac stem cell-based therapies. It will be possible only after pooled analysis of large-scale proof-of-concept studies, clinical trials and sufficient data analysis for validity/reliability measurements and success/failure rate of the applied methods. Identification of ideal stem cell type and dose-regimen, optimal timing for initiation of stem cell therapy, safe cell hunting method, proper patient selection and administration method, justified cell tracking strategies and directed follow-up sessions, makes this a very difficult task. Lack of trials with long follow-up period is potentially problematic. Thus far, trials with longest follow-up period were BOOST (5 year), ASTAMI and REPAIRE-AMI trials (both 12 months). Indeed, some cell-related endpoints as engraftment rate, cell retention and dose-response relations besides remodeling, regional and global LVEF, death, MI quality of life, symptom relief and hospitalization for heart failure should be considered in trials. This will mirror both technical and clinical success.

Candidate stem cell must have remarkable capacity for expansion and unquestioned potential for cardiogenesis. And only cells with true cardiac differentiation could likely effect scar regeneration. Candidate stem cell should posses the potential to form long-term stable grafts with no or less inflammation. Absolutely, it should be kept in mind that there can't be such a stem cell ranking. Appropriate stem cell selection is partly a function of patient's general conditions. Advance age and chronic illness are among factors with significant effect on the proper propagation of isolated stem cells due to their premature death. Stem-cell's age, a reflection of patient's age, is a determinant factor of stem-cell's plasticity. Although it can't be simply stated that younger is better, advanced age, old stem-cells or in the other terms octa- and nonagenarian stem cells might be unable to construct a virtually unexhausted cellular reserve pool. Apparently, stem cell therapy should be tried in patients with anticipated life expectancy. Underlying disease sates as cardiovascular diseases per se, could directly or indirectly affect functional activity of the endogenous progenitor cell reservoir. Diminished production and mobilization of EPCs from bone marrow demonstrated in the milieu conflicted by endothelial cell dysfunction [Hill et al., 2003, Tepper et al., 2002, Vasa et al., 2001, Schmidt-Lucke et al., 2005, Werner et al., 2005]. Short telomere length of CPCs has been observed in these circumstances [Dimmeler & Leri, 2008]. The positive or negative effects of ischemic preconditioning on stem cells of cases with cardiovascular diseases are unknown. Hence, the impact of extracellular tissues and signals derived from non-myocardial component on patterned cardiac differentiation should not be overlooked. In addition, some stem cells work better in the presence of underlying comorbidities. It has been demonstrated that BMCs are more effective in ageing and DM individuals but less effective in males [Bai et al., 2010]. So, selection of best cell or "cardiogenic cell preference" should be tailored to the patient's primary clinical ground. Certainly, the infarct size is also of paramount vale in determination of the best stem cell source and mode of delivery. Large amounts of infarct territory might need cell type with more restoring capacity. The hypothetical "patient-specific stem cells" might be adjoined into "patient's cardiac specific stem cell" in foreseeable future. The optimum dose should also be determined per case; larger infarcts might need more cells. Inadequate cell number leads to delayed recovery and decreased patient survival, but stem cell oversizing and heart-cell mismatch would not be free of risk. Sufficient number of individual stem cells for clinical benefits seems to be a function of its natural properties related to survival potential and capacity of mass production. In the other word, enough new myocyte mass with appropriate vascular density should restore sufficiently mechanical function of heart. Routinely, dose regimens contain notes regarding administration intervals. Thus, heart as a challenging organ for repair and integration of reparative stem cells might need more than one simple stem cell transplantation. Do booster cells engrafted at time intervals add more clinical benefits? Hypothetically, is it beneficial to primarily transplant one type of stem cell with superior cardiac benefits following by application of another cell type of stimulating agent with hours or days later? In addition, is there any difference between required doses for males and females? Generally, longer telomere length was observed in females' hematopoietic stem cells which might lead to lower senesce of these endogenous reparative stem cells [Sidorov et al., 2009].

Regarding optimal timing, some investigators demonstrated that BMCs applied up to four days after AMI had no benefits whereas later cell engraftment (4-8 days) showed beneficial effects [Dimmeler et al., 2008]. In the other hand, some investigators recommend early timing of cell administration due to microenvironment alteration at the first week after AMI which modulates functionality of the homed cells. It has been attributed to the initial edema formation as a consequence of inflammation which disrupts optimal stem cell homing. In contrast, some evidences support the clinical benefits of stem cells with early stem cell application in AMI. As a matter of fact, stem cell harvesting is not an immediate process. Since some culture-dependent cell hunting methods require days prior to application, it might not be possible to isolate cells on the patient arrival to the hospital during acute events. But at not too distant future, progress in cell banks may provide some facilities for having available stem cells at the hospital stem-cell rooms. And physicians can order one cell type based on the patients' clinical scenario. Perhaps, some day stem cells become as available as chewing aspirin in emergency rooms. Cells derived from sources like bone-marrow, peripheral or umbilical cord blood are not sufficient in number. Ex-vivo cell expansion provides enough number of required cells from clinical point of view, but a bit concerns remains regarding induced stem cell differentiation than self-renewal in cultures rather. Anyway, harvested autologous stem cells can be expanded in cultures in contamination-free ambient soon in life and stored for possible use in future. But the large number of cell banks needed for individual patients and the costly procedure for scaling-up of these cells are serious drawbacks should be solved. Reasonably, stem cells can be pre-preserved for patients recognized to be high risk for acute cardiac events. This risk would be assessed using perfect risk predictors in males and females more than 45 and 55 years old, respectively. The overhanging concept of stored allogenic stem cells is interesting from clinical point-of-view. But the elicited immune-mediated inflammatory reactions at the site of cell delivery might accelerate tissue damage and stem cell removal. Obviously, the cardiopoietic paracrine effects of allogenic stem cells might exceed the disadvantages of immune-mediated reactions but needs to be determined. In the case of allogenic stem cell harvesting, the eligible donor should be defined. Perhaps a donor with fresh stem cells without any underlying disease is better. Females with longer stem cells compared with age-matched males seem more suitable for this application but it is not as simple as a coin flip. However, the necessity of immune-matched cells at the time of application is a great obstacle for clinical utilities of allogenic stem cells. Cardiomyocytes derived from iPSC lines are promising in this context due to obviation of this necessity, but iPS technology can't merit the cost-benefit criteria for clinical usefulness. However, there might be some tricks bypassing these problems as isolation of stem cells from umbilical cord blood (UCB) as an accessible and less immunogenic source of stem cells. By the progress made in perseveration of human umbilical vein blood banks every person can have unlimited access to homologues stem cells for application in acute coronary syndrome. But the outcomes of the freshly used vs. stored or cultured cells needs to be clearly determined. LVEF enhancement with BMCs was inversely correlated with their storage duration [Jiang et al., 2010]. Anyway, since exerted beneficial effects of cells might be related to their basic characteristics, the optimal timing factor for each stem cell should be identified individually.

Patient subsets that stem cell application could be possibly beneficial need to be determined carefully. Ample evidences support the significant clinical benefits of applied stem cells in ACS case with viable hibernated myocardium, large regional wall motion abnormalities or depressed LVEF below median. Patients with these eligibility indices could be identified clinically using imaging modalities as echocardiography and myocardial perfusion imaging. Other factors as severity of symptoms, extent of jeopardized myocardium, percentage of scar tissue, number and extent of diseased vessels, left main diseases, involvement of proximal part of LAD, coronary flow characteristic, presence and grade of collateral arteries to the ischemic region, the percentage of downstream viable myocardium, clinical signs of heart failure, prior MI, history of angina, high-risk sub maximal exercise test, rhythm stability, age, gender and comorbidities might help physicians in decision making.

There is still lack of risk-stratification strategies based on low-, intermediate- or high-risk patient categories relied on the positive cardiac enzymes and diabetes. Current cell-based therapies for all patients are expensive and with a high risk of failure. Therefore, patients hospitalized for AMI predicted clinically that current therapies are modestly effective and or nature of their acute event seems to be vexing, benefit more from stem cell therapies. Indeed, subgroups of patients with limited options and "no-option" or incurable cases are also ideal candidate for cell-based therapies. Elderly patients, cases with contraindication for thrombolytic therapy, poor vascular anatomy for intervention and high risk patients for CABG will put in this group. However, knowledge about the decreased In-stent thromboses and restenosis by homed EPCs in the site of stent deployment tempt routine post-angioplasty stem cell application [Silber et al., 2011]. This would be also limited to the cases with reliable clinical predictors of high rate of In-stent restenosis and thrombosis.

Furthermore, it should be answered if hemodynamically unstable persons due to complicated ACS can undergo stem cell therapy or not? If the most clinical benefits of stem cells are within the first hours of ACS, are cooling-off periods spent for patient stabilization are still beneficial or not? Since heart is intrinsically an integrated organ with both vascular and muscular components, re-visualization and re-muscularization should be simultaneous and in-parallel. In the other word, enhanced neovascularization and neomyogenesis are both needed and any mismatch between these two arms will be associated with lack of sufficient success. Benefits of improved neomyogenesis in the territory of infarct related artery without optimal revascularization should always be scrutinized. Certainly, the restoring cardiac stem cells have their own nutritional requirements and the improvement process will down-hill in the case of deficient supply. Stem cell therapy as a risk-mitigating treatment and ad-on therapy or primary therapeutic choice should be well evaluated in the management of patients in acute setting. Trials should asses the benefits of initial stem cell therapies vs. initial conventional or invasive strategies. Peliotropic effects of Angiotensin-converting enzymes or Satins might be beneficial on stem cell functionality but the stem cell protective dose of these agents might differ from routinely used in emergency departments, which seeks to be determined. The optimal timing of beneficial medications on stem cells should be identified which could be even as early as ex-vivo stem cell processing. Do dual and triple anti-platelets exert effects on the ultimate benefits of applied regenerative cells? If invasive strategies are certainly needed, which of the upstream stem cell therapy (at present and before PCI) or deferred (at the time of PCI) are superior? Are all patients with ACS good candidate for stem cell therapy? Acute coronary *syndromes* encompass a wide spectrum from unstable angina pectoris to non-ST elevation MI and ST-elevation MI (transmural and non-transmural). Are stem cell-based therapies beneficial in medically or spontaneously relieved unstable angina? Like indications for thrombolytic therapy, should stem cell-based therapies restricted to transmural STEMIs? Do patients suffered from isolated right ventricular or posterior AMI benefit from stem cell therapies?

These questions need tight answers before widespread use of stem cells in clinical practice. Some considerations for complicated acute ischemic events by cardiogenic shock, with the need for cardiogenesis in its pure sense, should also be determined. These cases should be stabilized using bridge-to-treatment or bridge-to-transplant interventions. Simultaneous application of regenerative stem cells might be helpful in this case prospectively. Whether stem cell therapy would impact other complications of AMI as ventricular septal defect, aneurysms and free wall rupture is not yet demined. Stem cell therapy may move to be applied simultaneous with surgical ventricular repair.

Items in which clinicians can determine the success rate of treatment based on the pre-and post-test probabilities should be characterized. The advent of algorithms for stem cell therapies is necessary for future perspectives to determine selective stem cell application of routinely for "all comers" in the subset of ACS. Even if these caveats are solved and chart lines become available, physicians should not be boxed in chart cages. Short of that, recipients should be reviewed in cardiac stem cell clinics conversant with issues particular for patients undergoing such therapeutic measures. In aggregate, progression of these stem and progenitor cell-based cardiac repair, require close interaction between scientists, clinicians and patients. Stem cell encyclopedia needs question-directed state-of-science trails.

Challenges for finding appropriate cell source offers clues toward creation of more conductive myocardium through environmental modifiers with enhanced cell survival, persistence, differentiation and proliferation. Cardiac regeneration is not merely relied on stem cells and the underlying scaffold for applied stem cells, both mobilized and injected, should not be overlooked. Engagement and disengagement of stem cells to heart niche is a finely tuned dynamic process. This delicate balance is remarkably altered under stress conditions as ischemia. Physical contact of delivered stem cells with cardiac nascent niche and neighboring cells enhance cardiomyocyte differentiation. Stem cells decide to become incorporated physical elements of newly formed vessels or myocytes partly based on the niche they have exposed. Knowledge about stem cell microenvironment and trafficking mechanisms would lead to profound understanding of enhanced engagement and depressed stem cell regression to the desired organ. In acutely infracted myocardium, the dominant harsh ischemic and cytokine-rich microenvironment, infiltrated by inflammatory cells imposes a Strong challenge to the transplanted donor stem cells. Will stem cells in delivered in this niche fate with cardiac ischemic memory? With niche therapy, niche environment can be modified in such a way to boost stem cell homing, migration, engraftment, retention and commitment. Niche-based fate determination is possible by providing stromal matrix, physical contact and chemical dialogue for invited and activated resident stem cells. A prepared niche regulates mobilization of cells into the circulation and enhances stem cell recruitment, homing and cell retention. In the other word, a favored niche helps in maintenance of stem cell compartment. In contrast, a disturbed niche might lead to cell dysfunction probably by exhaustion. The clinical significance of niche-based strategies or niche-targeting is not yet clarified in the field of coronary artery disease and needs to be addressed. Cardiac niche therapy should be adjoined to cardiac stem cell-based therapies, in a mutually complementary manner.

15. Concluding remarks future recommendations

Despite of the remarkable advances in the care of ACS, missed opportunities are still troublesome. These mismanagements include failure to deliver any form of reperfusion in about 30% of patients or delayed application of reperfusion strategies related to perpetuation of inefficient system of care [Moon et al., 2002]. Pathologic remodeling, which evolves immediately after AMI, alters the contractile properties of non-infarct zone and consequently impairs systolic and diastolic performance of the LV. Thus, cases with missed reperfusion are at risk of suffering from complications of adverse remodeling. To modify the disease process, recapitulation of stem cells has been proposed to ameliorate adverse remodeling and consequently improve LV function and angiogenesis. Tremendous effort is being put to functionally revitalize scar, non-contractile myocardium. Stem cells added one new dimension for the treatment of AMI with multi-faceted nature. It can be applied singly or combined to boost the efficacy of other therapies. The final aim of SCT for myocardial regeneration has been directed to compensating myocardial loss and restoring myocardial deficits. Encourages due to the positive preliminary results and solved safety and tolerability issues paced cardiovascular stem cell therapies, but so far it has faced with contradictory results. This field is plagued by paucity of trials and trials with skepticism should definitely reinforce whether stem cell therapy should be augmented or not. Although emerging field stem cell based cardiac regenerative therapies are still limited, continued development in this field will impact this area in the very near future. Advent of magic stem cell bullet(s) or cocktails of stem cell with or without growth factors and homing agents might be revolutionary events achievable in future. As Feynman stated at 1959 "There is plenty of room at the bottom".

16. References

Abdel-Latif. A., Bolli. R., Zuba-Surma. EK., Tleyjeh. IM., Hornung. CA. & Dawn B. (2008). Granulocyte colony-stimulating factor therapy for cardiac repair after acute myocardial infarction: a systematic review and meta-analysis of randomized controlled trials. Am Heart J 156(2):216-226.e9.

Aggarwal. S. & Pittenger. MF. (2005). Human mesenchymal stem cells modulate allogeneic immune cell responses. Blood 105: 1815–22.

Amado. LC., Saliaris. AP., Schuleri. KH., St John. M., Xie. JS., Cattaneo. S., Durand. DJ., Fitton. T., Kuang. JQ., Stewart. G., Lehrke. S., Baumgartner. WW., Martin. BJ., Heldman. AW. & Hare. JM. (2005). Cardiac repair with intramyocardial injection of allogeneic mesenchymal stem cells after myocardial infarction. Proc Natl Acad Sci U S A 102(32):11474-9.

Arai. T., Kofidis. T., Bulte. JW., de Bruin. J., Venook. RD., Berry. GJ., Mcconnell. MV., Quertermous. T., Robbins. RC. & Yang. PC. (2006). Dual in vivo magnetic resonance evaluation of magnetically labeled mouse embryonic stem cells and cardiac function at 1.5 t. Magn Reson Med 55(1):203-9.

Assmus. B., Walter. DH., Lehmann. R., Honold. J., Martin. H., Dimmeler. S., Zeiher. AM. & Schächinger. V. (2006). Intracoronary infusion of progenitor cells is not associated with aggravated restenosis development or atherosclerotic disease progression in patients with acute myocardial infarction. Eur Heart J 27(24):2989-95.

Bai. Y., Sun. T. & Ye. P. (2010). Age, gender and diabetic status are associated with effects of bone marrow cell therapy on recovery of left ventricular function after acute myocardial infarction: a systematic review and meta-analysis. Ageing Res Rev 9(4):418-23.

Balbuena. J., Pachon. G., Lopez-Torrents. G., Aran. JM., Castresana. JS. & Petriz. J. (2011). ABCG2 is required to control the Sonic Hedgehog pathway in side population cells with stem-like properties. Cytometry A 19. doi: 10.1002/cyto.a.21103.

Banovic. M., Ostojic. MC., Bartunek. J., Nedeljkovic. M., Beleslin. B. & Terzic. A. (2011). Brachial approach to NOGA-guided procedures: electromechanical mapping and ransendocardial stem-cell injections. Tex Heart Inst J 38(2):179-82

Bersell. K., Arab. S., Haring. B. & Kühn. B. (2009). Neuregulin1/ErbB4 signaling induces cardiomyocyte proliferation and repair of heart injury. Cell 138(2):257-70.

Boheler. KR., Czyz. J., Tweedie. D., Yang. HT., Anisimov. SV. & Wobus. AM. (2002) Differentiation of pluripotent embryonic stem cells into cardiomyocytes. Circ. Res 91: 189-201

Burdon. T., Paul. A., Noiseux. N., Prakash. S. & Shum-Tim. D. (2011). Bone Marrow Stem Cell Derived Paracrine Factors for Regenerative Medicine: Current Perspectives and Therapeutic Potentialfor Regenerative Medicine: Current Perspectives and Therapeutic Potential. Bone Marrow Research 2011 Article ID 207326

Burridge. PW., Anderson. D., Priddle. H., Barbadillo Muñoz. MD., Chamberlain. S., Allegrucci. C, Young. LE. & Denning. C. (2007). Improved human embryonic stem cell embryoid body homogeneity and cardiomyocyte differentiation from a novel V-96 plate aggregation system highlights interline variability. Stem Cells 25(4):929-38.

Cao. F., Lin. S., Xie. X., Ray. P., Patel. M., Zhang. X., Drukker. M., Dylla. SJ., Connolly. AJ., Chen. X., Weissman. IL., Gambhir. SS. & Wu. JC. (2006). In vivo visualization of embryonic stem cell survival, proliferation, and migration after cardiac delivery. Circulation 21;113(7):1005-14.

Cao. F.., Drukker. M., Lin. S., Sheikh. AY., Xie. X., Li. Z., Connolly. AJ., Weissman. IL. & Wu. JC. (2007). Molecular imaging of embryonic stem cell misbehavior and suicide gene ablation. Cloning Stem Cells 9(1):107-17.

Carmeliet. P. (2005). VEGF as a key mediator of angiogenesis in cancer. Oncology 69 Suppl 3:4-10.

Chamuleau. SA., van Belle. E. & Doevendans. PA. (2009). Enhancing cardiac stem cell differentiation into cardiomyocytes. Cardiovasc Res 82(3):385-7.

Dambrot. C., Passier. R., Atsma. D. & Mummery. CL.(2011). Cardiomyocyte differentiation of pluripotent stem cells and their use as cardiac disease models. Biochem J 434(1):25-35.

David. L., Samavarchi-Tehrani. S., Golipour. A. &Wrana. J. (2011). Looking into the Black Box: Insights into the Mechanisms of Somatic Cell Reprogramming. Genes 2: 81-106

Dergilev. KV., Rubina. KA. & Parfenova. EV. (2011). Resident cardiac stem cells. Kardiologiia 51(4):84-92.

Dambrot. C., Passier. R., Atsma. D. & Mummery. CL. (2011). Cardiomyocyte differentiation of pluripotent stem cells and their use as cardiac disease models. Biochem J 27;434(1):25-35.

Dimmeler. S., Burchfield. J. & Zeiher. AM. (2008). Cell-based therapy of myocardial infarction. Arterioscler Thromb Vasc Biol 28(2):208-16.

Dimmeler. S. & Leri. A. (2008). Aging and disease as modifiers of efficacy of cell therapy. Circ Res 6;102(11):1319-30.

Dimmeler. S. (2010). Regulation of bone marrow-derived vascular progenitor cell mobilization and maintenance. Arterioscler Thromb Vasc Biol 30(6):1088-93.

Ding. DC., Shyu. WC. & Lin. SZ. (2011). Mesenchymal stem cells. Cell Transplant 20(1):5-14.

Ding. L., Poser. I., Paszkowski-Rogacz. M. & Buchholz. F. (2011). From RNAi Screens to Molecular Function in Embryonic Stem Cells. Stem Cell Rev 28. [Epub ahead of print]

Draper. JS., Smith. K., Gokhale. P., Moore. HD., Maltby. E., Johnson. J., Meisner. L., Zwaka. TP., Thomson. JA.,& Andrews. PW. (2004). Recurrent gain of chromosomes 17q and 12 in cultured human embryonic stem cells. Nat Biotechnol 22(1):53-4.

Freund, C., Ward-van Oostwaard, D., Monshouwer-Kloots, J., van den Brink, S., van Rooijen, M., Xu, X., Zweigerdt, R., Mummery, C. and Passier, R. (2008) Insulin redirects differentiation from cardiogenic mesoderm and endoderm to neuroectoderm in differentiating human embryonic stem cells. Stem Cells 26: 724-733

Gnecchi. M., He. H., Liang. OD., Melo. LG., Morello. F., Mu. H., Noiseux. N., Zhang. L, Pratt. RE., Ingwall. JS. & Dzau. VJ. (2005). Paracrine action accounts for marked protection of ischemic heart by Akt-modified mesenchymal stem cells. Nat Med 11:367–8.

Gnecchi. M., He. H., Noiseux. N., Liang. OD., Zhang. L., Morello. F., Mu. H., Melo. LG., Pratt. RE., Ingwall. JS. & Dzau VJ. (2006). Evidence supporting paracrine hypothesis for Aktmodified mesenchymal stem cell-mediated cardiac protection and functional improvement. FASEB J 20: 661–9.

Gnecchi. M., Zhang. Z., Ni. A. & Dzau. VJ. (2008). Paracrine mechanisms in adult stem cell signaling and therapy. Circ Res 21;103(11):1204-19.

Grieve. SM., Bhindi. R., Seow. J., Doyle. A., Turner. AJ., Tomka. J., Lay. W., Gill. A., Hunyor. SN. & Figtree. GA.(2010). Microvascular obstruction by intracoronary delivery of mesenchymal stem cells and quantification of resulting myocardial infarction by cardiac magnetic resonance. Circ Heart Fail 3(3):e5-6.

Guan. K. & Hasenfuss. G. (2007). Do stem cells in the heart truly differentiate into cardiomyocytes? J Mol Cell Cardiol;43(4):377-87.

Guan. K., Wagner. S., Unsöld. B., Maier. LS., Kaiser. D., Hemmerlein. B., Nayernia. K., Engel. W. & Hasenfuss. G.. (2007). Generation of functional cardiomyocytes from adult mouse spermatogonial stem cells. Circ Res 8;100(11):1615-25.

Wobus. AM. & Löser. P. (2011). Present state and future perspectives of using pluripotent stem cells in toxicology research. Arch Toxicol 85(2):79-117.

Harada. M., Qin. Y., Takano. H., Minamino. T., Zou. Y., Toko. H., Ohtsuka. M., Matsuura. K,. Sano. M, Nishi. J., Iwanaga. K., Akazawa. H., Kunieda. T., Zhu. W., Hasegawa. H., Kunisada. K., Nagai. T., Nakaya. H., Yamauchi-Takihara. K. & Komuro. I. (2005). G-CSF prevents cardiac remodeling after myocardial infarction by activating the Jak-Stat pathway in cardiomyocytes. Nat Med 11(3):305-11.

Hattori, F., Chen, H., Yamashita, H., Tohyama, S., Satoh, Y. S., Yuasa, S., Li, W., Yamakawa, H., Tanaka, T. and Onitsuka, T. (2010) Nongenetic method for purifying stem cell-derived cardiomyocytes. Nat. Methods 7: 61-66

He. JQ., Ma. Y., Lee. Y., Thomson. JA.,& Kamp. TJ. (2003). Human embryonic stem cells develop into multiple types of cardiac myocytes: action potential characterization. Circ Res 11;93(1):32-9.

Henning. RJ. (2011). Stem cells in cardiac repair. Future Cardiol 7(1):99-117

Hill. JM., Zalos. G., Halcox. JP., Schenke. WH., Waclawiw. MA., Quyyumi. AA. & Finkel. T. (2003). Circulating endothelial progenitor cells, vascular function, and cardiovascular risk. N Engl J Med 13;348(7):593-600.

Hofmann. M., Wollert. KC., Meyer. GP., Menke. A., Arseniev. L., Hertenstein. B., Ganser. A., Knapp. WH. & Drexler. H. (2005). Monitoring of bone marrow cell homing into the infarcted human myocardium. Circulation 3;111(17):2198-202.

Hong. H., Takahashi. K., Ichisaka. T., Aoi. T., Kanagawa. O., Nakagawa. M., Okita. K. & Yamanaka. S. (2009). Suppression of induced pluripotent stem cell generation by the p53-p21 pathway. Nature 27;460(7259):1132-5.

Hong. H., Takahashi. K., Ichisaka. T., Aoi. T., Kanagawa. O., Nakagawa. M., Okita. K. & Yamanaka. S. Lee. AS., Tang. C., Cao. F., Xie. X., van der Bogt. K., Hwang. A., Connolly. AJ., Robbins. RC. & Wu. JC. (2009). Effects of cell number on teratoma formation by human embryonic stem cells. Cell Cycle 15;8(16):2608-12.

Huangfu. D., Osafune. K., Maehr. R., Guo. W., Eijkelenboom. A., Chen. S., Muhlestein. W. & Melton. DA. (2008) Induction of pluripotent stem cells from primary human fibroblasts with only Oct4 and Sox2. Nat. Biotechnol. 26: 1269-1275

Huikuri. HV., Kervinen. K., Niemelä. M., Ylitalo. K., Saily. M., Koistinen P, Savolainen. ER., Ukkonen. H., Pietilä. M., Airaksinen. JK., Knuuti. J. & Mäkikallio. TH; FINCELL Investigators. (2008). Effects of intracoronary injection of mononuclear bone marrow cells on left ventricular function, arrhythmia risk profile, and restenosis after thrombolytic therapy of acute myocardial infarction (FINCELL trial). Eur Heart J 29:2723–32.

In 't Anker. PS., Scherjon. SA., Kleijburg-van der Keur. C., de Groot-Swings. GM., Claas. FH., Fibbe. WE. & Kanhai. HH. (2004). Isolation of mesenchymal stem cells of fetal or maternal origin from human placenta. Stem Cells 22(7):1338-1345.

Medvedev. SP., Grigor'eva. EV., Shevchenko. AI., Malakhova. AA., Dementyeva. EV., Shilov. AA., Pokushalov. EA., Zaidman. AM., Aleksandrova. MA., Plotnikov. EY., Sukhikh. GT. & Zakian. SM. (2011). Human induced pluripotent stem cells derived from fetal neural stem cells successfully undergo directed differentiation into cartilage. Stem Cells Dev 20(6):1099-112.

Janssens. S., Dubois. C., Bogaert. J., Theunissen. K., Deroose. C., Desmet. W., Kalantzi. M., Herbots. L., Sinnaeve. P., Dens. J., Maertens. J., Rademakers. F., Dymarkowski. S., Gheysens. O., Van Cleemput. J., Bormans. G., Nuyts. J., Belmans. A., Mortelmans. L., Boogaerts. M. & Van de Werf. F. (2006). Autologous bone marrow-derived stem-cell transfer in patients with Stsegment elevation myocardial infarction: double-blind, randomised controlled trial. Lancet 367:113–21.

Jiang. M., He. B., Zhang. Q., Ge. H., Zang. MH., Han. ZH., Liu. JP., Li. JH., Zhang. Q., Li. HB., Jin. Y., He. Q., Gong. XR. & Yin. XY. (2010). Randomized controlled trials on the therapeutic effects of adult progenitor cells for myocardial infarction: meta-analysis. Expert Opin Biol Ther 10(5):667-80.

Kalka. C., Masuda. H., Takahashi. T., Kalka-Moll. WM., Silver. M., Kearney. M., Li. T., Isner. JM. &, Asahara. T. (2000). Transplantation of ex vivo expanded endothelial progenitor cells for therapeutic neovascularization. Proc Natl Acad Sci USA 2000;97:3422-7.

Kanawaty. A. & Henderson. J. (2009). Genomic analysis of induced pluripotent stem (iPS) cells: routes to reprogramming. Bioessays 31(2):134-8.

Kang. HJ., Kim. HS., Koo. BK., Kim. YJ., Lee. D., Sohn. DW., Oh. BH. & Park. YB. (2007). Intracoronary infusion of the mobilized peripheral blood stem cell by G-CSF is better than mobilization alone by G-CSF for improvement of cardiac function and remodeling: 2-year follow-up results of the Myocardial Regeneration and Angiogenesis in Myocardial Infarction with G-CSF and Intra-Coronary Stem Cell Infusion (MAGIC Cell) 1 trial. Am Heart J 153: 237.e1–237.e8

Kawamoto. A., Gwon. HC., Iwaguro. H., Yamaguchi. JI., Uchida. S., Masuda. H., Silver. M., Ma. H., Kearney. M., Isner. JM. & Asahara. T.. (2001). Therapeutic potential of ex vivo expanded endothelial progenitor cells for myocardial ischemia. Circulation 103:634-7.

Kawamoto.. A. & Asahara. T. (2007). Role of progenitor endothelial cells in cardiovascular disease and upcoming therapies. Catheter Cardiovasc Interv 1;70(4):477-84.

Kehat. I., Kenyagin-Karsenti. D., Snir. M., Segev. H., Amit. M., Gepstein. A., Livne. E., Binah. O., Itskovitz-Eldor. J.,& Gepstein. L. (2001). Human embryonic stem cells can differentiate into myocytes with structural and functional properties of cardiomyocytes. J Clin Invest 108(3):407-14.

Keravala. A., Lee. S., Thyagarajan. B., Olivares. EC., Gabrovsky. VE., Woodard. LE. & Calos. MP. (2009). Mutational derivatives of PhiC31 integrase with increased efficiency and specificity. Mol Ther 17(1):112-20.

Kooreman. NG,& Wu. JC. (2010). Tumorigenicity of pluripotent stem cells: biological insights from molecular imaging. J R Soc Interface 6;7 Suppl 6:S753-63.

Kraitchman. DL., Heldman. AW., Atalar. E., Amado. LC., Martin. BJ., Pittenger. MF., Hare. JM. & Bulte. JW. (2003). In vivo magnetic resonance imaging of mesenchymal stem cells in myocardial infarction. Circulation 13;107(18):2290-3.

Kühn. B., del Monte. F., Hajjar. RJ., Chang. YS., Lebeche. D., Arab. S. & Keating MT. (2007). Periostin induces proliferation of differentiated cardiomyocytes and promotes cardiac repair. Nat Med 13(8):962-9.

Laflamme. MA., Chen. KY., Naumova. AV., Muskheli. V., Fugate. JA., Dupras. SK., Reinecke. H., Xu. C., Hassanipour. M. & Police. S. (2007) Cardiomyocytes derived from human embryonic stem cells in pro-survival factors enhance function of infarcted rat hearts. Nat. Biotechnol. 25: 1015-1024

Ieda. M., Fu. JD., Delgado-Olguin. P., Vedantham. V., Hayashi. Y., Bruneau. BG. & Srivastava. D. (2010) Direct reprogramming of fibroblasts into functional cardiomyocytes by defined factors. Cell 142: 375-386

Lee. RJ., Springer. ML., Blanco-Bose. WE., Shaw. R., Ursell. PC. & Blau. HM. (2000). VEGF gene delivery to myocardium: deleterious effects of unregulated expression. Circulation 22;102(8):898-901.

Leri. A., Kajstura. J. & Anversa. P. (2005). Cardiac stem cells and mechanisms of myocardial regeneration. hysiol Rev 85(4):1373-416.

Lemmens. K., Doggen. K. & De Keulenaer. GW. (2007). Role of neuregulin-1/ErbB signaling in cardiovascular physiology and disease: implications for therapy of heart failure. Circulation 21;116(8):954-60.

Lie-Venema. H., van den Akker. NM., Bax. NA., Winter. EM., Maas. S., Kekarainen. T., Hoeben. RC., deRuiter. MC., Poelmann. RE. & Gittenberger-de Groot. AC.(2007). Origin, fate, and function of epicardium-derived cells (EPDCs) in normal and abnormal cardiac development. ScientificWorldJournal 12;7:1777-98.

Limana. F., Capogrossi. MC. & Germani. A. (2011). The epicardium in cardiac repair: from the stem cell view. Pharmacol Ther129(1):82-96.

Lin. Q., Fu. Q., Zhang. Y., Wang. H., Liu. Z., Zhou. J., Duan. C., Wang. Y., Wu. K. & Wang. C.(2010). Tumourigenesis in the infarcted rat heart is eliminated through differentiation and enrichment of the transplanted embryonic stem cells. Eur J Heart Fail 12(11):1179-85

Liu. Y., Thyagarajan. B., Lakshmipathy. U., Xue. H., Lieu. P., Fontes. A., MacArthur. CC., Scheyhing. K., Rao. MS. & Chesnut. JD. (2009). Generation of platform human embryonic stem cell lines that allow efficient targeting at a predetermined genomic location. Stem Cells Dev 18(10):1459-72.

Lodi. D., Iannitti. T. & Palmieri. B. (2011). Stem cells in clinical practice: applications and warnings. J Exp Clin Cancer Res 17;30:9.

Lu. T., Pelacho. B., Hao. H., Luo. M., Zhu. J., Verfaillie. CM., Tian. J. & Liu. Z. (2010). Cardiomyocyte differentiation of rat bone marrow multipotent progenitor cells is associated with downregulation of Oct-4 expression. Tissue Eng Part A 16(10):3111-7.

Lunde. K., Solheim. S., Aakhus. S., Arnesen. H., Abdelnoor. M., Egeland. T., Endresen. K., Ilebekk. A., Mangschau. A., Fjeld. JG., Smith. HJ., Taraldsrud. E., Grøgaard. HK., Bjørnerheim. R., Brekke. M., Müller. C., Hopp. E., Ragnarsson. A., Brinchmann. JE. & Forfang. K.. (2006). Intracoronary injection of mononuclear bone marrow cells in acute myocardial infarction. N Engl J Med 355:1199–209.

Murohara. T., Ikeda. H., Duan. J., Shintani. S., Sasaki. K., Eguchi. H., Onitsuka. I., Matsui. K. & Imaizumi. T. (2000). Transplanted cord blood-derived endothelial precursor cells augment postnatal neovascularization. J Clin Invest 105:1527-36.

MacLaren. DC., Gambhir. SS., Satyamurthy. N., Barrio. JR., Sharfstein. S., Toyokuni T., Wu. L., Berk. AJ., Cherry. SR., Phelps. ME. & Herschman. HR. (1999). Repetitive, non-invasive imaging of the dopamine D2 receptor as a reporter gene in living animals. Gene Ther. 6(5):785-91.

Mangi. AA., Noiseux. N., Kong. D., He. H, Rezvani. M., Ingwall. JS. & Dzau. VJ.. (2003). Mesenchymal stem cells modified with Akt prevent remodeling and restore performance of infarcted hearts. Nat Med 9:1195–201.

Mathers, CD. & Loncar, D. (2006). Projections of global mortality and burden of disease from 2002 to 2030. PLoS Med 3(11):e442.

Matsumura. S., Iwanaga. S., Mochizuki. S., Okamoto. H., Ogawa. S.,& Okada. Y. (2005). Targeted deletion or pharmacological inhibition of MMP-2 prevents cardiac rupture after myocardial infarction in mice. J Clin Invest 115(3):599-609.

Meyer GP, Wollert KC, Lotz J, Steffens J, Lippolt P, Fichtner S, Hecker H, Schaefer A, Arseniev L, Hertenstein B, Ganser A, Drexler H. (2006). Intracoronary bone marrow cell transfer after myocardial infarction: eighteen months' follow-up data from the randomized, controlled BOOST (BOne marrOw transfer to enhance ST-elevation infarct regeneration) trial. Circulation 113:1287–94.

Meyer GP, Wollert KC, Lotz J, Pirr J, Rager U, Lippolt P Hahn A, Fichtner S, Schaefer A, Arseniev L, Ganser A, Drexler H. (2009). Intracoronary bone marrow cell transfer after myocardial infarction: 5-year follow-up from the randomized-controlled BOOST trial. Eur Heart J. 30:2978-84.

Mihu. CM., Mihu. D., Costin. N., Rus Ciuca. D., Susman. S. & Ciortea. R. (2008). Isolation and characterization of stem cells from the placenta and the umbilical cord. Rom J Morphol Embryol 49(4):441-446.

Mikkola. M., Olsson. C., Palgi. J., Ustinov. J., Palomaki. T., Horelli-Kuitunen. N., Knuutila. S., Lundin. K., Otonkoski. T. & Tuuri. T. (2006). Distinct differentiation characteristics of individual human embryonic stem cell lines. BMC Dev Biol 8 (6):40.

Minatoguchi. S., Takemura. G., Chen. XH., Wang. N., Uno. Y., Koda. M., Arai. M., Misao. Y., Lu. C., Suzuki. K., Goto. K, Komada A., Takahashi. T., Kosai. K., Fujiwara. T. & Fujiwara. H. (2004). Acceleration of the healing process and myocardial regeneration may be important as a mechanism of improvement of cardiac function and remodeling by postinfarction granulocyte colony-stimulating factor treatment. Circulation 109:2572-80.

Mingxia. Z., Jinyuan. Z., Guian.C. & Li. G. (2011). Early embryonic sensitivity to cyclophosphamide in cardiac differentiation from human embryonic stem cells. Cell Biol Int 12 [Epub ahead of print]

Miyagawa. M., Beyer. M., Wagner. B., Anton. M., Spitzweg. C., Gansbacher. B., Schwaiger. M.& Bengel. FM. (2005). Cardiac reporter gene imaging using the human sodium/iodide symporter gene. asc Res 1;65(1):195-202.

Mohr. JC., Zhang. J., Azarin SM., Soerens. AG., de Pablo. JJ., Thomson. JA., Lyons. GE., Palecek. SP. & Kamp, T. J. (2010) The microwell control of embryoid body size in order to regulate cardiac differentiation of human embryonic stem cells. Biomaterials 31: 1885-1893 Moreno. J., Quintanilla. JG., López-Farré. A., Archondo. T., Cervigón. R., Aragoncillo. P., Usandizaga. E., Silva. J., Rodríguez-Bobada. C., Rojo. JL., Pérez-Castellano. N., Mironov. S., Mont. L., Pérez de Prada. T., Macaya. C. & Pérez-Villacastín. J. (2010). Skeletal myoblast implants induce minor propagation delays, but do not promote arrhythmias in the normal swine heart. Europace 12(11):1637-44.

Moon. JC., Kalra. PR. & Coats. AJ. (2002). DANAMI-2: is primary angioplasty superior to thrombolysis in acute MI when the patient has to be transferred to an invasive centre? Int J Cardiol 85(2-3):199-201.

Mummery. C., Ward-van Oostwaard. D., Doevendans. P., Spijker. R., Van Den Brink. S., Hassink. R., van der Heyden. M., Opthof. T., Pera. M. & de la Riviere. AB. (2003) Differentiation of human embryonic stem cells to cardiomyocytes: role of coculture with visceral endoderm-like cells. Circulation 107: 2733-2740 Mummery. C., Van Der Heyden. MA., de Boer. TP., Passier. R., Ward. D., Van Den Brink. S., van Rooijen. M. & van de Stolpe. A. (2007) Cardiomyocytes from human and mouse embryonic stem cells. Methods Mol. Med 140: 249-272

Mummery. CL., Davis. RP. & Krieger. JE. (2010) Challenges in using stem cells for cardiac repair. Sci. Transl. Med 2: 27ps17

Nakagawa. M., Takizawa. N., Narita. M., Ichisaka. T., Yamanaka. S. (2010). Promotion of direct reprogramming by transformation-deficient Myc. Proc. Natl Acad. Sci. USA 107: 14 152–14 157

Nakamura T, Mizuno S, Matsumoto K, Sawa Y, Matsuda H, Nakamura T. (2000). Myocardial protection from ischemia/reperfusion injury by endogenous and exogenous HGF. J Clin Invest 106(12):1511-9.

Niebruegge. S., Bauwens. CL., Peerani. R., Thavandiran. N., Masse. S., Sevaptisidis. E., Nanthakumar. K., Woodhouse. K., Husain. M., Kumacheva. E. & Zandstra. PW. (2009). Generation of human embryonic stem cell-derived mesoderm and cardiac cells using size-specified aggregates in an oxygen-controlled bioreactor. Biotechnol Bioeng 102(2):493-507.

Ng. ES., Davis. RP., Azzola. L., Stanley. EG. & Elefanty. AG. (2005) Forced aggregation of defined numbers of human embryonic stem cells into embryoid bodies fosters robust, reproducible hematopoietic differentiation. Blood 106: 1601-1603

Ng. ES., Davis. R., Stanley. EG. & Elefanty. AG. (2008) A protocol describing the use of a recombinant protein-based, animal product-free medium (APEL) for human embryonic stem cell differentiation as spin embryoid bodies. Nat. Protoc 3: 768-776

Noiseux. N., Gnecchi. M., Lopez-Ilasaca. M., Zhang. L., Solomon. SD., Deb. A., Dzau. VJ. &Pratt. RE.. (2006). Mesenchymal stem cells overexpressing Akt dramatically repair infarcted myocardium and improve cardiac function despite infrequent cellular fusion or differentiation. Mol Ther 14:840–50.

Nordin. N., Lai. M., Veerakumarasivam. A., Ramasamy. R., Abdullah. S., Wendy-Yeo. W. & Rosli. R. (2011). Induced Pluripotent Stem Cells: History, Properties and Potential Applications. Med J Malaysia 66 (1)

Nuri. M. & Hafeez Sh (2011). Intracoronary administration of autologous bone marrow stem cell transplant in myocardial infarction. Jpma 61: 3

Passier. R., Oostwaard. DW., Snapper. J., Kloots. J., Hassink. RJ., Kuijk. E., Roelen. B., de la Riviere. A B. & Mummery. C. (2005) Increased cardiomyocyte differentiation from human embryonic stem cells in serum-free cultures. Stem Cells 23: 772-780

Passier. R., Denning. C. & Mummery, C. (2006) Cardiomyocytes from human embryonic stem cells. Handb. Exp. Pharmacol. 174, 101-122

Powell. TM., Paul. JD., Hill. JM., Thompson. M., Benjamin. M., Rodrigo. M., McCoy. JP., Read. EJ., Khuu. HM., Leitman. SF., Finkel. T. & Cannon. RO 3rd. (2005). Granulocyte colony-stimulating factor mobilizes functional endothelial progenitor cells in patients with coronary artery disease. Arterioscler Thromb Vasc Biol 25(2):296-301.

Okita. K. & Yamanaka.S. (2011). Induced pluripotent stem cells: opportunities and challenges. Philos Trans R Soc Lond B Biol Sci 366(1575):2198-207.

Orlic D, Kajstura J, Chimenti S, Jakoniuk I, Anderson SM, Li B, Pickel J, McKay R, Nadal-Ginard B, Bodine DM, Leri A, Anversa P. (2001). Bone marrow cells regenerate infarcted myocardium. Nature 410:701-5.

Otsuji. TG., Minami. I., Kurose. Y., Yamauchi. K., Tada. M. & Nakatsuji. N. (2010) Progressive maturation in contracting cardiomyocytes derived from human embryonic stem cells: qualitative effects on electrophysiological responses to drugs. Stem Cell Res 4: 201-213

Pal. R. & Khanna. A. (2007). Similar pattern in cardiac differentiation of human embryonic stem cell lines, BG01V and ReliCellhES1, under low serum concentration supplemented with bone morphogenetic protein-2. Differentiation 75(2):112-22.

Passier. R., van Laake. LW. & Mummery. CL. (2008) Stem-cell-based therapy and lessons from the heart. Nature 453: 322-329

Pfister. O., Mouquet. F., Jain. M., Summer. R., Helmes. M., Fine. A, Colucci. WS. & Liao. R. (2005). CD31−but Not CD31+ cardiac side population cells exhibit functional cardiomyogenic differentiation. Circ Res 97:52–61.

Pittenger. MF. & Martin (2004). BJ. Mesenchymal stem cells and their potential as cardiac therapeutics. Circ Res 95:9–20.

Polo. JM., Liu. S., Figueroa. ME., Kulalert. W., Eminli. S., Tan. KY., Apostolou. E., Stadtfeld. M., Li. Y., Shioda. T., Natesan. S., Wagers. AJ., Melnick. A., Evans. T. & Hochedlinger. K. (2010). Cell type of origin influences the molecular and functional properties of mouse induced pluripotent stem cells. Nat Biotechnol 28(8):848-55.

Psaltis. PJ., Zannettino. AC., Gronthos. S. & Worthley. SG. (2010). Intramyocardial navigation and mapping for stem cell delivery. J Cardiovasc Transl Res 3(2):135-46.

Rangappa. S., Makkar. R. & Forrester. J. (2010). Review article: current status of myocardial regeneration: new cell sources and new strategies. J Cardiovasc Pharmacol Ther 15(4):338-43.

Reinecke. H., Minami. E., Zhu. WZ. & Laflamme. MA. (2008). Cardiogenic differentiation and transdifferentiation of progenitor cells. Circ Res 103(10):1058-71.

Ren. J., Zhang. S., Kovacs. A., Wang. Y. & Muslin. AJ. (2005). Role of p38alpha MAPK in cardiac apoptosis and remodeling after myocardial infarction. J Mol Cell Cardiol 38(4):617-23.

Sawa. Y. (2010). [Myocardial regeneration for heart failure]. Nihon Rinsho 68(4):719-25.

Schächinger. V., Erbs. S., Elsässer. A., Haberbosch. W., Hambrecht. R., Hölschermann. H., Yu. J., Corti. R., Mathey. DG., Hamm. CW., Süselbeck. T., Assmus. B., Tonn. T., Dimmeler. S. & Zeiher. AM.; REPAIR-AMI Investigators. (2006). Intracoronary bone marrow derived progenitor cells in acute myocardial infarction (REPAIR-AMI trial). N Engl J Med 355:1210–21.

Schächinger. V., Assmus. B., Britten. MB., Honold. J., Lehmann. R., Teupe. C., Abolmaali. ND., Vogl. TJ., Hofmann. WK., Martin. H., Dimmeler. S. & Zeiher. AM. (2004). Transplantation of progenitor cells and regeneration enhancement in acute myocardial infarction: final one-year results of the TOPCARE-AMI Trial. J Am Coll Cardiol 19;44(8):1690-9.

Schaefer. A., Zwadlo. C., Fuchs. M., Meyer. GP., Lippolt. P., Wollert. KC. & Drexler. H. (2010). Long-term effects of intracoronary bone marrow cell transfer on diastolic function in patients after acute myocardial infarction: 5-year results from the randomized-controlled BOOST trial--an echocardiographic study. Eur J Echocardiogr 11(2):165-71.

Schmidt-Lucke. C., Rössig. L., Fichtlscherer. S., Vasa. M., Britten. M., Kämper. U., Dimmeler. S. & Zeiher. AM. (2005). Reduced number of circulating endothelial progenitor cells predicts future cardiovascular events: proof of concept for the clinical importance of endogenous vascular repair. Circulation 111(22):2981-7.

Scorsin. M., Hagège. A., Vilquin. JT., Fiszman. M., Marotte. F., Samuel. JL., Rappaport. L., Schwartz. K. & Menasché. P (2000). Comparison of the effects of fetal cardiomyocyte and skeletal myoblast transplantation on postinfarction left ventricular function. J Thorac Cardiovasc Surg119:1169–75.

Segers. VF&Lee. RT. (2008). Stem-cell therapy for cardiac disease. Nature;451(7181):937-42.

Segers. VF., Tokunou. T., Higgins. LJ., MacGillivray. C., Gannon. J. & Lee RT. (2007). Local delivery of protease-resistant stromal cell derived factor-1 for stem cell recruitment after myocardial infarction. Circulation 116(15):1683-92.

Segers. VF. & Lee. RT. (2010). Protein therapeutics for cardiac regeneration after myocardial infarction. J Cardiovasc Transl Res 3(5):469-77.

Si-Tayeb. K., Noto. FK., Sepac. A., Sedlic. F., Bosnjak. ZJ., Lough. JW.,& Duncan. SA. (2010). Generation of human induced pluripotent stem cells by simple transient transfection of plasmid DNA encoding reprogramming factors. BMC Dev Biol 3 (10): 81.

Sidorov. I., Kimura. M., Yashin. A. & Aviv. A. (2009). Leukocyte telomere dynamics and human hematopoietic stem cell kinetics during somatic growth. Exp Hematol;37(4):514-24.

Gurdon. JB. & Wilmut. I. (2011). Nuclear transfer to eggs and oocytes. Cold Spring Harb Perspect Biol 1;3(6).

Silber. S., Damman. P., Klomp. M., Beijk. MA., Grisold. M., Ribeiro. EE., Suryapranata. H., Wójcik. J., Hian Sim. K., Tijssen. JG. & de Winter. RJ. (2011). Clinical results after coronary stenting with the Genous™ Bio-engineered R stent™: 12-month outcomes of the e-HEALING (Healthy Endothelial Accelerated Lining Inhibits Neointimal Growth) worldwide registry. EuroIntervention 6(7):819-25.

Sinn. PL., Sauter. SL. & McCray. Jr. (2005). Gene therapy progress and prospects: development of improved lentiviral and retroviral vectors--design, biosafety, and production. Gene Ther 12(14):1089-98.

Škalamera. D., Ranall. MV., Wilson. BM., Leo. P., Purdon. AS., Hyde. C., Nourbakhsh. E., Grimmond. SM., Barry. SC., Gabrielli. B. & Gonda. TJ. (2011). A high-throughput platform for lentiviral overexpression screening of the human ORFeome. PLoS One 6(5):e20057.

Soejitno. A., Wihandani. DM. & Kuswardhani. RA. (2010). Clinical applications of stem cell therapy for regenerating the heart. Acta Med Indones 42(4):243-57

Sokolova. IB. & Pavlichenko. NN. (2010). Possible ways of MSCs influence on the ischemic tissue in the case of cardiovascular diseases. Tsitologiia 52(11):911-7.

Song. H., Hwang. HJ., Chang. W., Song. BW., Cha. MJ., Kim. IK., Lim. S., Choi. EJ., Ham. O., Lee. CY., Park. JH., Lee. SY., Choi. E., Lee. C., Lee. M., Lee. MH., Kim. SH., Jang. Y. & Hwang. KC. (2011). Cardiomyocytes from phorbol myristate acetate-activated mesenchymal stem cells restore electromechanical function in infarcted rat hearts. Proc Natl Acad Sci U S A 108(1):296-301.

Stadtfeld. M., Nagaya. M., Utikal. J., Weir. G. & Hochedlinger. K. (2008). Induced pluripotent stem cells generated without viral integration. Science 322(5903):945-9.

Stadtfeld. M. & Hochedlinger. K. (2010). Induced pluripotency: history, mechanisms, and applications. Genes Dev 24(20):2239-63.

Sun. J., Li. SH., Liu. SM., Wu. J., Weisel. RD., Zhuo. YF., Yau. TM., Li. RK. & Fazel. SS. (2009). Improvement in cardiac function after bone marrow cell thearpy is associated with an increase in myocardial inflammation. Am J Physiol Heart Circ Physiol 296(1):H43-50.

Sürder. D., Schwitter. J., Moccetti. T., Astori. G., Rufibach. K., Plein. S., Lo Cicero. V., Soncin. S., Windecker. S., Moschovitis. A., Wahl. A., Erne. P., Jamshidi. P., Auf der Maur. C., Manka. R., Soldati. G., Bühler. I,. Wyss. C., Landmesser. U., Lüscher. TF.& Corti. R. (2010). Cell-based therapy for myocardial repair in patients with acute myocardial infarction: rationale and study design of the SWiss multicenter Intracoronary Stem cells Study in Acute Myocardial Infarction (SWISS-AMI). Am Heart J 160(1):58-64.

Swelstad. B. & Kerr. C. (2009). Current protocols in the generation of pluripotent stem cells: theoretical methodological and clinical considerations. Stem Cells and Cloning: Advances and Applications 21:1009

Takahashi. K., Tanabe. K., Ohnuki. M., Narita. M., Ichisaka. T., Tomoda. K. & Yamanaka. S. (2007). Induction of pluripotent stem cells from adult human fibroblasts by defined factors. Cell 131(5):861-72.

Tan. JC., Li. Y., Qu. WY., Liu. LY., Jiang. L. & Sun. KL. (2008). Derivation of embryonic stem cell line from frozen human embryos and neural differentiation. Neuroreport 19(15):1451-5.

Taylor. DA., Atkins. BZ., Hungspreugs. P., Jones. TR., Reedy. MC., Hutcheson. KA., Glower. DD., Kraus. WE. (1998). Regenerating functional myocardium: improved performance after skeletal myoblast transplantation. Nat Med 4:929–33.

Tendera. M., Wojakowski. W., Ruzyłło. W., Chojnowska. L., Kepka. C., Tracz. W., Musiałek. P., Piwowarska. W., Nessler. J., Buszman. P., Grajek. S., Breborowicz. P., Majka. M. & Ratajczak. MZ; REGENT Investigators. (2009). Intracoronary infusion of bone marrow-derived selected CD34+CXCR4+ cells and non-selected mononuclear cells in patients with acute STEMI and reduced left ventricular ejection fraction: results of randomized, multicentre Myocardial Regeneration by Intracoronary Infusion of Selected Population of Stem Cells in Acute Myocardial Infarction (REGENT) Trial. Eur Heart J 30(11):1313-21.

Tepper. OM., Galiano. RD., Capla. JM., Kalka. C., Gagne. PJ., Jacobowitz. GR., Levine. JP. & Gurtner. GC. (2002). Human endothelial progenitor cells from type II diabetics exhibit impaired proliferation, adhesion, and incorporation into vascular structures. Circulation 106(22):2781-6.

Tesar. PJ., Chenoweth. JG., Brook, FA., Davies. TJ., Evans. EP., Mack. D L., Gardner. R L. & McKay. RD. (2007). New cell lines from mouse epiblast share defining features with human embryonic stem cells. Nature 448: 196–199

Theiss. HD., Brenner. C., Engelmann. MG., Zaruba. MM., Huber. B., Henschel. V., Mansmann. U., Wintersperger. B., Reiser. M., Steinbeck. G.& Franz. WM. (2010). Safety and efficacy of SITAgliptin plus GRanulocyte-colony-stimulating factor in patients suffering from Acute Myocardial Infarction (SITAGRAMI-Trial)--rationale, design and first interim analysis. Int J Cardiol 145(2):282-4.

van der Bogt. KE., Swijnenburg. RJ., Cao. F. & Wu. JC. (2006). Molecular imaging of human embryonic stem cells: keeping an eye on differentiation, tumorigenicity and immunogenicity. Cell Cycle 5(23):2748-52. Bone marrow cell therapy after acute myocardial infarction: the HEBE trial in perspective, first results.

van der Laan. A., Hirsch. A., Nijveldt. R., van der Vleuten. PA., van der Giessen. WJ., Doevendans. PA., Waltenberger. J., Ten Berg. JM., Aengevaeren. WR., Zwaginga. JJ., Biemond. BJ., van Rossum. AC., Tijssen. JG., Zijlstra. F. & Piek. JJ. (2008).Bone marrow cell therapy after acute myocardial infarction: the HEBE trial in perspective, first results. Neth Heart J 16:436–9.

van Ramshorst. J., Bax. JJ., Beeres. SL., Dibbets-Schneider. P., Roes. SD., Stokkel. MP., de Roos. A., Fibbe. WE., Zwaginga. JJ., Boersma. E., Schalij. MJ. & Atsma, D.E. (2009) Intramyocardial bone marrow cell injection for chronic myocardial ischemia: a randomized controlled trial. J. Am. Med. Assoc 301: 1997-2004

Vasa. M., Fichtlscherer. S., Aicher. A., Adler. K., Urbich. C., Martin. H., Zeiher. AM. & Dimmeler. S. (2001). Number and migratory activity of circulating endothelial progenitor cells inversely correlate with risk factors for coronary artery disease. Circ Res 89(1):E1-7.

Vassalli. G. &, Moccetti. T. (2011). Cardiac repair with allogeneic mesenchymal stem cells after myocardial infarction. Swiss Med Wkly 23;141.

Urbanek. K., Rota. M., Cascapera. S., Bearzi. C., Nascimbene. A., De Angelis. A., Hosoda. T., Chimenti. S., Baker. M., Limana. F., Nurzynska. D., Torella. D., Rotatori. F., Rastaldo. R., Musso. E., Quaini. F., Leri. A., Kajstura. J. & Anversa. P. (2005). Cardiac stem cells possess growth factor-receptor systems that after activation regenerate the infarcted myocardium, improving ventricular function and long-term survival. Circ Res 97(7):663-73.

Utikal. J., Polo. JM., Stadtfeld. M., Maherali. N., Kulalert. W., Walsh. RM., Khalil. A., Rheinwald. JG. & Hochedlinger. K. (2009). Immortalization eliminates a roadblock during cellular reprogramming into iPS cells. Nature 460(7259):1145-8.

Walsh. S., Pontén. A., Fleischmann. BK. & Jovinge. S. (2010). Cardiomyocyte cell cycle control and growth estimation in vivo--an analysis based on cardiomyocyte nuclei. Cardiovasc Res ;86(3):365-73.

Wang. W., Jiang. Q., Zhang. H., Jin. P., Yuan. X., Wei. Y. & Hu. S. (2011). Intravenous administration of bone marrow mesenchymal stromal cells is safe for the lung in a chronic myocardial infarction model. Regen Med 6(2):179-90.

Wang. X., Willenbring. H., Akkari. Y., Torimaru. Y., Foster. M., Al-Dhalimy. M., Lagasse. E., Finegold. M., Olson. S, & Grompe. M. (2003). Cell fusion is the principal source of bone-marrow-derived hepatocytes. Nature 422(6934):897-901.

Wang. Y., Ahmad. N., Wani. MA., Ashraf. M. (2004). Hepatocyte growth factor prevents ventricular remodeling and dysfunction in mice via Akt pathway and angiogenesis. J Mol Cell Cardiol 37(5):1041-52.

Werner. N., Kosiol. S., Schiegl. T., Ahlers. P., Walenta. K., Link. A., Böhm. M. & Nickenig. G. (2005). Circulating endothelial progenitor cells and cardiovascular outcomes. N Engl J Med 353(10):999-1007.

Westenbrink. BD., Lipsic. E., van der Meer. P., van der Harst. P., Oeseburg. H., Du Marchie Sarvaas. GJ., Koster. J., Voors. AA., van Veldhuisen. DJ., van Gilst. WH. & Schoemaker. RG. (2007). Erythropoietin improves cardiac function through endothelial progenitor cell and vascular endothelial growth factor mediated neovascularization. Eur Heart J 28(16):2018-27.

Winter. EM., Grauss. RW., Hogers. B., van Tuyn. J., van der Geest. R., Lie-Venema. H., Steijn. RV., Maas. S., DeRuiter. MC., deVries. AA., Steendijk. P., Doevendans. PA., van der Laarse. A., Poelmann. RE., Schalij. MJ., Atsma. DE. & Gittenberger-de Groot. AC. (2007). Preservation of left ventricular function and attenuation of remodeling after transplantation of human epicardium-derived cells into the infarcted mouse heart, Circulation 116 (8):917–927.

Wobus. AM. (2010). The Janus face of pluripotent stem cells--connection between pluripotency and tumourigenicity. Bioessays. 32(11):993-1002.

Wobus. AM. & Löser. P. (2011). Present state and future perspectives of using pluripotent stem cells in toxicology research. Arch Toxicol. 85(2):79-117.

Wojakowski. W., Kucia. M., Zuba-Surma. E., Jadczyk. T., Książek. B., Ratajczak. MZ. & Tendera. M. (2011). Very small embryonic-like stem cells in cardiovascular repair. Pharmacol Ther. 129(1):21-8.

Wollert. KC., Meyer. GP., Lotz. J., Ringes-Lichtenberg. S., Lippolt. P., Breidenbach. C., Fichtner. S., Korte T., Hornig. B., Messinger. D., Arseniev. L., Hertenstein. B., Ganser. A. & Drexler. H. (2004). Intracoronary autologous bone marrow cell transfer after myocardial infarction: the BOOST randomised controlled clinical trial. Lancet 364:141-8.

Xu. RH., Sampsell-Barron. TL., Gu. F., Root. S., Peck. RM., Pan. G., Yu. J., Antosiewicz-Bourget. J., Tian. S., Stewart. R. & Thomson, J. A. (2008) NANOG is a direct target of TGFβ/activin-mediated SMAD signaling in human ESCs. Cell Stem Cell 3: 196–206

Xu. C., Police. S., Rao. N. & Carpenter. MK.(2002). Characterization and enrichment of cardiomyocytes derived from human embryonic stem cells. Circ Res. 20;91(6):501-8.

Xu. C, Police. S., Hassanipour. M. & Gold. JD. (2006) Cardiac bodies: a novel culture method for enrichment of cardiomyocytes derived from human embryonic stem cells. Stem Cells Dev. 15: 631-639

Xu. RH., Sampsell-Barron. TL., Gu. F., Root. S., Peck. RM., Pan. G., Yu. J., Antosiewicz-Bourget. J., Tian. S., Stewart. R. & Thomson, J. A. (2008) NANOG is a direct target of TGFβ/activin-mediated SMAD signaling in human ESCs. Cell Stem Cell 3: 196–206

Yaghoubi. SS., Jensen. MC., Satyamurthy. N., Budhiraja. S., Paik. D., Czernin. J. & Gambhir. SS. (2009). Noninvasive detection of therapeutic cytolytic T cells with 18F-FHBG PET in a patient with glioma. Nat Clin Pract Oncol 6(1):53-8.

Yang. L., Soonpaa. MH., Adler. ED., Roepke. TK., Kattman. SJ., Kennedy. M., Henckaerts. E., Bonham. K., Abbott. GW. & Linden. RM. (2008) Human cardiovascular progenitor cells develop from a KDR^{+} embryonic-stem-cell-derived population. Nature 453: 524-528

Yoon. BS., Yoo. S. J., Lee. JE., You. S., Lee. HT. & Yoon. HS. (2006) Enhanced differentiation of human embryonic stem cells into cardiomyocytes by combining hanging drop culture and 5-azacytidine treatment. Differentiation 74: 149-159

Zhang. H., Song. P., Tang. Y., Zhang. XL., Zhao. SH., Wei. YJ. & Hu. SS. (2007). Injection of bone marrow mesenchymal stem cells in the borderline area of infarcted myocardium: heart status and cell distribution. J Thorac Cardiovasc Surg 134(5):1234-40.

Zhu. WZ., Xie. Y., Moyes. KW., Gold. JD., Askari. B & Laflamme. MA. (2010) Neuregulin/ErbB signaling regulates cardiac subtype specification in differentiating human embryonic stem cells. Circ. Res 107: 776-786

Zimmermann. WH. (2011). Embryonic and embryonic-like stem cells in heart muscle engineering. J Mol Cell Cardiol 50(2):320-6.

Zwi. L., Caspi. O., Arbel. G., Huber. I., Gepstein. A., Park. IH. & Gepstein. L. (2009) Cardiomyocyte differentiation of human induced pluripotent stem cells. Circulation 120: 1513-1523

Part 4

Coronary Artery Disease and Comorbidities

12

Impact of Thyroid Dysfunction on Natural Course of Coronary Artery Disease

Nataliia N. Sydorova
Ukrainian Military Medical Academy,
Kiev,
Ukraine

1. Introduction

Cardiovascular diseases have similar pathophysiologic mechanisms which lead patient from risk factors, such as dyslipidemia, smoking, high blood pressure etc. to congestive heart failure and finally - to death (Fig. 1.). This global approach to the natural history of cardiac pathology has been proposed at the end of the twentieth century and remains current till now (Cheung, 2006). Thyroid dysfunction is a common clinical problem which plays a key role in the regulation of the cardiovascular system and can contribute to the clinical course of coronary artery disease (CAD). As it was shown on Fig.1 thyroid dysfunction can affect almost all chains of this continuum and its influence should be taken into account when treating patients with CAD.

In several studies the presence of predominantly adverse cardiac effects of thyroid dysfunction on the natural history of CAD has been shown (Iervasi et al., 2007). Thyroid diseases are associated with systolic and diastolic cardiac dysfunction, hypertension, heart rhythm disorders etc. Overt hypo- as well as hyperthyroidism affect outcomes in patients with CAD. As it has been recently shown in numerous studies, even subclinical hyperthyroidism can be an independent risk factor for all-cause and cardiovascular mortality (Sgarbi et al., 2010). Previously subclinical hypothyroidism was recognized as an independent risk factor for atherosclerosis and myocardial infarction in elderly women (Hak et al., 2000). But results of these studies are sometimes controversial (Biondi, 2010; Cappola et al., 2006; Iervasi et al., 2007; Ittermann et al., 2010)

Thyroid hormone excess causes a lot of cardiovascular changes due to both direct and indirect effects on the cardiovascular system (Table 1), and results in neurohormonal activation, including sympathetic nervous system activation. The latter determines increased heart rate and appearance of arrhythmia, especially atrial fibrillation. Hyperthyroidism is also associated with hypertension and CAD clinical manifestation.

With aging, physiological changes in thyroid homeostasis interact with different cardiovascular risk factors (Mariotti, 2008). Hypothyroidism is frequently found in the elderly, may cause several functional cardiovascular abnormalities and increases the risk of atherosclerosis and CAD manifestation (Mariotti & Cambuli, 2007). Hypothyroidism alters lipid metabolism, which contributes to the natural course of CAD. Hypertension can be also a clinical sign of thyroid hypofunction. Hypothyroidism may result in diastolic and systolic cardiac dysfunction, i.e. heart failure. Other its potential cardiovascular risk factors are increased circulating C-reactive protein and homocysteine levels, increased arterial stiffness, endothelial dysfunction, and altered coagulation parameters (Mariotti & Cambuli, 2007). On the contrary, some investigators had found that hypothyroidism is not associated with an increased risk of carotid atherosclerosis (Chiche et al., 2009). On the other hand, Mazzeffi et al. (2010) confirmed the association between hypothyroidism and lower extremity arterial disease as an atherosclerosis display. So, after years of research there are still unexplored facts waiting to be resolved.

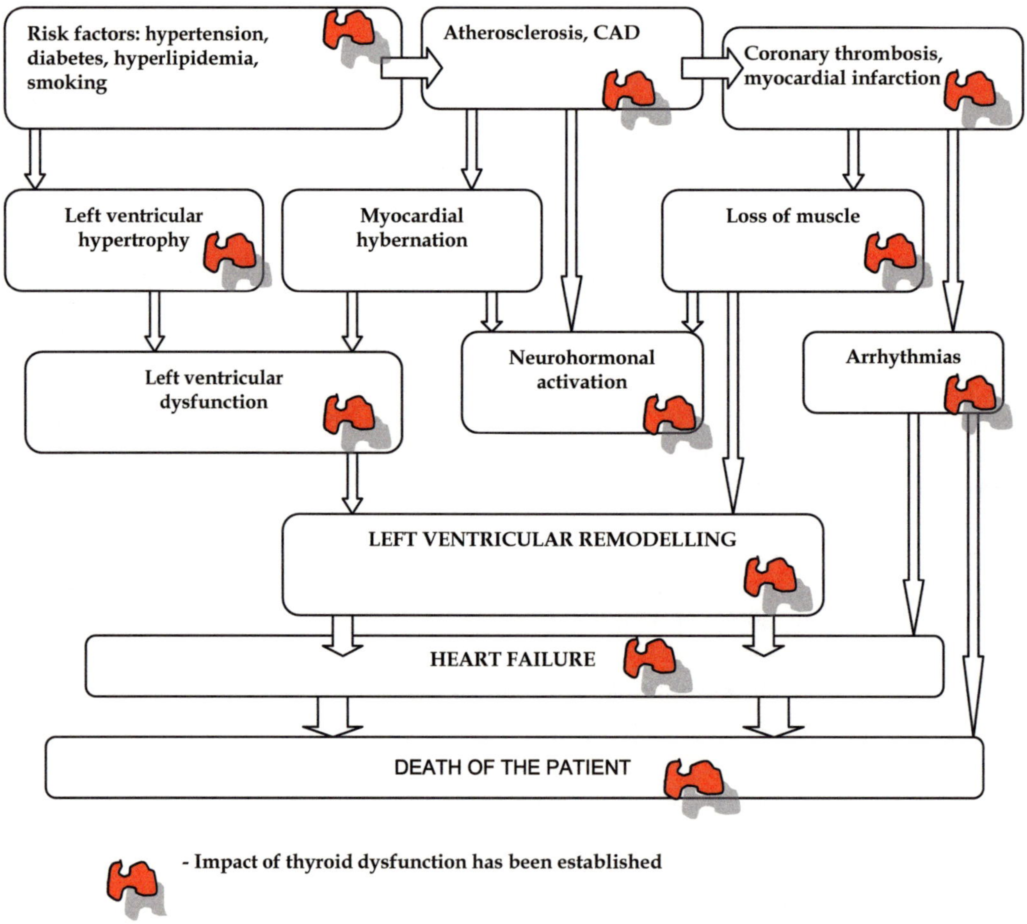

Fig. 1. Cardiovascular continuum and thyroid dysfunction (modified from Dzau & Braunwald, 1991).

Pathways	Clinical manifestations
Effects predominantly on cardiomyocytes:	
1. On the genome level (prolonged effects): in the nucleus triiodthyronine interacts with specific transcriptional activators or repressors and alters the transcription modality of specific target genes (Brent, 1994). Triiodthyronine contributes to: -protein synthesis and thus transcriptional activation of α-isoform of myosin heavy chain, sarcoplasmic reticulum calcium-activated adenosine triphosphatase, β_1-adrenergic receptors, guanine-nucleotide-regulatory proteins, Na^+/K^+-adenosine triphosphatase, some of voltage-gated K^+ channels (Fazio et al, 2004; Kahaly & Dillmann, 2005) -transcriptional repression of β-isoform of myosin heavy chain, phospholamban, nuclear receptor α_1, adenylyl-cyclase types V & VI, Na^+/Ca^{2+} exchanger (Fazio et al., 2004; Kahaly & Dillmann, 2005)	
2. Extranuclear cellular mechanisms (short-term effects):	
Effects on membrane	
Augmented activity of the sinoatrial node (Sun et al., 2001) through increasing the conductance density of I(f)-channels (Renaudon et al., 2000)	Increased heart rate and myocardial oxygen demand
Activation of transmembrane transfer of sodium and potassium (Kahaly & Dillmann, 2005), calcium (Kiss et al, 1994) and glucose (Chidakel et al., 2005)	Activation of cardiomyocytes' metabolism
Effects on sarcoplasmic reticulum	
Activation of calcium reuptake during diastole, up-regulation of calcium-activated adenosine triphosphatase, down-regulation of phospholamban expression (Fazio et al., 2004; Kiss et al., 1994; Ojamaa et al., 2002)	Augmented contraction of cardiomyocytes, enhancing myocardial relaxation
Effects on mitochondria	
Activation of oxidative phosphorylation (Verhoeven et al., 1985)	Activation of cardiomyocytes' metabolism
Activation of adenine nucleotide translocase (Sterling, 1986)	Activation of cardiomyocytes' metabolism
Effects on heart:	
Increased density of cardiac β_1-adrenoreceptors (Kahaly & Dillmann, 2005) and, thus, response to catecholamines	Elevation of cardiac output
Effects on vascular wall:	
Relaxation effect on vascular smooth-muscle cells (Ojamaa et al., 1996)	Vasodilatation, decreased preload as well as afterload on the heart, decreased peripheral vascular resistance
Other effects of thyroid hormone, which have influence on the natural course of cardiovascular diseases:	
Activation of metabolism	Increased myocardial oxygen demand
Effects on lipid profile (Rizos et al., 2011)	Maintaining serum very low-, low- and high-density lipoprotein cholesterol, triglyceride and apo-B 100 levels within normal range
Modulation of glucose production and glycogen storage in the liver and heart (Boelen, 2009; Forhead et al., 2009; Klieverik et al., 2009)	Activation of cardiomyocytes' metabolism
Increase sodium reabsorbtion in the kidney (Capasso et al., 1999)	Increase circulation blood volume

Table 1. The most important effects of thyroid hormone on the cardiovascular system.

There are also several challenges of CAD treatment in patients with coexisting thyroid dysfunction. Usage (especially long-term, with high doses) of amiodarone *per se* can result in amiodarone-induced thyroiditis and thyroid dysfunction (Iervasi et al., 1997; Martino et al. 2001). Different β-blockers show dissimilar effects on thyroid hormone levels, and these responses should be taken into account when treating patients with CAD and coexisisting thyroid dysfunction. There is a wide discussion about safety of levothyroxine replacement treatment in patients with CAD. It is known that this therapy can improve results of cardiac function measurements in subjects with hypothyroidism, however in the presence of CAD levothyroxine replacement treatment may result in manifestation or worsening of the CAD symptoms (Mariotti & Cambuli, 2007).

New data emerged about association between thyroid dysfunction and CAD natural history, which will be discussed hereafter. During the last decades interest to the influence of subclinical thyroid dysfunction on CAD progression rises significantly, but findings are still too controversial to make definitive decision. By now even definition for normal serum thyroid hormone and thyrotropin range is still not completely established. This chapter will be dedicated to the main problems of coexisting CAD and overt thyroid dysfunction. Influence of subclinical thyroid dysfunction on CAD will not be discussed in this chapter because of the immensity and complexity of the issue.

2. Impact of hypothyroidism on the natural history of CAD

Hypothyroidism can influence the natural course of CAD in different ways. In patients with overt hypothyroidism hyperlipidemia, coagulation abnormalities, endothelial dysfunction, hypertension, hypertrophy and diastolic dysfunction of heart ventricles, and abnormalities of insulin resistance had been found. Most of these factors can alter atherosclerotic process and modify morbidity and mortality rates for CAD. But after decades of research implication of thyroid hypofunction in CAD progression is still unclear and needs to be reassessed.

2.1 Effects of overt hypothyroidism on the most important cardiovascular risk factors: hyperlipidemia and hypertension

2.1.1 Hypothyroidism and hyperlipidemia

The role of lipid metabolism disorders in pathophysiologic mechanisms of atherosclerosis, following CAD and its complications is well established. Hyperlipidemia is a first step of the cardiovascular continuum; it is widely known as an independent cardiovascular risk factor. Clear and exact recommendations addressed to the lipid levels control, especially in patients with CAD and those at high cardiovascular risk were developed. It is also generally accepted that hypothyroidism accelerates development of CAD by its impairment action on lipid metabolism (Jung et al., 2003; Rizos et al., 2011). Hyperlipidemia is more often observed in patients with serum concentration of thyrotropin more than 10 mIU/L (Biondi & Klein, 2004).

The most important mechanisms of thyroid hormone action on lipid metabolism are shown in Table 2.

Mechanism	Result	Impact on the course of CAD in case of hypothyroidism
Inducing the HMG-CoA reductase	Cholesterol biosynthesis	Theoretically depressed cholesterol production, but in practice increased total cholesterol and LDL cholesterol levels due to decreased catabolism of LDL and IDL cholesterol
Controlling the LDL receptor gene activation (for T_3) by: -the direct binding to specific thyroid hormone responsive elements (Rizos et al., 2011) -controlling the sterol regulatory element-binding protein-2 (Shin & Osborne, 2003)	Up-regulation of LDL receptors	Decreased catabolism of LDL and IDL cholesterol, increased total cholesterol and LDL cholesterol, acceleration of atherosclerosis and CAD
Controlling the TG levels by hypotriglyceridemic gene *APOA5* regulation (Prieur et al., 2005)	Inhibition of TGs production	Increased TG levels, acceleration of atherosclerosis and CAD
T_3 and its acetic derivative protect LDL from oxidation (Faureet al., 2004)	Protection from oxidation of LDL	Burden of oxidative stress, acceleration of atherosclerosis and CAD
Increased cholesteryl ester transfer protein activity	Increased exchange of cholesteryl esters from HDL_2 to VLDL and TGs to the opposite direction (Rizos et al., 2011)	Not definitely established, due to this mechanism plasma HDL levels may be elevated
Stimulation of lipoprotein lipase	Activation of TG-rich lipoproteins catabolism (Rizos et al., 2011)	Decreased clearance of TG-rich lipoproteins, hypertriglyceridemia, acceleration of atherosclerosis and CAD
Stimulation of hepatic lipase	Activation of hydrolyzation HDL_2 to HDL_3, conversion of IDL to LDL and in turn LDL to small dense LDL (Rizos et al., 2011)	Increased levels of HDL_2, IDL and LDL. Impact on the natural history of CAD is controversial
Up-regulation of apoAV	Decreased hepatic TGs, VLDL production, increased both plasma lipoprotein lipase levels and activity, enhanced affinity for the LDL receptor, greater clearance of lipoprotein core remnants (Rensen et al., 2005)	Increased plasma TG and VLDL levels; acceleration of atherosclerosis and CAD

Table 2. The most important mechanisms of thyroid hormone action on lipid metabolism and their impact on the course of CAD in case of hypothyroidism. HMG-CoA = 3-hydroxy-3-methylglutaryl-coenzyme A; LDL = low-density lipoprotein; IDL = intermediate-density lipoprotein; T_3 = triiodthyronine; TG = triglyceride; HDL = high-density lipoprotein; VLDL = very low-density lipoprotein

Therefore overt thyroid hypofunction primarily leads to elevated plasma total cholesterol and low-density lipoprotein cholesterol levels. Elevation of triglyceride levels is also possible as well as increased concentration of high-density lipoprotein cholesterol (mainly because of increased concentration of high-density lipoprotein-2 particles). So, lipid profile in patients with hypothyroidism has atherogenic properties, and may be characterized by unusual condition with simultaneously elevated triglycerides and high-density lipoprotein cholesterol levels despite it is widely accepted that hypothyroidism is associated with decreased high-density lipoprotein cholesterol levels (Cappola & Ladenson, 2003) and that there is an inverse relation between these two measures. Thus, atherogenic lipid profile in patients with overt hypothyroidism may be partly diminished by this elevated plasma concentration of high-density lipoprotein cholesterol. It was also shown that patients with hypothyroidism have increased concentration of lipoprotein (a) - known by its atherogenic facilities and associated with atherosclerotic artery lesion, particularly CAD (Rizos et al., 2011; Tzotzas et al., 2000).

2.1.2 Hypothyroidism and hypertension

Hypertension is another strong cardiovascular risk factor and the starting point of the cardiovascular continuum. Hypertension has a great influence on the natural course of CAD resulting in an increase in cardiac afterload, ventricular hypertrophy, impairment of diastolic function of ventricles as well as endothelial dysfunction and neurohormonal activation (Dzau & Braunvald, 1991). Hypothyroidism prevalence among general population of patients with hypertension reaches 3-4%, and it was established that patients with hypothyroidism and hypertension represent higher blood pressure levels compared with those without thyroid dysfunction (Fommei & Iervasi, 2002; Saito, 1983). At the same time hypertension is more common in hypothyroid population - its prevalence reaches 20-40% (Klein & Ojamaa, 1995; Streeten et al., 1988). So, hypertension is a frequent symptom of hypothyroidism and independent risk factor for cardiovascular events, morbidity and mortality, particularly CAD-associated. As it was shown in several studies, thyroid hypofunction is associated with predominantly diastolic hypertension as a result of increased systemic vascular resistance, increased arterial stiffness and impaired endothelial function (Biondy & Klein, 2004; Dernellis & Panaretou, 2002; Kanbay et al., 2007; Obuobie et al., 2002).

Hypothyroid patients have significantly higher diastolic blood pressure levels in the fifth and sixth decades of life (time of CAD manifestation in most cases) compared with measures in euthyroid controls (Aronow et al., 2011). Iqbal et al. (2006) have shown in their study of 5,872 subjects (2,623 male subjects) without antihypertensive or replacement levothyroxine treatment, that even within the normal serum thyrotropin range (0.20–4.00 mIU/L) there was a modest, but significant and positive association between serum thyrotropin and both systolic and diastolic blood pressure levels. Serum thyrotropin levels were higher in the hypertensive subjects, but differences were significant only for diastolic hypertension. The same trend was found by group of Norwegian scientists (Åsvold et al., 2007a).

2.2 Hypothyroidism, atherosclerosis and CAD

In one of the recent reviews addressed to the problem of the association between CAD and hypothyroidism Cappola & Ladenson (2003) mentioned: "...today's clinicians managing patients with hypothyroidism and atherosclerosis are still guided more by medical folklore than evidence-based medicine". It is widely accepted that hypothyroidism adverse contributes to the natural course of CAD (Miller & Gambert, 2008), but most of the studies, aimed to proof this postulate, are outdated, not large enough and have serious limitations. Most of them have been conducted in patients with subclinical hypothyroidism and/or predominantly in women. For example, findings of Vanhaelst et al. (1967) have been based on autopsy data of 25 patients with myxoedema and suggest that intensity of atherosclerotic disease was significantly higher in hypothyroid compared with euthyroid patients. But results of the Cardiovascular Health Study of 3,678 men and women didn't establish any prepotency of angina, myocardial infarction, transient ischemic attack, stroke and peripheral arterial disease in patients with subclinical hypothyroidism compared with such prevalence in euthyroid people (Ladenson et al, 1994). In the frequently cited study, performed by Perk & O`Neill and published in 1997, the authors found angiographic CAD progression differences for only 10 participants with hypothyroidism compared with those on adequate replacement therapy.

Interestingly, the evidence body of the association between overt hypothyroidism and CAD was proposed mostly by studies of not overt, but subclinical hypothyroidism, possibly because of its wider prevalence. The Wickham Survey, first large-scale examination of the relationship between thyroid function and cardiovascular outcomes, enrolled 2,779 men and women. Overt hypothyroidism was an exclusion criteria, 132 persons have subclinical thyroid hypofunction (Vanderpump et al., 1996). In a 20-yr follow-up of this population-based cohort study any relationship between incident CAD or mortality and composite variable of hypothyroidism on replacement therapy, presence of circulating antithyroid antibodies, and/or thyrotropin level more than 6 mIU/L was not established in both men and women. But replacement treatment was the most important limitation, which could cause shift in indexed results (Cappola & Ladenson, 2003). The Rotterdam Study of 1,149 women (age 55 years or older) was another study of subclinical hypothyroidism which proves the possibility of hypothyroidism to affect the natural course of atherosclerosis and to increase CAD-morbidity (Hak et al., 2000). It was shown after adjustment for age, smoking status, body weight index, blood pressure, and high-density lipoprotein cholesterol levels, that women with subclinical hypothyroidism had higher prevalence of aortic atherosclerosis on chest radiograms (odds ratio [OR] 1.9; 95% confidence interval [CI] 1.2-3.1) and higher prevalence of myocardial infarction (OR 2.3; 95% CI 1.3-4.2) compared with euthyroid ones.

Prevalence of obstructive CAD in patients with diabetes mellitus depending on the presence of hypothyroidism was shown in the study, conducted by Pierre-Louis et al. (2008). In this study totally 352 patients with diabetes mellitus underwent coronary angiography because of recent myocardial infarction or unstable angina or chest pain with a positive stress test. More than 50% narrowing of 1 or more major coronary arteries was present in 145 of 173 patients (84%) with diabetes mellitus and hypothyroidism and in 132 of 179 patients (74%) with diabetes mellitus without hypothyroidism ($p<0.025$). More than 50% narrowing of 3 major coronary arteries was present in 69 of 173 patients (40%) with diabetes mellitus and hypothyroidism and in 39 of 179 patients (22%) with diabetes mellitus without hypothyroidism ($p<0.001$). So, these findings represent evidence that patients with diabetes mellitus and hypothyroidism have higher prevalence and intensity of CAD compared with patients with diabetes mellitus without hypothyroidism.

One recent study provides some kind of confirmation of the association between hypothyroidism and lower extremity arterial disease as an atherosclerosis display (Mazzeffi et al., 2010). Six hundred fourteen patients and 529 control cases were enrolled, and gender was found to be a significant confounder. In men there was a positive independent association between hypothyroidism and lower extremity arterial disease (adjusted OR 2.65; 95% CI 1.19-5.89), whereas in women there was a negative independent association (adjusted OR 0.22; 95% CI 0.11-0.46).

Thus, despite of widely accepted opinion about ability of hypothyroidism to accelerate the natural course of CAD, carefully designed large controlled studies are still needed to prove this point of view conclusively.

3. Impact of hyperthyroidism on the natural history of CAD

Hyperthyroidism can alter the natural course of CAD in several ways. First of all it increases myocardial oxygen demand together with sinus and/or supraventricular tachycardia (as well as atrial fibrillation) – these factors can contribute to decompensation of underlying CAD and lead to manifestation of angina pectoris and heart failure (mostly with high cardiac output). Furthermore, systolic blood pressure is usually increased, while diastolic blood pressure – decreased in patients with hyperthyroidism. Due to this pulse pressure becomes wider and mean blood pressure – moderately decreased. These changes are associated with an increase in cardiac output and reduction in peripheral vascular resistance, resulting in the classic hyperdynamic cardiovascular status (Fazio, et al., 2004). Cardiac preload is increased and blood volume is enlarged in patients with hyperthyroidism, there are also conditions for diastolic dysfunction of heart ventricles due to above-listed factors and tachycardia. Hyperthyroidism affects one more chain of the cardiovascular continuum: renin-angiotensin-aldosterone system is activated in patients with thyroid hyperfunction (Resnick & Laragh, 1982). It was also shown that hyperthyroidism is associated with elevation of von Willebrand factor levels as well as enhanced platelet function and therefore shortened collagen-epinephrine-induced closure time (platelet plug formation measure) (Homoncik et al., 2007). The presence of CAD may compromise the ability of myocardium to respond to the metabolic demands of hyperthyroidism (Kahaly & Dillman, 2005). Hyperthyroidism may cause myocardial infarction even in subjects without coronary stenosis (Cowda et al., 2003; Jaber et al., 2010; Moliterno et al., 1992). There were also described such changes which can influence the natural course of CAD as necrosis of myocytes, small areas of fibrosis or round-cell infiltration in the hearts of patients with hyperthyroidism (Kahaly & Dillman, 2005).

The prevalence of cardiac decompensation in hyperthyroid patients with advancing age was established (Davis & Devis, 1975; Kahaly & Dillman, 2005; Trivalle et al., 1996). In patients over 50 years of age cardiovascular complications are the leading cause of death after treatment of hyperthyroidism (Franklyn et al., 1998). Supraventricular arrhythmias in older patients may contribute to some of the excess cardiovascular mortality as it was shown in several long-term follow-up studies (Franklyn et al., 1998; Parle et al., 2001; Osman et al., 2002). In one population-based study (Franklyn et al., 1998) of mortality with standardized mortality ratio (SMR) as a measure of relative risk in a cohort of 7,209 patients with hyperthyroidism treated with radioiodine it was shown, that during 105,028 person-years of follow-up, 3,611 subjects died; the expected number of deaths was 3,186 (SMR 1.1; 95% CI 1.1-1.2; $p<0.001$). The risk was increased for deaths due to cardiovascular disease (240 excess deaths; SMR 1.2; 95% CI 1.2-1.3; $p<0.001$), and cerebrovascular disease (159 excess deaths; SMR 1.4; 95% CI 1.2-1.5; $p<0.001$). Rheumatic disease (46 excess deaths, SMR 3.2; 95% CI 2.5-4.2; $p<0.001$) and hypertensive heart disease (31 excess deaths, SMR 2.1; 95% CI 1.6-2.7; $p<0.001$) had the highest SMRs. On the other hand, SMR for ischemic heart disease was modest (SMR 1.1; 95% CI 1.0-1.1; $p=0.03$) with 55 excess deaths. Intriguingly, in this study after separate analyses for men and women the excess deaths due to the cardiovascular disease was established for women but not for men (women: SMR 1.3; 95% CI 1.2-1.4; men: SMR 1.0; 95% CI 0.9-1.2; $p<0.001$ for the comparison between men and women).

So, the most important confounders for cardiovascular morbidity and mortality of hyperthyroid patients are dysrhythmias (especially atrial fibrillation) with tromboembolic complications, and hypertension. Gender of the patient may also have some influence on the clinical course of cardiovascular diseases in patients with hyperthyroidism.

4. Cardiovascular risk factors in patients with different thyroid status: Our findings

Recently we conducted a retrospective study, which took place in two medical centres in Kiev (Ukraine), aimed to establish prevalence of the main cardiovascular risk factors in 464 consecutive patients with CAD depending on their thyroid status, stratified into 3 groups: euthyroid (n=115, mean age 57.4±0.8 years, 76.5% female, mean thyrotropin level 1.6±0.12 mIU/L), hypothyroid (n=108, mean age 56.8±1.1 years, 76% female, mean thyrotropin level 12±1.7 mIU/L), and hyperthyroid (n=241, mean age 55.4±0.6 years, 86.7% female, mean thyrotropin level 0.16±0.03 mIU/L). Medical records were estimated and all patients, who met inclusion criteria (registered CAD and/or prescribed antiischemic therapy together with defined thyroid status), were included in our study. During statistical analysis continuous variables were expressed as mean±error of mean, categorical variables were expressed as frequency and percentage. Comparison between variables was performed using analysis of variance and the Student *t* test. A *p* value less than 0.05 was considered statistically significant.

The prevalence of hypertension was high in all groups with the highest rate for hypothyroid group (Fig.2). For hyperthyroid patients there was a trend for the increased prevalence of grade 1-2 hypertension, and less prevalent (approximately 2.1 times) grade 3 hypertension compared with rates in the euthyroid group. There was also significantly increased rate of grade 1-2 hypertension in hypothyroid patients compared with rate in the euthyroid group (see Fig.2).

We didn't find any significant differences in lipid profile among these 3 groups: total cholesterol, low-density lipoprotein and triglyceride levels were somewhat elevated in all groups, the only difference was obtained for high-density lipoprotein level, which was 26.6% lower in hypothyroid compared with euthyroid group of patients (Fig.3), but still within the normal range. These findings are consistent to the results of several studies (Cappola & Ladenson, 2003), but disagree with statement of Rizos et al. (2011) about possibility of high-density lipoprotein levels increasing in hypothyroid patients, likely due to mild-to-moderate hypothyroidism in our study (mean thyrotropin level 12±1.7 mIU/L). On the other hand, our results didn't show any significant differences in lipid profile between patients with CAD depending on thyroid status. This finding suggests that these changes were determined by alternative mechanisms, and their consequences are almost irrespective of thyroid status when it comes to moderate but overt thyroid dysfunction.

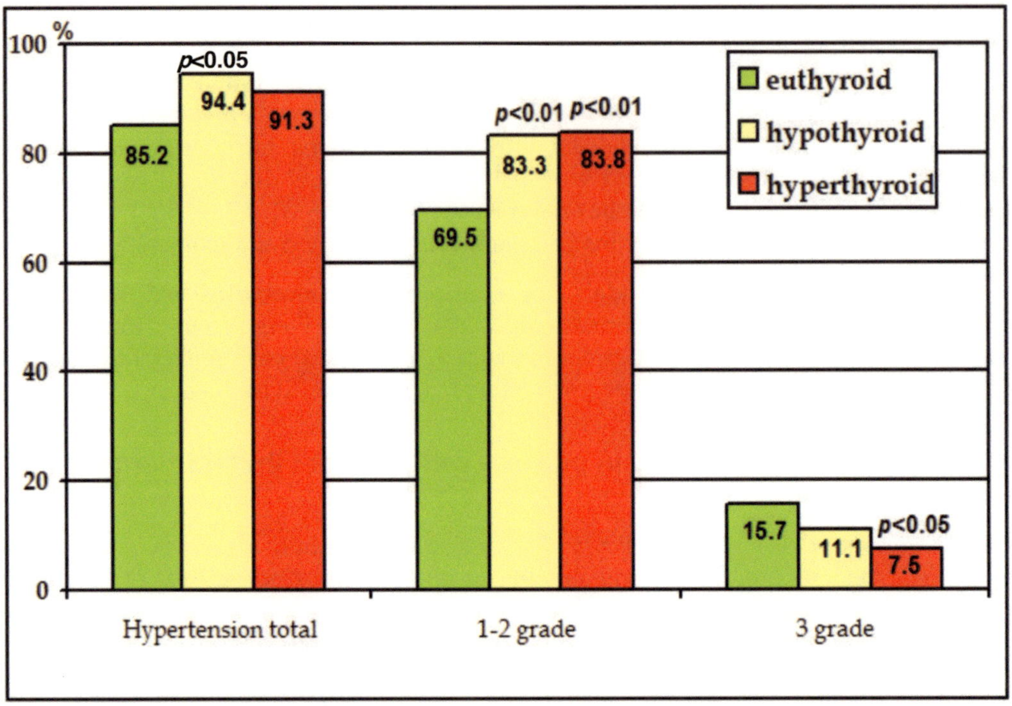

Fig. 2. Prevalence of hypertension in patients with CAD depending on thyroid status. *p* indicates statistical significance for comparison with euthyroid group.

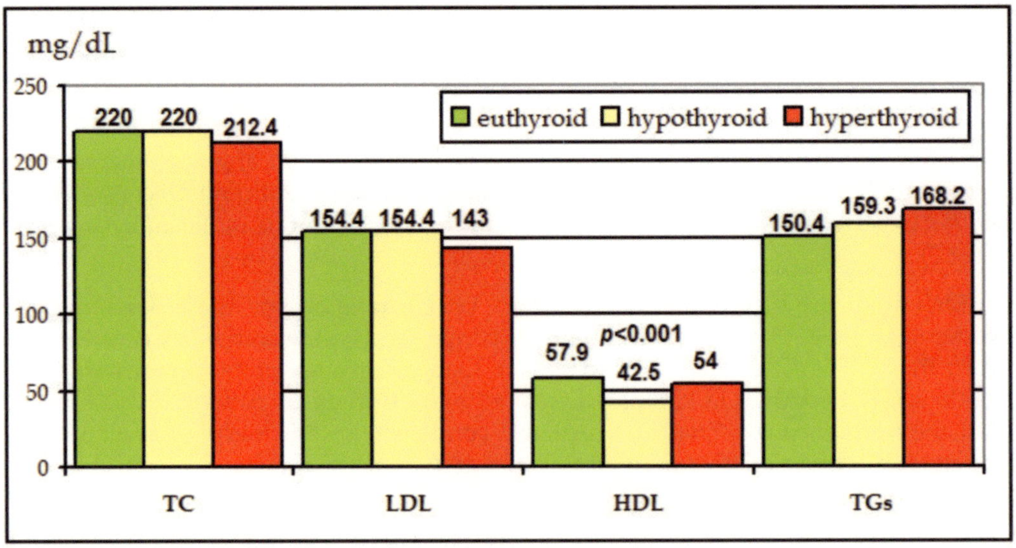

Fig. 3. Lipid profile in patients with CAD depending on thyroid status. *p* indicates statistical significance for comparison with euthyroid group. TC = total cholesterol, LDL = low-density lipoprotein, HDL = high-density lipoprotein, TGs = triglycerides.

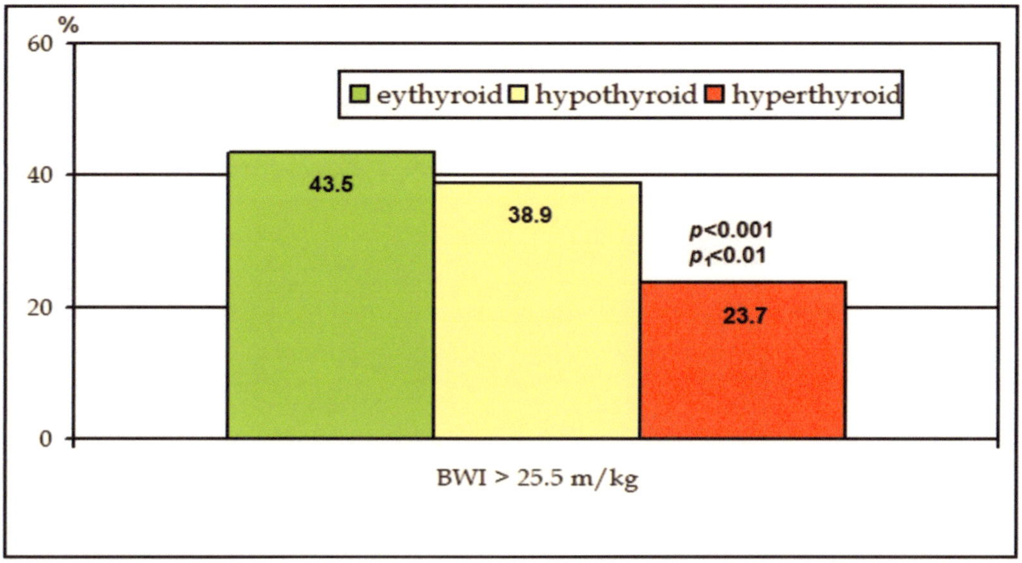

Fig. 4. Proportion of patients with body weight index more than 25.5 m/kg among those with CAD depending on thyroid status. *p* indicates statistical significance for comparison with euthyroid group, p_1 – statistical significance for comparison with hypothyroid group. BWI = body weight index.

In the course of body weight index estimation we had obtained expected results: patients with hyperthyroidism had better measures compared with other groups. Less than ¼ subjects of the hyperthyroid group had body weight index > 25.5 m/kg (Fig.4). In our study proportion of overweight patients in the hypothyroid group was more than ⅓ and in the euthyroid group – a little less than ½. We couldn't estimate waist circumference and waist-to-hip ratio, both the definite cardiovascular risk factors, because of the retrospective design of the study and lack of these data in medical records.

Our results regarding glycaemic status of the patients with CAD and thyroid dysfunction were surprising enough (Fig.5 & 6). Despite of being within normal limits, mean fasting plasma glucose level for patients in hyperthyroid group was significantly lower compared with such in euthyroid group (see Fig.5). This result was consistent to another one: in our study proportion of patients with fasting plasma glucose level > 102 mg/dL (5.6 mmol/L) was the smallest for hyperthyroid population (16.2%) compared with euthyroid (33%, $p<0.001$) and hypothyroid (25.9%, $p>0.05$) groups (see Fig.6). Fasting plasma glucose level >102 mg/dL is known cardiovascular risk factor influencing prognosis of the patients with hypertension (Mancia et al., 2007), and is important for patients with hyperthyroidism and CAD associated with increased prevalence of hypertension. This relatively lower level of fasting plasma glucose is probably linked to both activation of metabolism (particularly carbohydrate metabolism) and sensitivity to insulin, and reflects more intense glucose uptake by cells. There weren't any significant differences in diabetes prevalence between study groups (all $p>0.05$).

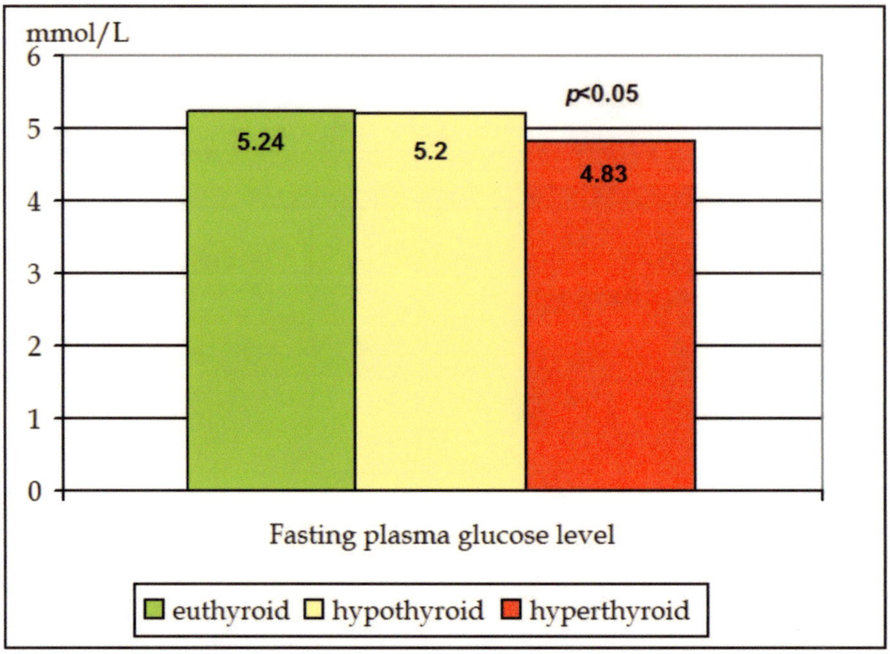

Fig. 5. Fasting plasma glucose levels in patients with CAD depending on thyroid status. p indicates statistical significance for comparison with euthyroid group.

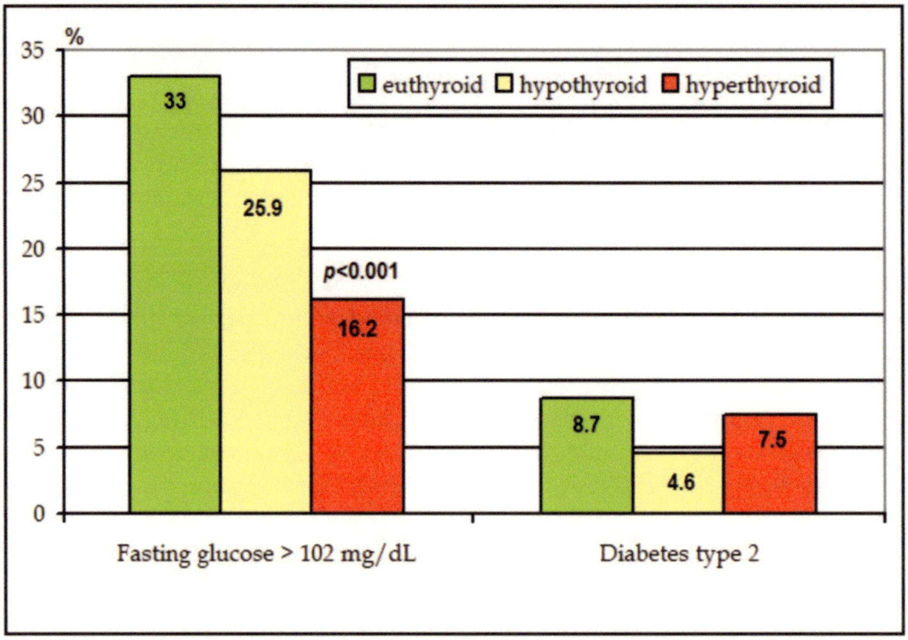

Fig. 6. Glycaemic status and prevalence of cardiovascular risk factors in patients with CAD depending on thyroid status. p indicates statistical significance for comparison with euthyroid group.

We also investigated the prevalence of previous main cardiovascular events: myocardial infarction and stroke in patients with CAD and different thyroid status (Fig.7). According to our data, in the euthyroid group prevalence of previous myocardial infarction was more than 2 times higher compared with such in hyperthyroid group (13.9% *vs.* 5%, respectively, $p<0.01$). In our study there weren't any statistically significant differences in the rates of stroke between study groups, which was really unexpected because of general opinion, that hyperthyroidism is strongly associated with stroke as a thromboembolic complication of atrial fibrillation (Franklyn et al., 1998). The lowest rate of previous myocardial infarction in this hyperthyroid group partly denies assumption that mild but not subclinical thyroid hyperfunction can definitely cause serious worsening of the natural course of CAD, and this hypothesis still needs careful and well designed investigation.

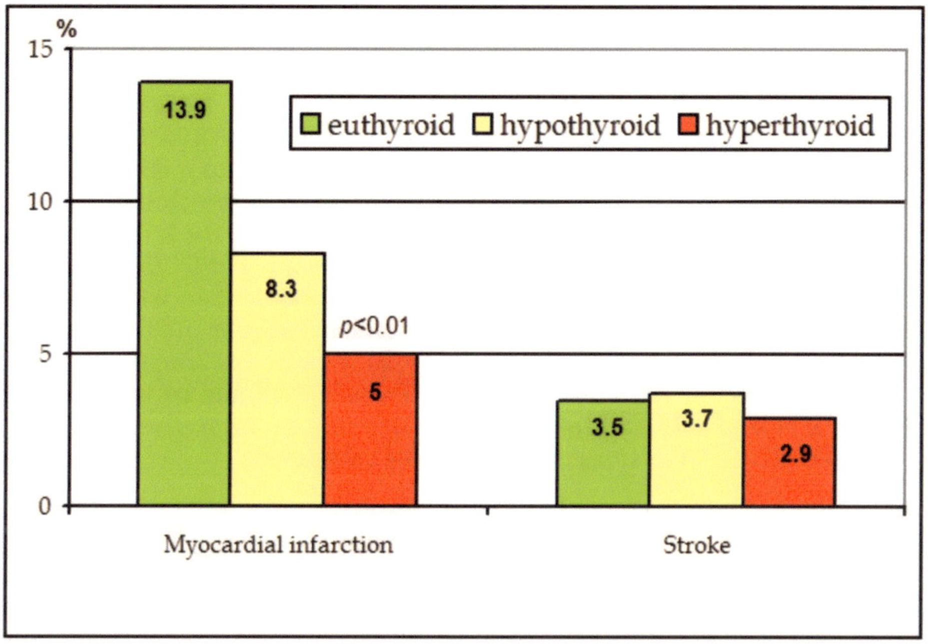

Fig. 7. Prevalence of previous cardiovascular events in patients with CAD depending on thyroid status. *p* indicates statistical significance for comparison with euthyroid group.

5. Conclusion

Despite numerous studies dedicated to the interaction between cardiovascular system and thyroid, a lot of issues are still unclarified. The results of different authors are often controversial first of all because of extreme difficulties in designing of such studies. The most problem of thyroid status identification and evaluation is its instability within the natural course of thyroid diseases. During years of illness thyroid function can be changed from activated to moderate activated, "normal" by results of several screening tests, and then - decreased. But if thyroid tissue is relatively preserved, it's absolutely possible, that thyroid function at times may become increased or "normal" again necessary amount of thyroid cells are available. This instability may cause selection bias during studies.

There is also a wide discussion about normal range of main markers of thyroid dysfunction: serum thyrotropin, triiodthyronine, thyroxine levels (Surks et al., 2004). Taking into consideration current complex classification of thyroid disorders, which is based on these marker levels, a new question arises: do we use the proper criteria for definition of thyroid dysfunction and dysfunction of different organs due to thyroid hormone changes, particularly cardiovascular system? What about tissue sensibility to thyroid hormone in patients with CAD? It is still unclear, how works thyroid hormone in people with cardiovascular diseases: atherosclerosis and CAD? Is this mechanism similar or not to such in healthy subjects? What are the differences? Can genetic features of the patients with cardiovascular disease, which predispose a person to atherosclerosis and CAD, influence normal or pathological thyroid?

Recently emerging evidence indicates that 45–65% of the inter-individual variation in serum thyroid hormone levels is due to genetic factors (Medici et al., 2011). In one study 68 genes (1512 polymorphisms) were studied in relation to serum thyrotropin and thyroxine levels in 1,121 Caucasian subjects. It was shown that for thyrotropin 8 *PDE8B* polymorphisms ($p=4\times10^{-17}$) and for thyroxine 2 *DIO1* ($p=8\times10^{-12}$) and 1 *FOXE1* ($p=0.0003$) polymorphisms remained significant in the meta-analysis (Medici at al., 2011). In the meta-analysis of 2,557 patients Taylor et al. (2011) have clarified associations between the rs4704397 single nucleotide polymorphism in *PDE8B* and thyrotropin, triiodothyronine and thyroxine levels. This meta-analysis confirmed presence of genetic variation in *PDE8B* associated with thyrotropin ($p=1.64\times10^{-10}$) and identified a possible new association with free thyroxine ($p=0.023$). Taylor et al. (2011) suggest that common genetic variation in *PDE8B* is associated with reciprocal changes in thyrotropin and free thyroxine levels that are consistent over time and lost in individuals on levothyroxine therapy. These both results are intriguing because they display possible genetic markers of variation in serum thyroid hormone levels that will be helpful in designing and carrying out epidemiological studies.

Treatment of both thyroid and cardiovascular diseases can contribute to pathways and outcomes, but till now we know little about this. Some studies were dedicated to the evaluation of influence of hyperthyroidism treatment strategies on cardiovascular outcomes (Hall et al., 1993; Franklyn et al, 1998), but precise mechanisms of their action are still unclear. One of the recent treatment approaches for hyperthyroidism is so called "suppress and replace" management with complete suppression of thyroid function (marker – thyrotropin levels) and simultaneously replacement therapy with thyroid hormone (Kahaly & Dillmann, 2005). This condition and its possibility to influence the cardiovascular system should be carefully established. In some cases of treatment with levothyroxine it is possible even in previously hypothyroid patients appearance of "tissue hyperthyroidism" on cardiac level (normal thyroxine and triiodthyronine and suppressed thyrotropin) (Banovac et al., 1989). The fact that euthyroid due to the replacement therapy hearts are not similar to those euthyroid without such therapy were discussed elsewhere (Bengel et al., 2000; Biondi et al., 1996), but we need more evidence.

It is also widely known that cardiovascular diseases may contribute to the thyroid function predominantly causing its down-regulation. In one study it was shown, that patients with CAD during acute phase of myocardial infarction demonstrated a rapid and sustained fall in serum total triiodothyronine concentration, a rise in reverse triiodothyronine concentration, and a transient fall in total thyroxine concentration. This observed fall in triiodothyronine concentration wasn't accompanied by significant changes in basal thyrotropin concentrations (Franklyn et al., 1984). In another study of 47 consecutive euthyroid patients with acute myocardial infarction thyroid status also was evaluated (Friberg et al., 2002) with mostly similar results. The study had demonstrated that thyroid hormone was rapidly down-regulated with maximal development by 24-36 hours after onset of symptoms. The mean of serum total triiodothyronine concentration decreased by 19% (p=0.02), the mean of serum reverse triiodothyronine concentration increased by 22% (p=0.01), while serum thyrotropin concentration decreased by 51% (p<0.001) between the first 6-hour of myocardial infarction and 24-36-hour time interval. Notably, patients with severe heart dysfunction or more intense inflammatory reaction showed more pronounced down-regulation of the thyroid function. Interestingly, serum free thyroxine levels was predominantly unchanged in both studies (Franklyn et al., 1984; Frieberg et al., 2002). This adaptive reaction provides reduction of myocardial oxygen demand and relieves emerged mismatch between myocardial oxygen demand and oxygen delivery in patients with CAD. On the other hand, in several studies association between thyrotropin levels (even within reference range) and body weight index, the occurrence of obesity (Knudsen et al., 2005), and serum lipid concentrations (Åsvold et al., 2007b) was found. In 2008 Åsvold et al. had published their new results from the Nord-Trøndelag Health study (the HUNT study) about association between CAD mortality and relatively low thyroid function within the clinical reference range. Total 25,313 patients without history of thyroid disease, angina, myocardial infarction, stroke or diabetes mellitus at baseline were enrolled. At the end of follow-up (median 8.3 years) 228 women (1.3%) and 182 men (2.3%) died of CAD (192 women and 164 men of them had thyrotropin levels within the reference range). The presence of positive association of thyrotropin level within the reference range with risk of fatal CAD was shown (p for trend=0.01 in the total population and p for trend=0.007 in non-smokers), especially in women (p for trend=0.005). Compared with women in the lower part of reference range (thyrotropin level 0.5-1.4 mIU/L) hazard ratios were 1.41 (95% CI 1.02-1.96) and 1.69 (95% CI 1.14-2.52) for women in the intermediate (thyrotropin level 1.5-2.4 mIU/L) and higher (thyrotropin level 2.5-3.5 mIU/L) parts of the reference range, respectively (Åsvold et al., 2008). These results suggest that relatively low but clinically normal thyroid function may increase the risk of fatal CAD, especially in non-smoking women.

In Czech Republic Mayer et al. (2006) conducted a study aimed to ascertain the prevalence of hypothyroidism in 410 patients (303 men and 107 women) with manifest CAD and to establish its association with cardiovascular risk factors. The prevalence of hypothyroidism (overt & subclinical) in the total sample and among male and female patients was 11.2, 6.9 and 23.4%, respectively. Overt hyperthyroidism (thyrotropin level> 3.65 mIU/L and free thyroxine <9 pmol/L and/or levothyroxine substitution) in this study was detected in 4.1% of total sample, 2.6% male and 8.4% female patients. Interestingly, there weren't any differences in hyperthyroidism prevalence: for total sample and separately male and female patients it was 5.6%. On the other hand, in this study the high prevalence of diabetes type 2 was found for the total sample (was not shown) with mean of fasting plasma glucose levels ranged from 6.7 to 7.6 mmol/L in euthyroid and hypothyroid groups without statistical difference. This finding is somewhat controversial to our results, but it can be explained by differences in the study samples: Mayer et al. (2006) enrolled only those who had survived after acute coronary episode in their study, while we didn't use this selection approach.

A lot of issues must be investigated before we can understand all mechanisms of interaction between thyroid and cardiovascular system, especially the natural course of CAD. It seems there is a great influence of individual differences of our patients with CAD and thyroid dysfunction on cardiovascular outcomes, and we should determine them in new large carefully designed controlled studies.

6. References

Aronow, W. S., Fleg, J.L., Pepine, C. J. et al. (2011) ACCF/AHA 2011 Expert Consensus Document on Hypertension in the Elderly. A Report of the American College of Cardiology Foundation Task Force on Clinical Expert Consensus Documents Developed in Collaboration With the American Academy of Neurology, American Geriatrics Society, American Society for Preventive Cardiology, American Society of Hypertension, American Society of Nephrology, Association of Black Cardiologists, and European Society of Hypertension, *J Am Coll Cardiol* Vol.57:2059.

Åsvold, B.O., Bjøro, T., Nilsen, T.I. et al. (2007a) Association between blood pressure and serum TSH concentration within the reference range: a population-based study, *J Clin Endocrinol Metab* Vol.92(3):841-845.

Åsvold, B.O., Bjøro, T., Nilsen, T.I.L., et al. (2008) Thyrotropin levels and risk of fatal coronary heart disease: the HUNT study, *Arch Intern Med* Vol.168(8):855-860.

Åsvold, B.O., Vatten, L.J., Nilsen, T.I. et al. (2007b) The association between TSH within the reference range and serum lipid concentrations in a population-based study: the HUNT Study, *Eur J Endocrinol* Vol.156(2):181-186.

Banovac. K., Papic, M., Bilkser, M.S. et al. (1989) Evidence of hyperthyroidism in apparently euthyroid patients treated with levothyroxine, *Arch Intern Med* Vol.149:809–812.

Bengel, F.M., Nekolla, S.G., Ibrahim, T. et al. (2000) Effect of thyroid hormones on cardiac function, geometry, and oxidative metabolism assessed noninvasively by positron emission tomography and magnetic resonance imaging, *J Clin Endocrinol Metab* Vol.85:1822–1827.

Biondi, B. & Klein I. (2004) Hypothyroidism as a risk factor for cardiovascular disease, *Endocrine* Vol.24:1–13.

Biondi, B. (2010) Cardiovascular mortality in subclinical hyperthyroidism: an ongoing dilemma, *Eur J Endocrinol* Vol.162 (3):587–589.

Biondi, B., Fazio, S., Cuocolo, A. et al., (1996) Impaired cardiac reserve and exercise capacity in patients receiving long-term thyrotropin suppressive therapy with levothyroxine, *J Clin Endocrinol Metab* Vol.81:4224–4228.

Boelen, A. (2009) Thyroid hormones and glucose metabolism: the story begins before birth, *Experimental Physiology*, Vol.94:1050-1051.

Brent, G.A. (1994) The molecular basis of thyroid hormone action, *N Engl J Med* Vol.331: 847–853.

Capasso, G., De Tommaso, G., Pica, A., et al. (1999) Effects of Thyroid Hormones on Heart and Kidney Functions, *Mineral Electrolyte Metab* Vol. 25:56-64.

Cappola, A.R. & Ladenson, P.W. (2003) Hypothyroidism and atherosclerosis, *J Clin Endocrinol Metab* Vol.88:2438–2444.

Cappola, A.R., Fried, L.P., Arnold, A.M., et al. (2006) Thyroid status, cardiovascular risk, and mortality in older adults, *JAMA* Vol.295:1033–1041.

Cheung, B.M.Y. (2006) The new cardiovascular continuum, *Hong Kong Med J* Vol.12:161-163.

Chiche, F., Jublanc, C., Coudert M. et al. (2009) Hypothyroidism is not associated with increased carotid atherosclerosis when cardiovascular risk factors are accounted for in hyperlipidemic patients, *Atherosclerosis* Vol.203(1):269-276.

Chidakel, A., Mentuccia, D. & Celi, F.S. (2005) Peripheral metabolism of thyroid hormone and glucose homeostasis, *Thyroid* Vol.8:899–903.

Cowda, R.M., Khan, I.A., Soodini, G., et al. (2003) Acute myocardial infarction with normal coronary arteries associated with iatrogenic hyperthyroidism, *Int J Cardiol* Vol.90:327-329.

Davis, P.J. & Davis, F.B. (1974) Hyperthyroidism in patients over the age of 60 years. Clinical features in 85 patients, *Medicine* Vol.53:161–181.

Dernellis, J. & Panaretou, M. (2002) Effects of thyroid replacement therapy on arterial blood pressure in patients with hypertension and hypothyroidism, *Amer Heart J* Vol.143(4):718-724.

Dzau, V. & Braunvald, E. (1991) Resolved and unresolved issues in the prevention and treatment of coronary artery disease: a workshop consensus statement, *Am Heart J* Vol.121:1244-1263.

Faure, O., Oziol, L., Artur, Y., et al. (2004) Thyroid hormone (T3) and its acetic derivative (TA3) protect low density lipoprotein cholesterol from oxidation by different mechanisms, *Biochemie* Vol.86:411-418.

Fazio, S., Palmieri, E.A., Lombardi, G., et al. (2004) Effects of Thyroid Hormone on the Cardiovascular System, *Recent Progress in Hormone Research* Vol. 59:31-50.

Fommei, E. & Iervasi, G. (2002) The role of thyroid hormone in blood pressure homeostasis: evidence from short-term hypothyroidism in humans, *J Clin Endocrinol Metab* Vol.87:1996 -2000.

Forhead, A.J., Cutts, S., Matthews, P.A., et al. (2009) Role of thyroid hormones in the developmental control of tissue glycogen in fetal sheep near term, *Exp Physiol* Vol.94:1079–1087.

Franklyn, J.A., Gammage, M.D., Ramsden, D.B. et al. (1984) Thyroid status in patients after acute myocardial infarction, *Clin Sci* Vol.67:585–590.

Franklyn, J.A., Maisonneuve, P., Sheppard, M.C., et al. (1998) Mortality after the treatment of hyperthyroidism with radioactive iodine, *N Engl J Med* Vol.338:712–718.

Friberg, L., Werner, S., Eggertsen, G. et al. (2002) Rapid down-regulation of thyroid hormones in acute myocardial infarction, *Arch Intern Med* Vol.162:1388–1394.

Hak, A.E., Pols, H.A., Visser, T.J. et al. (2000) Subclinical hypothyroidism is an independent risk factor for atherosclerosis and myocardial infarction in elderly women: the Rotterdam Study, *Ann Intern Med* Vol.132: 270–278.

Hall, P., Lundell, G. & Holm, L.E. (1993) Mortality in patients treated for hyperthyroidism with iodine-131, *Acta Endocrionol* Vol.128:230-234.

Homoncik, M., Gessl, A., Ferlitsch, A., et al., (2007) Altered Platelet Plug Formation in Hyperthyroidism and Hypothyroidism, *the Journal of Clinical Endocrinology and Metabolism* Vol.92(8):3006-3012.

Iervasi, G., Clerico, A., Bonini, R. et al. (1997) Acute effects of amiodarone administration on thyroid function in patients with cardiac arrhythmia, *J Clin Endocrinol Metab* V.82:275-280.

Iervasi, G., Molinaro, S., Landi, P. et al. (2007) Association between increased mortality and mild thyroid dysfunction in cardiac patients, *Arch Intern Med* Vol.167(14):1526-1532.

Iqbal, A., Figenschau, Y. & Jorde, R. (2006) Blood pressure in relation to serum thyrotropin: the Tromso study, *J Hum Hypertens* Vol.20:932-936.

Ittermann, T., Haring, R., Sauer, S. et al. (2010) Decreased serum TSH levels are not associated with mortality in the adult northeast German population, *Eur J Endocrinol* Vol.162(3):579–585.

Jaber, J., Haque, S., Noor, H., et al. (2010) Thyrotoxicosis and Coronary Artery Spasm: Case Report and Review of the Literature, *Angiology* Vol.61(8):807-812.

Jung, C.H., Sung, K.C., Shin, H.S., et al. (2003) Thyroid dysfunction and their relation to cardiovascular risk factors such as lipid profile, hsCRP, and waist hip ratio in Korea, *The Korean Journal of Internal Medicine* Vol.18:146-153.

Kahaly, G.J. & Dillmann, W.H. (2005) Thyroid Hormone Action in the Heart, *Endocrine Reviews* Vol.26:704-728.

Kanbay, M., Turgut, F., Karakurt, F., et al. (2007) Relation between serum thyroid hormone and "nondipper" circadian blood pressure variability, *Kidney Blood Press Res* Vol.30:416-420.

Kiss, E., Jakab, G., Kranias, E.G., et al. (1994) Thyroid hormone induced alteration in phospholamban protein expression: regulatory effects on sarcoplasmic reticulum Ca2+ transport and myocardial relaxation, *Circ Res* Vol.75 : 245 –251.

Klein, I. & Ojamaa, K. (1995) Thyroid hormone and blood pressure regulation, in Laragh, J.H. & Brenner, B.M. (eds). *Hypertension: Pathophysiology, Diagnosis and Management, 2d ed.*, Raven Press, Ltd, New York, p.2247.

Klieverik, L.P., Janssen, S.F., van Riel, A., et al. (2009). Thyroid hormone modulates glucose production via a sympathetic pathway from the hypothalamic paraventricular nucleus to the liver, *Proc Natl Acad Sci USA* Vol.106:5966–5971.

Knudsen, N., Laurberg, P., Rasmussen, L.B. et al. (2005) Small differences in thyroid function may be important for body mass index and the occurrence of obesity in the population, *J Clin Endocrinol Metab* Vol.90(7):4019-4024.

Ladenson, P.W., Wilson, M.C., Gardin, J., et al. (1994) Relationship of subclinical hypothyroidism to cardiovascular risk factors and disease in an elderly population, *Thyroid* Vol.4:S-18.

Mancia, G., De Backer, G., Dominiczak, A., et al. (2007) Guidelines for the management of arterial hypertension. The Task Force for the management of arterial hypertension of the European Society of hypertension (ESH) and the European Society of Cardiology (ESC), *Eur Heart J* Vol.28:1462-1536.

Mariotti, S. & Cambuli, V.M. (2007) Cardiovascular risk in elderly hypothyroid patients, *Thyroid* Vol.17:1067–1073.

Mariotti, S. (2008) Mild hypothyroidism and ischemic heart disease: is age the answer? *J Clin Endocrinol Metab* Vol.93:2969-2971.

Martino, E., Bartalena, L., Bogazzi, F. et al. (2001) The effects of amiodarone on the thyroid, *Endocrine Reviews* V.22:240–254.

Mayer, O., Šimon, J., Filipovský, J. et al. (2006) Hypothyroidism in coronary heart disease and its relation to selected risk factors, *Vasc Health Risk Manag* Vol.2(4): 499-506.

Mazzefi, M.A., Lin, H.-M., Flynn, B.C., et al. (2010) Hypothyroidism and the risk of lower extremity arterial disease, *Vascular Health and Risk Management* Vol.6:957-962.

Medici, A., van der Deure, W. M., Verbiest M. et al. (2011) A large-scale association analysis of 68 thyroid hormone pathway genes with serum TSH and FT4 levels, *Eur J Endocrinol* Vol.164:781-788.

Miller, M. & Gambert, S.R. (2008) Thyroid heart disease in the elderly, *in* Aronov, W.S., Fleg, J.L., Rich, M.W. (eds). *Cardiovascular Disease in the Elderly, 4th ed.,* Informa Healthcare, New York, pp. 517-540.

Moliterno, D., Debold, C.R. & Robertson, R.M. (1992) Case report: coronary vasospasm—relation to the hyperthyroid state, *Am J Med Sci* Vol.304:38–42.

Obuobie, K., Smith, J., Evans, L.M., *et al.* (2002) Increased central arterial stiffness in hypothyroidism, *J Clin Endocrinol Metab* Vol.87:4662 -4666.

Ojamaa, K., Kenessey, A. & Klein, I. (2002) Thyroid hormone regulation of phospholamban phosphorylation in the rat heart, *Endocrinology* Vol.141:2139 -2144.

Ojamaa, K., Klemperer, J.D. & Klein, I. (1996) Acute effects of thyroid hormone on vascular smooth muscle, *Thyroid* Vol.6:505 -512.

Osman, F., Gammage, M.D. & Franklyn, J.A. (2002) Hyperthyroidism and cardiovascular morbidity and mortality, *Thyroid* Vol.12:483–488.

Parle, J.V., Maisonneuve, P., Sheppard, M.C., et al. (2001) Prediction of all cause and cardiovascular mortality in elderly people from one low serum thyrotropin result: a 10-year cohort study, *Lancet* Vol.358:861–865.

Perk, M. & O'Neill, B.J. (1997) The effect of thyroid hormone therapy on angiographic coronary artery disease progression, *Can J Cardiol* Vol.13:273–276.

Pierre-Louis, B., Aronow, W.S., Palaniswamy, C., et al. (2008) Prevalence of obstructive coronary artery disease in patients with diabetes mellitus with and without hypothyroidism, *Open Longevity Science* Vol.2:104-106.

Prieur, X., Huby, T., Coste, H. et al. (2005) Thyroid hormone regulates the hypotriglyceridemic gene APOA5, *J Biol Chem* Vol.280(30):27533-27543.

Renaudon, B., Lenfant, J., Decressac S., et al. (2000) Thyroid hormone increases the conductance density of f-channels in rabbit sino-atrial node cells, *Receptors Channels* Vol.7(1):1-8.

Rensen, P.C., van Dijk, K.W. & Havekes, L.M. (2005) Apolipoprotein AV: low concentration, high impact, *Arterioscler Tromb Vasc Biol* Vol.25:2445-2447.

Resnick, L.M. & Laragh, J.H. (1982) Plasma renin activity in syndromes of thyroid hormone excess and deficiency, *Life Sci* Vol.30:585-586.

Rizos, C.V., Elisaf, M.S. & Lieberopoulos, E.N. (2011) Effects of thyroid dysfunction on lipid profile, *The Open Cardiovascular Medicine Journal* Vol.5: 76-84.

Saito, I., Ito, K. & Saruta, T. (1983) Hypothyroidism as a cause of hypertension, *Hypertension* Vol.5:112-115.

Sgarbi, J.A., Matsumura, L.K., Kasamatsu, T.S. et al. (2010) Subclinical thyroid dysfunctions are independent risk factors for mortality in a 7,5-year follow-up: the Japanese-Brazilian thyroid study, *Eur J Endocrinol* Vol.162:569–577.

Shin, D. J. & Osborne, N.F. (2003) Thyroid hormone regulation and cholesterol metabolism are connected through Sterol Regulatory Element-Binding Protein-2 (SREBP-2), *J Biol Chem* Vol.278:34114-341148.

Sterling, K. (1986) Direct thyroid hormone activation of mitochondria: the role of adenine nucleotide translocase, *Endocrinology* Vol.119(1):292-295.

Streeten, D.H., Anderson, Jr. G.H., Howland, T., et al. (1988) Effects of thyroid function on blood pressure: recognition of hypothyroid hypertension, *Hypertension* Vol.11:78-83.

Sun, Z.Q., Ojamaa, K., Nakamura, T.Y., et al. (2001) Thyroid hormone increases pacemaker activity in rat neonatal atrial myocytes, *J Mol Cell Cardiol* Vol.33:811-824.

Surks, M.I., Ortiz, E., Daniels, G.H. et al. (2004) Subclinical thyroid disease: scientific review and guidelines for diagnosis and management, *JAMA* Vol.291:228–238.

Taylor, P.N., Panicker, V., Sayers, A. et al. (2011) A meta-analysis of the associations between common variation in the *PDE8B* gene and thyroid hormone parameters, including assessment of longitudinal stability of associations over time and effect of thyroid hormone replacement, *Eur J Endocrinol* Vol.164: 773-780.

Trivalle, C., Doucet, J., Chassagne, P., et al. (1996) Differences in the signs and symptoms of hyperthyroidism in older and younger patients, *J Am Geriatr Soc* Vol.44:50–53.

Tzotzas, T., Krassas, G.E., Konstantinidis, T., et al. (2000) Changes in lipoprotein (a) levels in overt and subclinical hypothyroidism before and during treatment, *Thyroid* Vol.10:803-808.

Vanderpump, M.P., Tunbridge, W.M., French, J.M., et al. (1996) The development of ischemic heart disease in relation to autoimmune thyroid disease in a 20-year follow-up study of an English community, *Thyroid* Vol.6:155–160.

Vanhaelst, L., Neve, P., Chailly, P., et al. (1967) Coronary artery disease in hypothyroidism. Observations in clinical myxoedema, *Lancet* Vol.2:800–802.

Verhoeven, A., J., Kamer, P., Groen, A.K., et al. (1985) Effects of thyroid hormone on mitochondrial oxidative phosphorylation, *The Biochemical Journal* Vol. 226(1):183-192.

13

Coronary Artery Disease and Systemic Vasculitis: Case Report and Review

Damianos Eleftheriadis and Nikolaos Eleftheriadis
Aristotle's University of Thessaloniki, Cardiology Department, 'Bodosakio' Hospital, Ptolemaida Greece

1. Introduction

Chronic systemic inflammation and immune dysregulation, as a consequence of primary or secondary vasculitis, has been emphasized in pathogenesis of coronary artery disease. (Gasparyan & Ugurlucan, 2008; Mukhtyar et al., 2009; Turesson et al., 2008). Severe coronary artery disease in absence of obvious serious risk factors, especially in young age, remains a challenge to modern cardiology. In these cases, possible relation of ischemic heart disease to systemic vasculitis or thrombophilic predisposition should be also examined. (Kaplan 2009; Knockaert 2007; Tenedios et al., 2006).

Henoch-Schonlein Purpura is a rare disease characterized by systemic vasculitis (Agraharkar et al., 2000; Satoh et al., 1991). It is rarely related with acute myocardial infarction or multivessel disease. (Abdel-Hadi et al., 1981; Eleftheriadis, 2007a; Lutz et al., 2009; Osman & McCreery, 2000). (Table 1)

An atypical presentation of severe acute myocardial infarction in a young male with Henoch-Schonlein Purpura in remission and no other risk factors for coronary artery disease is reported and discussed. After meticulous investigation, including complete blood examinations for thrombophilic diathesis, antiphospholipid antibodies and autoimmunity, it was concluded that severe acute myocardial infarction in this case was a consequence of latent systemic vasculitis in the setting of Henoch-Schonlein Purpura.

The relation of coronary artery disease with primary or secondary vasculitides is also reviewed. Early suspicion and recognition of vasculitis in atypical cases and early initiation of appropriate treatment, including corticosteroids and immunosuppressives, may become the only optional strategy for prevention of vasculitis-related coronary lesions and life-threatening infarctions on the ground of undiagnosed systemic vasculitis.

Key Words: coronary artery disease, acute myocardial infarction, coronary aneurysms, systemic vasculitis, Henoch-Schonlein Purpura, Kawasaki disease, polyarteritis nodosa, systemic lupus erythematosis, Wegener's granulomatosis, antiphospholipid syndrome, polyangiitis overlap syndrome, Churg-Strauss syndrome, Takayasu arteritis.

2. Severe coronary artery disease in the setting of Henoch-Schoenlein purpura: Case report

2.1 Case report

A 49-year-old male with acute myocardial infarction and Henoch-Schoenlein purpura in remission for 10-years, is reported. The patient was admitted with chest pain. Laboratory examination showed elevation of cardiac enzymes, while the 12-lead electrocardiogram demonstrated ST elevation (up to five mm) in leads II, III, and aVF.

He had a previous history of acute glomerulonephritis for ten-years, which was finally attributed to Henoch-Schonlein Purpura, after detailed clinico-laboratory investigation in tertiary center. At that time, total immunological examination did not reveal any other autoimmune disease, neither systemic lupus erythematosis nor other known vasculitis. Thereafter, he was totally asymptomatic with normal renal function. During ten-year follow-up, he had no other admissions, used no medications and had no personal or family history of thrombotic events.

Except for b-blockers use for arterial hypertension, he reported no other medications, smoking or alcohol use. All other personal and family history was negative for coronary artery disease.

Clinical examination revealed: blood pressure: 120/80 mmHg, heart rate 50/1min. Urine examination showed mild haematuria. Laboratory examination showed: urea 42mg/dl, creatinin 1.1mg/dl (normal<1.3), cholesterol: 197mg/dl, (normal<200mg/dl), LDL 135mg/dl (normal <150), triglycerides 96mg/dl (normal <150mg/dl), HDL 47mg/dl (normal >35mg/dl), ESR 54/1h (normal <8/1h), CRP 16.22 mg/dl, (normal <0.8). All other hematological, blood chemistry results and thorax photo were normal.

The patient was successfully treated in intensive care unit for acute myocardial infarction, while no thrombolysis was given due to delay arrival. Angiography showed three-vessel disease (right coronary artery 100%, middle circumflex artery 75% and left anterior descending artery 50%) and angioplasty was performed in two vessels.

Blood examinations for thrombophilic diathesis were performed. All known risk factors associated with increased risk of thrombosis, such as antiphospholipid antibodies, coagulation factors, protein C, protein S, factor V Leiden, mutation G20210A of prothrombin [PTHR A(20210)], and mutation TT677 of methylenetetrahydrofolate reductase [MTHFR C677-->T]), were within normal.

Thereafter, the patient is under continuous combined anticoagulation with low dose aspirin plus clopidogrel. During five-year follow-up post-infarction the patient is totally asymptomatic and he is under continuous antianginal agents. No corticosteroids or immunosuppressive drugs were administered.

2.2 Discussion

Henoch-Schonlein Purpura is a rare disease, characterized by systemic vasculitis of the skin and other abdominal organs (Agraharkar et al., 2000; Satoh et al., 1991). It has good prognosis, except if it is complicated by severe glomerular disease (Watanabe et al., 2003).

Although, it has been extensively studied in children, its natural history in adults is less known, with outcome worse in adults than in children. (Pillebout et al., 2002). Correlation with acute myocardial infarction or multivessel disease has been rarely reported (Abdel-Hadi et al., 1981; Eleftheriadis, 2007; Lutz et al., 2009; Osman & McCreery, 2000). (Table 1)

An interesting finding of the present case, is the discrepancy between absence of serious risk factors for coronary artery disease in a young patient and severity of infarction (three-vessel disease), which was also reported in two similar cases, with thrombotic thrombocytopenic purpura. (Dhawan & Tak, 2004; Hasper et al., 2006).

Only the previous history of Henoch-Schoenlein purpura and its vasculitis-related coronary lesions, could explain the premature infarction of this case. However, Henoch-Schonlein purpura and its nephritis regressed and stabilized the last ten years, which is also another interesting finding of the present case.

Co-existence of other predisposing factors for ischemic heart disease, such as thrombophilic disorders or potential superimposition of other systemic vasculitis, could also be a possible explanation of the unusual severe premature infarction, in the present case. (Eleftheriadis, 2007b; Shin & Lee, 2007).

Antiphospholipid syndrome should be excluded in cases of Henoch-Schonlein Purpura, and antiphospholipid antibodies should be measured to determine whether prophylactic antithrombotic measures are needed to prevent additional thrombotic manifestations. (Espinosa & Gervera, 2010; Monastiri et al. 2002; Sullivan et al., 1999).

However, repeated and meticulous examinations for thrombophilic diathesis, including antiphospholipid antibodies, as well as immunological examinations for other secondary systemic vasculitis, did not reveal any additional diagnosis in this case. (Eleftheriadis, 2007b). Moreover, the possibility of polyangitis overlap syndrome was also excluded.

Although vasculitis is classified according to the size of involved vessels, some patients do not belong to a single disease entity and show the symptoms seen in more than two diseases. (Tanimoto, 1994; Zaidi et al, 2008).

The incidence of polyangitis overlap syndrome in patients with cardiac vasculitis is unknown, because this overlap has often been diagnosed by postmortem autopsy. (Freddo et al., 1999; Kimura et al, 2011; Kumar et al., 2002; Wegner & Schneider, 1996). Therefore, when a patient presents with atypical presentation of Henoch-Schonlein Purpura, the overlap of other vasculitis should also be examined to prevent unexpected fatal situations. (Watanabe et al., 2003; Zaidi et al., 2008).

Latent vasculitis in the setting of Henoch-Scoenlein purpura was the only obvious cause for the severe infarction in this case. No other alarm symptoms for years and no previous signs of active vasculitis were reported, which could had lead to preventive measures for coronary thrombosis.

In conclusion, this case is of interest due to rarity of Henoch-Schonlein Purpura as a cause of severe coronary artery disease and the atypical presentation with latent course of Purpura-related vasculitis.

3. Coronary artery disease and primary systemic vasculitis

Primary systemic vasculitides are a group of autoimmune conditions characterized by occlusion, stenosis or aneurysmal dilatation of blood vessels, including coronary arteries, secondary to intramural inflammation. Increased prevalence of premature cardiovascular disease has been observed in chronic inflammatory disorders, such as systemic vasculitis. Coronary abnormalities may also be the only manifestations of many vasculitides. (Bijl, 2003; Kaplan, 2009; Knockaert, 2007; Mukhtyar et al., 2009; Nabatian et al., 2006; Reinhold-Keller et al, 2005).

Skin biopsy, showing mural fibrin deposition in arterioles or venules and angiocentric inflammatory cell infiltration, in cases with suspicion of vasculitis, is important for early diagnosis. (Magro & Crowson, 1999). (Figure 1)

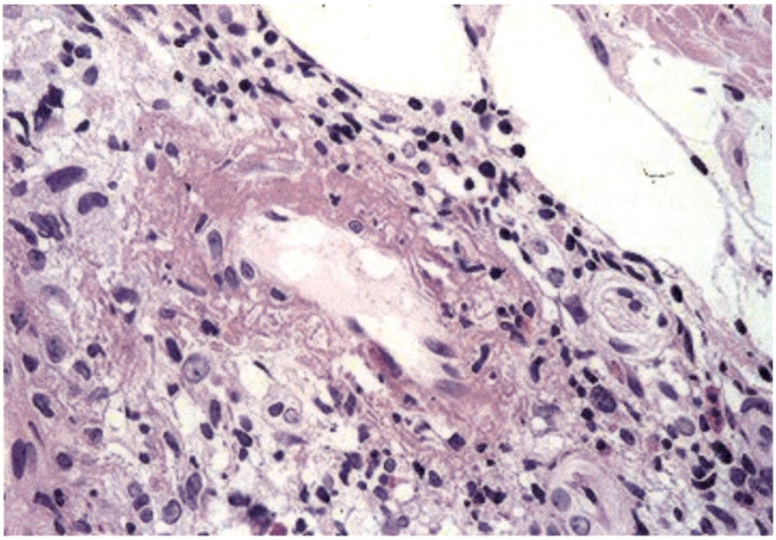

Fig. 1. Skin biopsy from a patient with leukocytoclastic vasculitis showing mural fibrin deposition in a venule and angiocentric mixed meutrophilic and lymphocytic infiltration. (Magro & Crowson, 1999).

Although the mechanisms of accelerated atherosclerosis in systemic vasculitis have not been fully clarified and may differ in the different vasculitic syndromes, direct injury to arteries, arterial intimal –media calcification, pro-atherogenic changes in lipid and fibrin metabolism, and systemic hypertension due to alterations in carotid baroreceptor sensitivity, as a consequence to vasculitis, have been proposed.(Agarwal et al., 2010; Donald et al., 1976; Kane & Keogh, 2009; Mukhtyar, et al., 2009).

Endothelial cell activation through autoantibodies, resulting in endothelial cell dysfunction, complement-dependent and antibody-dependent cytotoxicity, cytokines and direct effect of adhesion molecules have all been also implicated in vasculitis-related premature atherosclerosis. (Bijl, 2003; Savage, 2002).

Current therapy has changed the natural history of these diseases from death or severe morbidity to a remitting-relapsing condition in most instances. However, despite major immunosuppressive care, systemic vasculitis may lead to potential fatal complications and death, through diffuse vessel fibrinoid necrosis and interstitial hemorrhages, attaching multiple organs. (Andersson, 2000; Bossert, et al. 2011; Eberhardt & Dhadly, 2007; Freddo et al., 1999; Lin, et al., 2007; Osman & McCreery, 2000; Wegner & Schneider, 1996).

What is more, longer survival, relapsing course and complications related to chronic corticosteroid therapy (hypertension, diabetes mellitus and change in lipid profile), may further contribute to an increase in cardiovascular events and morbidity. (Lin et al., 2007; Mukhtyar et al., 2009).

On the other hand, there is evidence that glycocorticoid therapy in combination with immunosuppressive may improve endothelial dysfunction and prevent myocardial ischemia as a consequence of vasculitis in some cases. (Cocco & Gasparyan, 2010; Gonzalez-Juanatey et al., 2006; Lutz et al., 2009; Oates-Whitehead, et al. 2003).

Primary systemic vasculitides are categorized according to the vessel size, into large-vessel and medium- to small-vessel vasculitis, while the mode and incidence of cardiac involvement vary within the different vasculitic syndromes. (Agarwal et al., 2010; Hata & Onouchi, 2009; Hewins & Jane, 2010; Kane & Keogh, 2009; Mukhtyar et al., 2009). The relation of coronary artery disease with different categories of primary vasculitides are reviewed.

3.1 Cardiovascular involvement in large vessel vasculitis

3.1.1 Coronary artery disease and giant cel arteritis

Giant cell arteritis is a relatively common large vessel vasculitis, which affects, predominantly cranial nerves, especially temporal artery, occasionally aorta and rarely coronary arteries or other visceral or peripheral arteries. (Andersson, 2000). Stroke, aortic aneurysm or dissection, and even aortic rupture, visual loss due to ischemic optic neuropathy, secondary to temporal arteritis, are tragic manifestations of giant cell arteritis. (Andersson, 2000; Eberhardt & Dhadly, 2007; Lin et al., 2007).

Coronary artery disease is most commonly occurred in the long-term course, but it is also reported at disease presentation, in atypical cases. (Bossert et al., 2011; Eberhardt & Dhadly, 2007; Kimura et al., 2011; Lin, et al., 2007). Giant cell-related early myocardial infarction, often with fatal outcome, is more commonly reported than previously appreciated. (Freddo et al., 1999; Lin et al., 2007; Bossert et al., 2011; Wegner & Schneider, 1996).

Although, most of the complications of giant cell arteritis can be effectively prevented by early initiation of corticosteroid treatment, severe myocardial infarction, even fatal, can still occur despite high-dose corticosteroid therapy. (Andersson, 2000; Bossert et al., 2011; Eberhardt & Dhadly, 2007; Freddo et al., 1999; Lin et al., 2007; Wegner & Schneider, 1996).

Furthermore, in unusual cases of coronary giant arteritis, precise diagnosis was done antemortem at autopsy. (Freddo, T., et al., 1999; Kimura, T., et al. 2011; Kumar, P., et al., 2002; Wegner, M., & Schneider, J. 1996).

Modern imaging techniques, including positron emission tomography and magnetic resonance imaging should be considered in atypical cases of giant cell aortitis and coronary giant arteritis, which are more common than previously thought. (Bossert et al., 2011; Kimura et al., 2011; Lin et al., 2007; Mavrogeni et al., 2009). Directional coronary atherectomy can also be an alternative diagnostic method for coronary giant arteritis. ;Saito et al., 1994).

3.1.2 Coronary artery disease and Takayasu arteritis

Takayasu arteritis is a large vessel vasculitis that usually involves the large cardiac vessels, predominantly the aorta and its main branches. Approximately 10% of cases are associated with ostial or proximal coronary artery stenosis, necessitating bypass. (Amano & Suzuki, 1992; Ouali et al., 2011; Park et al., 2010, Sheikhzadeh et al., 2002).

Angiographically Takayasu arteritis was classified as cervicobranchial (I), thoracoabdominal (II), peripheral type (III) and generalized type (IV), which was the most frequent. (Sheikhzadeh, A. et al. 2002). Atypical presentation of Takayasu arteritis, with acute myocardial infarction in young patients, which could not be fully classified, was also reported. (Araszkiewicz et al., 2007).

Coronary artery disease as a consequence of Takayasu arteritis, is relatively rare, resulting however in severe life-threatening complications. It is also associated with aneurysmal dilation of other arteries such as carotid, vertebral and renal arteries. (Amano & Suzuki, 1992; Araszkiewicz et al., 2007; Ouali et al., 2011; Sheikhzadeh et al., 2002).

3.2 Cardiovascular involvement in medium and small vessel vasculitis

Coronary vasculitis is an uncommon but catastrophic clinical presentation of small and medium vessel vasculitis. Inflammation and damage of the coronary arteries lead to aneurysm formation and subsequently to stenosis and coronary thrombosis. (Agarwal et al., 2010; Hata & Onouchi, 2009; Hewins &Jayne, 2010; Kane & Keogh, 2009).

Prompt diagnosis and early treatment with corticosteroid and immunosuppressives in combination to anti-anginic therapy is usually effective and reduced the frequency of cardiovascular complications. However, vasculitis relapse although rare, may result in an increased risk of cardiovascular disease later in life despite aggressive therapy. (Hewins & Jayne, 2010; Kane & Keogh, 2009).

3.2.1 Coronary artery disease and Kawasaki disease

Kawasaki disease is an acute systemic vasculitis of childhood, of unknown origin, that particularly affects the coronary arteries. It is complicated by coronary arterial aneurysms (Figure 2) and stenosis in approximately 20 to 25% of untreated patients and subsequently can lead to myocardial infarction and/or sudden death. (De Castro et al., 2009; La Pellegrin et al., 2011; Tsuda et al., 2011; Wood & Tulloh, 2009).

Kawasaki disease has an incidence of approximately 8 per 100000 children in the western countries, while it is more frequent in Japan. (Fukazawa & Ogawa, 2009; Hata & Onouchi, 2009). It is considered one of the most common causes of acquired heart disease in children in developed countries. (Caballero-Mora et al., 2011; De Castro et al 2009; Fukazawa & Ogawa, 2009; La Pellegrin et al., 2011; Tsuda et al., 2011; Wood & Tulloh, 2009).

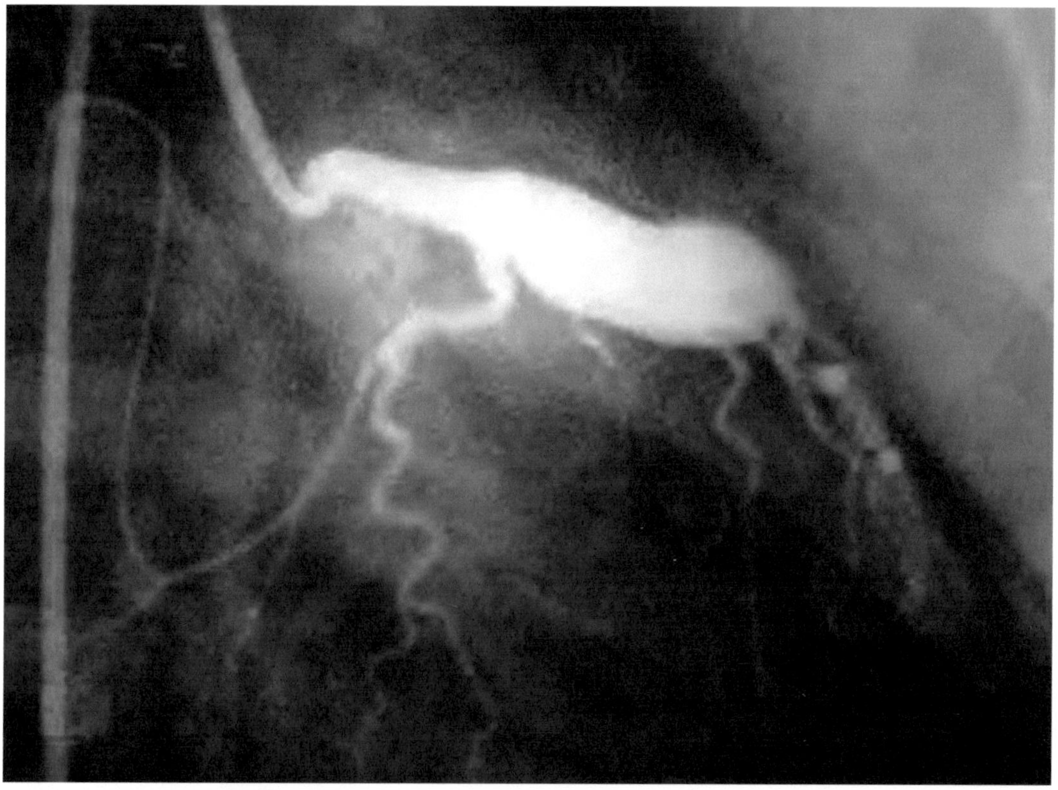

Fig. 2. Coronary-artery aneurysm in a patient with Kawasaki disease (Hewins & Jayne, 2010).

Despite treatment of acute phase with intravenous immunoglobulin and aspirin, up to 5% of Kawasaki disease patients, still continued to develop serious cardiac life-threatening complications, mainly giant coronary aneurysms and thrombotic stenoses, resulted in myocardial infarction and/or death. (Caballero-Mora et al., 2011; De Castro et al., 2009; Hata & Onouchi, 2009; LaPellegrin et al., 2011; Lin et al., 2011; Tsuda et al., 2011; Wood & Tulloh, 2009).

Atypical presentation or incomplete form is presented in one third of all Kawasaki disease patients, characterized by an older age at onset and diagnostic delay. (La Pellegrin et al., 2011; Gomard-Mennesson et al., 2010).

Acute coronary syndrome in adults caused by Kawasaki disease is rarely reported. (LaPellegrin et al., 2011, Tsuda E et al., 2011). Older age, male sex, higher C-reactive protein levels, urticarial exanthema, lack of response to the first intravenous immunoglobulin (IVIg) infusion and IVIg dosage < 2 g/kg, were reported as risk factors for the development of atherosclerosis in adults with Kawasaki disease. (La Pellegrin et al., 2011, Caballero-Mora et al 2011). C-reactive protein, oxidative stress, and inflammatory cytokines, are also increased in the remote phase of Kawasaki disease (Fukazawa & Ogawa, 2009).

Despite intensive research the cause remains unknown. It is generally accepted that an as yet undefined infectious trigger in a genetically predisposed individual results in Kawasaki disease. (Eleftheriou et al., 2009).

A strong genetic influence on Kawasaki disease susceptibility has been indicated from epidemiological studies. (Hata & Onouchi, 2009). Advances in molecular genetic analysis, have permitted the identification of inositol 1,4,5-triphosphate 3-kinase C (ITPKC), as a predisposing gene associated with Kawasaki disease. (Eleftheriou et al., 2009; Hata & Onouchi, 2009; Lin et al., 2011; Rowley, 2011).

Early detection and initiation of therapy is substantial for good outcome in Kawasaki patients with coronary lesions. The combination of aspirin, corticosteroids and/or intravenous immunoglobulin, started early after the onset of symptoms, has reduced the frequency of coronary artery aneurysms in Kawasaki disease. (Oates-Whitehead et al., 2003; Wooditch & Aronoff, 2005).

Although there are no clear specific recommendations regarding thrombolytic therapy in Kawasaki pediatric patients, there are reports of the use of all known thrombolytics, in children with myocardial infarction related to Kawasaki disease. (Paredes et al., 2000). Close collaboration between pediatric cardiologists and coronary interventional cardiologists is necessary. (Akagi, 2011).

3.2.2 Coronary artery disease and Henoch Schoenlein Purpura

Henoch Schoenlein Purpura is one of the most common forms of leukocytoclastic vasculitis in children, which is self-limited in the majority of cases. (Lutz et al., 2009; Pillebout et al., 2002; Polizzotto et al., 2006; Zaidi et al., 2008).

Infectious triggers are still implicated in the aetiopathogenesis of Henoch-Schoenlein purpura, while several genetic polymorphisms have been described that may be relevant in disease predisposition or development of disease complications. (Eleftheriou et al., 2009; Lutz et al., 2009). In adults clinical presentation of Henoch Schoenelin purpura is severe, with relatively poor outcome, worse than in children, which is mainly related to renal impairment and glomerulonephritis. (Eleftheriou et al., 2009; Lutz et al., 2009).

Coronary artery disease in adults with Henoch Schoenelin purpura is rarely reported as main manifestation and only in case reports. (Table 1). It should be distinguished from secondary Henosch Schoenelin purpura caused for example by rheumatic fever. (Lutz et al., 2009; Pillebout et al., 2002).

Patient Sex/Age (y)	Cardiac Involvement	Treatment	Outcome
Male/71 (Polizzotto, M.N., et al., 2006)	Complete atrioventricular block, no myocardial necrosis	Methylprednisolone, pulse therapy	Complete resolution
Male/69 (Carmichael, P. et al., 2002)	Creatinine kinase increase, left bundle branch block	Methylprednisolone	Death within 11 d
Male/63 (Agraharkar, M., et al 2000)	Escape rhythm and myocardial infarction	Methylprednisolone	Death within 10 d
Male/14 (Osman, A., 2000)	Junctional rhythm, troponin T increase	Prednisone, azathioprine, ventricular pacemaker	Death within a few days

Patient Sex/Age (y)	Cardiac Involvement	Treatment	Outcome
Male/24 (Kereiakes DJ, et al., 1984)	Congestive heart failure (biopsy-proven immunoglobulin A deposits in myocardium)	Prednisone, cyclophosphamide	Persistent congestive heart failure with low ejection fraction (18%)
Male/29 (Abdel-Hadi, O., et al., 1981)	Myocardial infarction without macroangiopathy	–	Persistent apical dyskinesia
Male/11 (Lecutier, M.A., 1952)	Myocardial necrosis, likely secondary HSP	Penicillin	Death 1 mo after first admission
Male/64 (Satoh, M., et al., 1991)	Cardiac dysfunction and dilatation	–	Unknown
Male/9 (Guven, H., et al., 2006)	Mobitz type 2 atrioventricular block, likely secondary HSP	Salicylate, penicillin	Complete resolution
Male/13 (Kalyoncu, M., et al., 2006)	Severe mitral insufficiency with dilatation of the left ventricle, likely secondary HSP	Methylprednisolone, cyclophosphamide	Death 1 mo after admission from cardiac arrest
Male/17 (Zaidi, M., et al., 2008)	Left ventricular dilatation, likely secondary HSP	Methylprednisolone pulse therapy	Kidney function normal at 3-mo follow-up, cardiac outcome unknown
Male/19 (Lutz, H., et al., 2009)	Myocardial involvement, arrhythmia (atrioventricular blocking type 2)	Methylprednisolone pulse therapy, Cyclophosphamide pulse therapy	Complete resolution
Male/49 (Eleftheriadis, D., 2007)	Acute myocardial infarction	Salicylate, antianginal therapy	Complete resolution

Abbreviation: HSP, Henoch-Schönlein purpura.

Table 1. Published case reports of coronary artery disease related to Henoch-Schoenlein Purpura. (Lutz et al., 2009).

Although immunosuppressive therapy, mainly with steroids and/or cyclophosphamide, is reported to be insufficient in diminishing the incidence of renal insufficiency, they may prevent infarction and deleterious outcome. (Lutz et al., 2009). Different immunosuppressive medications and newer therapeutic approaches such as biologic agents have been also reported as alternative options for better management. (Eleftheriou et al., 2009; Lutz et al., 2009; Pillebout et al, 2002;).

3.2.3 Coronary artery disease and antineutrophilic cytoplasmic antibodies (anca) associated vasculitis

Wegener's granulomatosis, microscopic polyangiitis and Churg-Strauss syndrome are small-to medium vessel vasculitides, with strong association with the presence of anti-neutrophil cytoplasm antibodies (ANCAs). There are several reports of extensive myocardial infarction in young patients, as a consequence of coronary aneurysms, related to an ANCA-positive vasculitis. (Mukhtyar et al., 2009; Musuruana et al., 2011). According to similar reported cases early treatment with high doses of immunosuppressives such as corticosteroids and cyclophosphamide, resulted in aneurysm resolution and may prevent myocardial infarction. (Musuruana et al., 2011).

Churg-Strauss syndrome is a vasculitis associated with asthma and eosinophilia. There are two subsets of patients with different pathogenetic mechanisms, with ANCA mediated process in ANCA positive patients and tissue infiltration by eosinophils in ANCA negative patients. Heart diseases related to Churg-Strauss syndrome include coronary vasculitis, myocarditis, valvular heart abnormalities, congestive heart failure and pericarditis. Coronary artery disease is significantly more common in ANCA-negative cases and is the leading cause of mortality in Churg-Strauss syndrome. (Churg & Strauss, 1951; Keogh & Specks, 2003; Sable-Fourtassou et al., 2005; Sinico & Bottero, 2009).

3.2.3.1 Coronary artery disease and Wegener granulomatous disease

Wegener's granulomatosis is one of the most common small-and medium sized necrotizing vasculitis that mainly affects the respiratory tract and kidneys. Cardiac manifestations, although they are increasingly recognized, are relatively rare and in most cases silent. Coronary arteries, pericardium, myocardium, endocardium, valves, conduction system and great vessels may be involved. (Korantzopoulos et al., 2004; Suppiah et al., 2011).

According to substantially increased number of reports Wegener's vasculitis can manifest as myocardial ischemia and infarction. Cardiovascular complications without previous history will be also reported in 14% of patients within five years of newly diagnosed Wegener's granulomatosis. (Suppiah et al., 2011). The presence of proteinase 3 (PR3) antineutrophil cytoplasmic antibodies (ANCA) is associated with reduced cardiovascular risk in patients with vasculitis. (Phillip & Luqmani, 2008; Suppiah et al., 2011).

Coronary angiography failed to reveal atheroscletotic disease or thrombotic occlusion in some reported cases. In similar cases magnetic resonance imaging with adenosine test may become the alternative examination to reveal myocardial ischemia, especially subendocardial ischemia. (Cocco & Gasparyan, 2010).

Immunosuppressive therapy with steroids and cyclophosphamide resulted in disappearance of myocardial ischemia in reported cases. (Cocco & Gasparyan, 2010; Phillip & Luqmani, 2008; Suppiah et al., 2011).

3.2.4 Coronary artery disease and polyarteritis nodosa

Polyarteritis nodosa is an ANCA-negative medium and small vessel vasculitis that commonly affects kidneys, gastrointestinal tract, skin, nerves, joints and muscles. There are no specific serological markers and diagnosis depends on clinical presentation, angiography and tissues biopsy. It can pursue a relapsing course, although treatment with corticosteroids and immunosuppressive is usually effective. It is now rarely associated with hepatitis B infection. (Hewins & Jayne, 2010).

Premature coronary artery disease, presenting multiple progressive coronary lesions and necessitating repeated percutaneous interventions and/or bypass, has been described in several case reports in the context of polyarteritis nodosa. (Maillard-Lefebvre ey al., 2008; Yanagawa et al., 2010; Yuce et al., 2011).

4. Coronary artery disease and secondary systemic vasculitis

Coronary artery disease as a consequence of secondary systemic vasculitis on the ground of autoimmune diseases such as systemic lupus erythematosis, rheumatoid arthritis, primary antiphospholipid syndrome etc is the leading cause of morbidity and mortality in these cases. It may occur in younger age, it is often asymptomatic and it may be clinically silent in early phases. (Caracciolo et al., 2004; Salmon & Roman, 2008; Sitia et al., 2009; Yildiz, 2010; Yiu et al., 2011). Arterial compliance and arterial distensibility may be altered via systemic inflammation and may lead to accelerated atherosclerosis in secondary systemic vasculitis. (Yildiz, 2010).

Although coronary angiography remains the cold standard for diagnosing coronary stenosis, non invasive and more reliable methods, such as magnetic resonance imaging and PET scan, have been proposed in order to detect subclinical microcirculation abnormalities. (Pennell, & Keenan, 2011; Sitia et al., 2009).

4.1 Coronary artery disease and systemic lupus erythematosis

Systemic lupus erythematosis is a chronic autoimmune disease involving multiple organ systems, characterizing by flares and remissions and presence of antinuclear autoantibodies. Early symptoms most frequently involve the skin and joints. (Kalunian & Merill, 2009).

Severe lupus morbidity and mortality however, is usually associated with cardiovascular events and major organ damage, particularly kidneys. Coronary artery disease was found to be the main cause of death in systemic lupus erythematosis in all studies. (Caracciolo et al., 2004; Gilboe, 2008; Kalunian & Merill, 2009).

Improved understanding of systemic lupus erythematosis pathogenesis and immunology has lead to target treatments, such as this provided by biologic agents, which resulted in disease stabilization or even reverse of the disease course. (Kalunian & Merill, 2009;).

4.2 Coronary artery disease and rheumatoid arthritis

Secondary vasculitis in the setting of rheumatoid arthritis can affect small as well as large vessels, contributing to renal, neurological, gastrointestinal and cardiac complications. High rheumatoid factor levels and cryoglobulins were associated with multi-organ complications of rheumatoid vasculitis. (Albada-Kuipers et al., 1986; Solomon, et al., 2003).

Chronic systemic inflammation contributed to accelerated atherosclerosis in rheumatoid arthritis. (Ku et al., 2009; Solomon et al., 2003). Coronary rheumatoid vasculitis although rare, is increasingly recognized, can be subclinical, has high mortality rate and in some cases can be found only post-mortem. (Abu-Fadel et al., 2011; Albada-Kuipers et al., 1986; Jeffery, 2010; Solomon et al., 2003). Rapid progression from an ectatic to an aneurysmatic coronary artery leading to acute coronary syndrome in rheumatoid vasculitis has been also reported and only in case reports. (Abu-Fadel et al., 2011; Wang, K.Y., et al., 1999).

Other cardiac manifestations of rheumatoid arthritis reported, were valvular disease, pericarditis and rarely myocarditis and aortitis. (Solomon, 2003; Abu-Fadel et al., 2011).

Early diagnosis and prompt initiation of immunosuppressive therapy in coronary rheumatoid vasculitis, is crucial in prevention of further coronary aneurysmal expansion and rupture. (Abu-Fadel et al., 2011; Wang, K.Y., et al., 1999). According to recent reports, a comprehensive cardiac magnetic resonance imaging is considered an effective and less-invasive method for assessing the microvascular and/or subendocardial ischemic lesions of asymptomatic patients with rheumatoid vasculitis. (Kobayashi, Y., et al., 2010; Mavrogeni et al., 2009).

4.3 Coronary artery disease and antiphospholipid syndrome

Antiphospholipid syndrome is an autoimmune disorder characterized by hypercoagulability, arterial and venous thrombosis, recurrent fetal loss and the presence of antiphospholipid antibodies. (Kaynar et al., 2007; Benzarouel et al., 2007; Levine et al., 2000; Silbiger, 2009).

It may be primary, without other signs of autoantibodies, besides antiphospholipid antibodies or secondary in the setting of underlying disease e.g. malignancy or autoimmune diseases, mainly systemic lupus erythematosis. (Kaynar et al., 2007; Sullivan et al., 1999). Antiphospholipid antibodies also include the lupus anticoagulant and anticardiolipin antibody. (Sullivan et al., 1999; Espinosa & Gervera, 2010).

Coronary artery disease, especially myocardial infarction in young patients, even silent, has been reported in antiphospholipid syndrome, with or without systemic lupus erythematosis. (Kaynar et al., 2007; Benzarouel et al., 2007). In similar cases simultaneous multiple organ thrombotic signs, including renal vein thrombosis, portal vein thrombosis, pulmonary emboli and myocardial infarction, must be excluded by tomographic angiography. (Kaynar et al., 2007; Levine et al., 2000; Silbiger, 2009; Tenedios et al., 2006). Transesophageal echocardiography is also important for detection of leaflet thickening, vegetations and intramural thrombosis in patients with antiphospholipid syndrome and vasculitis. (Silbiger, 2009).

In all cases of coronary artery disease and vasculitis, especially in young patients with no other risk factors for heart disease, hypercoagulability should be excluded, mainly antiphospholipid syndrome. (Eleftheriadis, D., 2007a; Shin & Lee, 2007; Sullivan et al., 1999). Intensive anticoagulation therapy in combination with immunosuppressives is the therapy of choice in antiphospholipid syndrome and vasculitis-related thrombosis. This strategy results in disease stabilization and prevention of recurrent thrombotic events. (Kaynar et al., 2007; Sullivan et al., 1999).

5. Conclusions

Primary or secondary systemic vasculitides, although rare and diverse chronic inflammatory diseases, resulted in severe and often life-threatening complications, with coronary artery disease being the leading cause of morbidity and mortality in these cases. Chronic inflammation related to vasculitis resulted in coronary aneurysms, coronary stenosis, intramural thrombosis and microcirculation abnormalities, with subsequent cardiovascular events, which may occur at younger age and they are often silent in early phases.

In some reported cases the exact diagnosis can be only made postmortem. Severe acute myocardial infarction and/or sudden death could also be the first manifestation of coronary artery disease related to undiagnosed vasculitis.

Although coronary angiography remains the gold standard for diagnosing coronary lesions, modern non-invasive and more reliable sophisticated imaging techniques, including MRI with adenosine test and PET scan, have been introduced into clinical practice. In order to detect subclinical intramural thrombosis, coronary micro-aneurysms and microcirculation abnormalities, these imaging techniques should be recommended in evaluation of vasculitis-related cardiovascular disease.

Early diagnosis of vasculitis and immediate initiation of therapy with corticosteroids and immunosuppressives, in addition to intensive anticoagulation, is the only optional strategy for good outcome, prevention of further vasculitis progression, regression of early lesions and prevention of further thrombotic events. However, despite intensive therapy in some reports the coronary lesions could not be regressed.

The close collaboration between cardiologist, rheumatologist, pediatrician and radiologist is essential for optional outcome in atypical cases of coronary artery disease related to vasculitis.

6. References

Abdel-Hadi, O., Greenstone, M.A., Hartley, R.B., & Kidner, P.H. (1981). Myocardial infarction - a rare complication in Henoch-Schonlein purpura. *Postgraduate Medical Journal,* Vol.57, No.668, (1981), pp. 390-392, ISSN: 00325473.

Abu-Fadel, M.S., Pappy, R., Wayangankar, S., & Kalapura, T. (2011). Rapidly evolving coronary aneurysm in a patient with rheumatoid arthritis. *Cardiology Research and Practice,* Vol. 1, No. 1, (February 2011), article number:659439, ISSN: 20900597.

Agarwal, M.P., Dwivedi, S., Chaudhary, S.C., Khanna, S., & Agarwal, S. (2010). Small vessel vasculitis associated with myocardial infarction. *Journal, Indian Academy of Clinical Medicine,* Vol.11, No.1, (January 2010), pp. 54-58, ISSN:09723560.

Agraharkar, M., Gokhale, S., Le, L., Rajaraman, S., & Campbell. G.A. (2000). Cardiopulmonary manifestations of Henoch-Schonlein purpura. *American Journal of Kidney Diseases,* Vol.35, No.2, (2000), pp. 319-322, ISSN: 02726386.

Akagi, T. (2011). Catheter interventions for Kawasaki disease : Curent concepts and future directions. *Korean Circulation Journal,* Vol.41, No.2, (February 2011), PP. 53-57, ISSN: 17385520.

Albada-Kuipers, G.A., Bruijn, J.A, Westedt, M.-L., Breedveld, F.C. &Eulderink, F. (1986). Coronary arteritis complicating rheumatoid arthritis. *Annals of the Rheumatic Diseases,* Vol.45, No. 11, (November 1986), pp. 963-965, ISSN: 00034967.

Amano, J., & Suzuki, A. (1992). Surgical treatment of cardiac involvement in Takayasu Arteritis. *Heart and Vessels,* Vol. 7, No. 7 suppl., (1992), pp 168-178. ISSN: 09108327.

Andersson, R. (2000). Giant cell arteritis as a cause of death. Clinical and Experimental Rheumatology, Vol. 18, No. suppl. 20, (2000), pp. S27-S28. ISSN: 0392856X.

Araszkiewicz, A., Prech, M., Hrycaj, P., Lesiak, M., Grajek, S., Cieslinski, A. (2007). Acute myocardial infarction and rapid development of coronary aneurysms in a young woman-Unusual presentation of Takayasu arteritis? *Canadian Journal of Cardiology,* Vol.23, No. 1, (January 2007). Pp. 61-63, ISSN: 0828282X.

Benzarouel, D., Benyass, A., Rabhi, M., Chaari, J., Boukili, A., & Hamani, A. (2007). Silent myocardial infarction and antiphospholipid antibody syndrome. *Annales de Cardiologie et d'Angeiologie,* Vol.56, No. 6, (December 2007), pp. 313-315, ISSN: 00033928.

Bijl, M. (2003). Endothelial activation, endothelial dysfunction and premature atherosclerosis in systemic autoimmune disease. *Netherlands Journal of Medicine,* Vol.61, No.9, (September 2003), pp.273-277, ISSN: 03002977.

Bossert, M., Clement, P., Balblanc, J.-C., Lohse, A., & Wendling, D. (2011). Aortic involvement in giant cell arteritis: Current data. *Joint Bone Spine,* Vol. 78, No.3, (May 2011), pp. 246-251, ISSN: 1297319X.

Caballero-Mora, F.J., Alonso-Martin, B., Tamariz-Martel-Moreno, A., Cano-Fernandez, J., & Sanchez-Bayle, M. (2011).Kawasaki disease in 76 patients. Risk factors for coronary artery aneurysms. *Anales de Pediatria,* Vol.74, No.4, (April 2011), pp. 232-238, ISSN: 16954033.

Caracciolo, E.A, Marcu, C.B., Chantous, A., Donohue, T.J., Hutchinson, G. (2004). Coronary vasculitis with acute myocardial infarction in a young woman with systemic lupus erythematosis. *Journal of Clinical Rheumatology,* Vol. 10, No.2, (april 2004), pp. 66-68, ISSN: 10761608.

Carmichael, P., Brun, E., Jayawardene, S., Abdulkadir, A., & O'Donnell, P.J. (2002). A fatal case of bowel and cardiac involvement in Henoch-Schonlein Purpura. *Nephrology Dialysis Transplantation,* Vol.17, No.3, (2002), pp.497-499, ISSN: 09310509.

Churg, J., & Strauss, J. (1951). Allergic granulomatosis, allergic angiitis and periarteritis nodosa. The *American Journal of Pathology,* Vol. 27, No.2, (March 1951), pp. 277-301, ISSN: 00029440.

Cocco, G., & Gasparyan, A.Y. (2010). Myocardial ischemia in Wegener's granulomatosis: Coronary atherosclerosis versus vasculitis. *Open Cardiovascular Medicine Journal,* Vol.4, No.1, (specific issues 2010), pp.57-62, ISSN: 18741924.

De Castro, P.A, Urbano, L.M.F., & Costa, I.M.C. (2009). Kawasaki disease. *Anais Brasileiros de Dermatologia,* Vol.84, No.4, (July 2009), pp. 317-329, ISSN: 03650596.

Dhawan, S., & Tak, T. (2004). Myocardial infarction in a patient with thrombotic thrombocytopenic purpura. *International Journal of Cardiology,* Vol.95, No.(2-3), (June 2004), pp.339-341, ISSN: 01675273.

Donald, K.J., Edwards, R.L., & McEvoy, J.D. (1976) An ultrastructural study of the pathogenesis of tissue injury in limited Wegener's granulomatosis. *Pathology*, Vol.8, No.2, (April 1976), pp.161–169, ISSN: 00313025.

Eberhardt, R.T., & Dhadly, M. Giant cell arteritis: Diagnosis, management and cardiovascular implications. *Cardiology in Review*, Vol.15, No.2, (March 2007), pp. 55-61, ISSN: 10615377.

Eleftheriadis, D. (2007a). Severe coronary artery disease in the setting of Henoch-Schoenlein Purpura. *International Journal of Cardiology*, Vol.118, No. 2, (May 2007), pp. 262-263, ISSN: 01675273.

Eleftheriadis, D. (2007b). Severe coronary artery disease in the setting of Henoch-Schoenlein Purpura: Superimposition of antiphospholipid or polyangitis overlap syndrome?. *International Journal of Cardiology*, Vol.122, No. 2, (November 2007), pp. 184, ISSN: 01675273.

Eleftheriou, D., Dillon, M.J., & Brogan, P.A. (2009). Advances in childhood vasculitis. *Current Opinion in Rheumatology*, Vol.21, No.4, (July 2009), pp.411-418, ISSN:10408711.

Espinosa, G., & Gervera, R. (2010). Cardiac and pulmonary manifestations in the antiphospholipid syndrome. *Current Rheumatology Reviews*, Vol.6, No.1, (February 2010), pp. 3-11, ISSN: 15733971.

Freddo, T., Price, M., Kase, C., & Goldstein, M.P. (1999). Myocardial infarction and coronary artery involvement in giant cell arteritis. *Optometry and Vision Science*, Vol.76, No.1, (January 1999), pp. 14-18, ISSN: 10405488.

Fukazawa, R., & Ogawa, S. (2009). Long-term prognosis of patients with Kawasaki disease: At risk for future atherosclerosis? *Journal of Nippon Medical School*, Vol.76, No.3, (June 2009), pp. 124-133, ISSN: 13454676.

Gasparyan, A.Y., & Ugurlucan, M. The emerging issue of cardiovascular involvement in familial Mediterranean fever. *Archives of Medical Science*, Vol. 4, No.4, (2008), pp. 465-467, ISSN: 17341922.

Gilboe, J-M. (2008). The epidemiology of systemic lupus Erythematosis. *Norsk Epidemiologi*, Vol. 18, No.1, (February 2008), pp.31-36, ISSN: 08032491.

Gomard-Mennesson, E., Landron, C., Dauphin, C., Epaulard, O., Petit, C., Green, L., Roblot, P., Lusson, J.R., Broussolle, C., & Seve, P. (2010). Kawasaki disease in adults: report of 10 cases. *Medicine*, Vol.89, No. 3, (May 2010), pp. 149-158, ISSN::00257974.

Gonzalez-Juanatey, C., Llorca, J., Garcia-Porrua, C., Sancher-Andrade, A., Martin, J., & Gonzalez-Gay, M.A. (2006). Steroid therapy improves endothelial function in patients with biopsy-proven giant cell arteritis. *Journal of Rheumatology*, Vol.33, No.1, (January 2006), pp. 74–78, ISSN: 0315162X.

Guven, H., Ozhan, B., Bakiler, A.R., Salar, K., Kozan, M., & Bilgin, S. (2006). A case of Henoch-Schönlein purpura and rheumatic carditis with complete atrioventricular block. *European Journal of Pediatrics*, Vol. 165, No.6, (June 2006), pp.395-397, ISSN:03406199.

Hasper, D., Schrage, D., Niesporek, S., Knollmann, F., Barckow, D., & Oppert, M. (2006). Extensive coronary thrombosis in thrombotic-thrombocytopenic purpura. *International Journal of Cardiology*, Vol.106, No.3, (January 2006), pp. 407-409, ISSN:01675273.

Hata, A., & Onouchi, Y. (2009). Susceptibility genes for Kawasaki disease: Toward implementation of personalized medicine. *Journal of Human Genetics,* Vol.54, No.2, (February 2009), pp. 67-73, ISSN: 14345161.

Hewins, P., & Jayne, D. (2010). Medium vessel vasculitis. *Medicine,* Vol. 38, No.2, (February 2010), pp.93-96, ISSN:13573039.

Jeffery, R.C. (2010). Clinical features of rheumatoid arthritis. *Medicine,* Vol.38, No.4, (April 2010), pp. 167-171, ISSN: 13573039.

Kalunian, K., & Merill, J.T. (2009). New directions in the treatment of systemic lupus erythematosus. *Current Medical Research and Opinion,* Vol.25, No.6, (June 2009), pp.1501-1514, ISSN: 03007995.

Kalyoncu, M., Cakir, M., Erduran, E., & Okten, A. (2006) Henoch-Schönlein purpura: A case with atypical presentation. *Rheumatology International,* Vol. 26, No.7, (May 2006), pp.669-671, ISSN: 01728172.

Kane, G.C., & Keogh, K.A. (2009). Involvement of the heart by small and medium vessel vasculitis. *Current Opinion in Rheumatology,* Vol.21, No.1, (January 2009), pp. 29-34, ISSN:10408711.

Kaplan, M.J. (2009). Management of cardiovascular disease risk in chronic inflammatory disorders. *Nature Reviews Rheumatology,* Vol. 5, No.4, (April 2009), pp. 208-217, ISSN: 17594804.

Kaynar, K., Ulusoy, S., Gul, S., Kilicarslan, F, Oztuna, F., Ahmetoglou, A., & Omay, S.B. (2007). Antiphospholipid syndrome with lupus erythematosus presenting with myocardial infarction. *Scottish Medical Journal,*Vol. 52, No.2, (May 2007), ISSN: 00369330.

Keogh, K.A., & Specks, U. (2003). Churg-Strauss syndrome. Clinical presentation, antineutrophil cytoplasmic antibodies and leukotriene receptor antagonists. *American Journal of Medicine,* Vol. 115, No.4, (September 2003), pp. 284-290, ISSN:00029343.

Kereiakes, D.J., Ports, T.A., & Finkbeiner, W. (1984). Endomyocardial biopsy in Henoch-Schönlein purpura. *American Heart Journal,* Vol. 107, No.2, (1984), pp. 382-385, ISSN:00028703.

Kimura, T., Komura, M., & Okubo, Y. (2011). Atypical giant cell arteritis predominantly involving intramural coronary arteries: a case showing refractory dialysis-related hypotension. *Heart and Vessels,* (2011), pp.1-5. ISSN: 09108327, (article in press).

Knockaert, D.C. (2007). Cardiac involvement in systemic inflammatory diseases. *European Heart Journal,* Vol.28, No. 15, (August 2007), pp. 1797-1804, ISSN: 0195668.

Korantzopoulos, P., Papaioannides, D., & Siogas, K. (2004). The heart in wegener's granulomatosis. *Cardiology,* Vol. (102), No.1, (2004), pp. 7-10, ISSN: 00086312.

Kobayashi, Y., Giles, J.T.Hirano, M., Yokoe, I., Nakajima, Y., Bathon, J.M., Lima, J.A.C., & Kobayashi, H. (2010). Assessment of myocardial abnormalities in rheumatoid arthritis using a comprehensive cardiac magnetic resonanve approach: A pilot study. *Arthritis Research & Therapy,* Vol.12, No. 5, (September 2010), pp.R171, ISSN: 14786354.

Ku, I.A., Imboden, J.B., Ysue, P.Y., & Ganz, P. (2009). Rheumatoid arthritis-A model of systemic inflammation driving atherosclerosis. *Circulation Journal,* Vol.73, No.6, (June 2009), pp. 977-985, ISSN:13469843.

Kumar, P., Velissaris, T., Sheppard, M.N., & Pepper, J.R. (2002). Giant cell arteritis confined to intramural coronary arteries. Journal of Cardiovascular Surgery, Vol. 43, No. 5, (October 2002), pp. 647-649, ISSN: 00219509.

Lecutier, M.A. (1952). A case of the Schönlein-Henoch syndrome with myocardial necrosis. *Journal of Clinical Pathology,* Vol.5, No.4, (November 1952), pp. 336-338, ISSN:00219746.

Levine, J.S., Branch, D.W., & Rauch, J. (2002). The antiphospholipid syndrome. *The New England Journal of Medicine,* Vol. 346, No. 10, (March 2000), pp. 752-763, ISSN: 00284793.

Lin, L.-W., Wang, S.-S., & Shun, C.T. (2007). Myocardial infarction due to giant cell arteritis: A case report and literature review. Kaohsiung Journal of Medical Sciences, Vol. 23, No. 4, (April 1007), pp. 195-198, ISSN: 1607551X.

Lin, M.-T., Wang, J.-K., Yeh, J.-I., Sun, L.-C., Chen, P.-L., Wu, J.-F., Chang, C.-C., Lee, W-L, Shen, C.-T., Wang, N.-K., Wu, C.-S., Yeh, S.-Z., Chen, C.-A., Cjiu, S.-N., & Wu, M.-H. (2011). Clinical implication of the C allele of the ITPKC gene SNP rs28493229 in Kawasaki disease: Association with disease susceptibility and BCG scar reactivation. *Pediatric Infectious Disease Journal,* Vol.30, No.2, (February 2011), pp. 148-152, ISSN:08913668.

Lutz, H., Ackermann, T., Krombach, G.A., Groene, H-J., Rauen, T., Floege, J., Mertens, P.R. (2009). Henoch-Schönlein Purpura complicated by cardiac involvement: Case report and review of the literature. *American Journal of Kidney Diseases,* Vol.54, No.5, (November 2009), pp. e9-e15, ISSN: 02726386.

Magro, C.M., & Crowson, A.N. (1999). A clinical and histologic study of 37 cases of immunoglobulin A-associated vasculitis. *American Journal of Dermatology,* Vol. 21, No.3, (June 1999), pp. 234-240, ISSN: 01931091.

Maillard-Lefebvre, H., Launay, D., Mouquet, F., Gaxotte, V., Hachulla, E., De Groote, P., Lambert, M., Queyrel, V., Morell-Dubois, S., Beregi, J.-P., Bauters, C., Hatron, P.-Y. (2008). Polyarteritis nodosa-related coronary aneurysms. *Journal of Rheumatology,* Vol. 35, No. 5, (May 2008), pp. 933-934, ISSN: 0315162X.

Mavrogeni, S., Manoussakis, M.N., Karagiorga, T.C., Douskou, M., Panagiotakos, D., Bournia, V., Cokino, D.V, & Moutsopoulos, H.M. (2009). Detection of coronary artery lesions and myocardial necrosis by magnetic resonces in systemic necrotizing vasculitides. Arthritis Care and Research, Vol.61, No.8, (August 2009), pp.1121-1129, ISSN: 00043591.

Monastiri, K., Selmi. H., Tabarki, B., Yacoub, M., Mahjoub, T., & Essoussi, A.S. (2002). Primary antiphospholipid syndrome presenting as complicated Henoch-Schonlein purpura. *Archives of Disease in Childhood,* Vol.86, No.2, (month 2002), pp. 132-133, ISSN:00039888.

Mukhtyar, C., Brogan, P., & Luqmani, R., (2009). Cardiovascular involvement in primary systemic vasculitis. *Best Practice and Research Clinical Rheumatology,* Vol.23, No. 3, (June 2009), pp. 419–428, ISSN: 15216942.

Musuruana, J.L., Cavallasca, J.A., Berduc, J., & Vicario, J. (2011). Coronary artery aneurysms in wegener's granulomatosis. Case report. *Joint Bone Spine,* Vol.78, No.3, (May 2011), pp. 309-311, ISSN:1297319X.

Nabatian, S., Quinn, P., DuBrow, I., Rosenberg, M., & Lakier, J. (2006). Suspected vasculitis in an adolescent female with cardiomyopathy, myocardial infarction and heart failure requiring heart transplantation. *Journal of Adolescent Health,* Vol. 38, No.1, (January 2006), pp. 60-64. ISSN:1054139X.

Oates-Whitehead, R.M., Baumer, J.H., Haines, L., Love, S., Maconochie, I.K., Gupta, A., Roman, K., Dua, J.S., & Flyn I. (2003). Intravenous immunoglobulin for the treatment of Kawasaki disease in children. *Cochrane Database Syst Review,* Vol. 4, (2003), CD004000,

Osman, A., & McCreery, C.J. (2000). Cardiac vasculitis in Henoch-Schönlein purpura. *Circulation,* Vol.101, No.5, (February 2000), pp. E69-E70, ISSN 0009-7322. Online ISSN: 1524-4539.

Ouali, S., Kacem, S., Fradj, F.B., Gribaa, R., Naffeti, E., Remedi, F., Laaoueni, S., & Boughzela, E. (2011). Takayasu arteritis with coronary aneurysms: Causing acute myocardial infarction in a young man. *Texas Heart Institute Journal,* Vol. 38, No.2, (2011), pp. 183-186. ISSN: 07302347.

Paredes, N., Mondal, T., Brandao, L.R., & Chan, A.K. (2010). Management of myocardial infarction in children with Kawasaki disease. *Blood Coagulation & Fibrinolysis,* Vol.21, No.7, (October 2010), pp. 620-631, ISSN: 09575235.

Park, J.-S., Lee, H.C., Lee, S.-K., Kim, S.-P., Kim,Y.D., Ahn, M.S., & Hong, T.J. (2009). Takayasu's arteritis involving the ostia of three large coronary arteries. *Korean Circulation Journal*, Vol. 39, No. 12, (December 2009), pp.551-555, ISSN: 17385520.

Pellegrin, M.C., Taddio, A., Ventura, A., & Lepore, L. (2011). Kawasaki disease: A retrospective study on 45 patients. *Medico e Bambino*, Vol.30, No.4, (April 2011), pp. 236-241, ISSN: 15913090.

Pennel, D.J., & Keenan, N.G. (2011). Coronary microvascular dysfunction in systemic lupus erythematosis identified by CMR imaging. *JACC: Cardiovascular Imaging,* Vol.4, No.1, (January 2011), pp.34-36, ISSN:1936878X.

Pilletout, E., Thervet, E., Hill, G., Alberti, C., Vanhille, P., Nochy, D. (2002). Henoch-Schoenlein Purpura in adults: outcome and prognostic factors. *Journal of the American Society of Nephrology,* Vol.13, No.5, (May 2002), pp. 1271-1278, ISSN: 10466673.

Phillip, R., & Luqmani, R. (2008). Mortality in systemic vasculitis: A systematic review. *Clinical and Experimental Rheumatology,* Vol. 26, No. 5 suppl, (September 2008), pp. S94-S104, ISSN: 0392856X.

Polizzotto, M.N., Gibbs, S.D., Beswick, W., & Seymour, J.F. (2006). Cardiac involvement in Henoch-Schönlein purpura. *Internal Medicine Journal,* Vol.36, No. 5, (May 2006), pp.328-331, ISSN:14440903.

Reinhold-Keller, E., Herlyn, K., Wagner-Bastmeyer, R., & Gross, W.L. (2005). Stable incidence of primary systemic vasculitides over five years: results from the German vasculitis register. *Arthritis Rheum*, Vol.53, No.1, (February 2005), pp. 93-99, ISSN:

Rowley, A.H. (2011). Kawasaki disease: Novel insights into etiology and genetic susceptibility. *Annual Review of Medicine*, Vol.62, No.18, (February 2011), pp. 69-77, ISSN:00664219.

Sable-Fourtassou, R., Cohen, P., Mahr, A., Pagnoux, C., Mouthon, L., Jayne, D., Blockmans, D., Cordier, J.-F., Delaval, P., Puechal, X., Lauque, D., Viallard, J.-F., Zoulim, A., Guillevin, L. (2005). Antineutrophil cytoplasmic antibodies and the Churg-Strauss syndrome. *Annals of Internal Medicine,* Vol.143, No.9, (November 2005), pp.632-638, ISSN :00034819.

Saito, S., Arai, H., Kim, K. & Aoki, N. (1994). Acute myocardial infarction in a young adult due to solitary giant cell arteritis of the coronary artery diagnosed antemortemly by primary directional coronary atherectomy. *Catheterication and Cardiovascular Diagnosis*. Vol. 33, No. 3, (1994), pp. 245-249, ISSN: 00986569.

Salmon, J.E. & Roman, M.J. (2008). Subclinical atherosclerosis in rheumatoid arthritis and systemic lupus erythematosis. American Journal of Medicine, Vol.121, No. 10 suppl 1, (October 2008), pp. S3-S8, ISSN:00029343.

Satoh, M., Mikuniya, A., Mikami, M., Higashiyama, A., Sasaki, N., Tahkahashi, M., Fukushi, K., Onodera, K., & Oike, Y. (1991). A case of Schönlein -Henoch purpura with myocardial complications. *Respiration and Circulation,* Vol.39, No.3, (March 1991), pp. 273-277, ISSN:04523458.

Savage, C.O.S. (2002). The evolving pathogenesis of systemic vasculitis. *Clinical Medicine,* Vol.2, No.5, (September 2002), pp. 458–464, ISSN:14702118.

Sheikhzadeh, A., Tettenborn, I., Eftekharzadeh, M., Schnabel, A. (2002). Occlusive thromboaortopathy (Takayasu Disease): Clinical and angiographic features and a brief review of literature. *Angiology,* Vol.53, No.1, (2002), pp. 29-40, ISSN: 00033197.

Shin, J.I.,& Lee J.S. (2007). Severe coronary artery disease in Henoch-Schoenlein purpura: superimposition of antiphospholipid or polyangitis overlap syndrome? *International Journal of Cardiology,* Vol.122, No. 2, (November 2007), pp. 182-183, ISSN:01675273.

Silbiger, J.J. (2009). The cardiac manifestations of antiphospholopid syndrome and their echocardiographic recognition. *Journal of the American Society of echocardiography,* Vol. 22, No.10, (October 2009), pp.1100-1108, ISSN: 08947317.

Sinico, R.A., & Bottero, P. (2009). Churg-Strauss angiitis. *Best Practice & Research: Clinical Rheumatology,* Vol.23, No.3 (June 2009), pp.355-366, ISSN:15216942.

Sitia, S., Atzeni, F., Sarzi-Puttini, P., Di Bello, V., Tomasoni, L., Delfino, L., Antonini-Canterin, F., Di Salvo, G., De Gennaro Colonna, V., La Carrubba, S., Carerj, S., & Turiel, M. (2009). Cardiovascular involvement in systemic autoimmune diseases. *Autoimmunity Reviews,* Vol. 8, No.4, (February 2009), pp. 281-286, ISSN:15689972.

Solomon DH, Karlson EW, Rimm EB, Cannuscio, C.C., Mandl, L.A., Manson, J.E., Stampfer, M.J., & Curhan, G.C. (2003). Cardiovascular morbidity and mortality in women diagnosed with rheumatoid arthritis. *Circulation,* Vol. 107, No.9, (March 2003), pp.1303-1397, ISSN:00097322.

Sullivan, M.A., De Pasquale, N.P., & Coplan, N.L. (1999). Antiphospholipid antibodies and coronary arterial thrombosis. *Cardiovascular Reviews and Reports,* Vol. 20, No. 6, (June 1999).pp. 315+325+335, ISSN: 01973118.

Suppiah, R., Judge, A., Batra, R., Flossman, O., Harper, L., Höglund, P., Javaid, M.K., Jayne, D., Mukhtyar, C., Westman, K., Davis Jr., J.C., Hoffman, G.S., McCune, W.J., Merkel, P.A., StClar, E.W., Seo, P., Spiera, R., Stone, J.H. Luqmani, R. (2011). A model to predict cardiovascular events in patients with newly diagnosed Wegeners's granulomatosis and microscopic polyangiitis. *Arthritis Care & Research,* Vol. 63, No.4, (April 2011), pp. 588-596, ISSN: 21514658.

Tanimoto, K. (1994). Polyangiitis overlap syndrome. *Nippon Rinsho, Japanese Journal of Clinical Medicine,* Vol.52, No.8, (August 1994), pp. 2123-2126, ISSN:00471852.

Tenedios, F., Erkan, D., & Lockshin, M.D. (2006). Cardiac manifestations in the antiphospholipid syndrome. Rheumatic Disease Clinics of North America, Vol. 32, No.3, (August 2006), pp.491-507, ISSN:0889857X.

Tsuda, E., Abe, T., & Tamaki, W. (2011). Acute coronary syndrome in adult patients with coronary artery lesions caused by Kawasaki disease: Review of case reports. *Cardiology in Young,* Vol.21, No.1, (February 2011), pp. 74-82, ISSN: 10479511.

Turesson, C., Jacobsson, L.T., Matteson, E.L. (2008). Cardiovascular comorbidity in rheumatic diseases. *Vascular Health and Risk Management,* Vol. 4, No.3, (2008), pp.605-614, ISSN: 11766344.

Wang, K.-Y., Ting, C.-T., Sutton, M.St.J., & Chen, Y.T. (1999). Coronary artery aneurysms: A 25-patient study. Catheterization and Cardiovascular Interventions, Vol.48, No.1, September 1999), pp.31-38, ISSN: 15221946.

Watanabe, K., Abe, H., Mishima, T., Ogura, G., & Suzuki, T. (2003). Polyangitis overlap syndrome: a fatal case combined with adult Henoch-Schonlein purpura and polyarteritis nodosa. *Pathology International,* Vol.53, No.8, (August 2003), pp. 569-573, ISSN : 13205463.

Wenger, M., & Schneider, J. (1996). Coronary infarction due to giant cell arteritis. *Vasa-Journal of Vascular Diseases,* Vol.25, No.4, (1996), pp. 373-377, ISSN:03011526.

Wood, L.E., & Tulloh, R.M.R. (2009). Kawasaki disease in children. *Heart,* Vol.95, No.10, (May 2009), pp. 787-792, ISSN:13556037.

Wooditch, A.C. & Aronoff, S.C. (2005). Effect of initial corticosteroid therapy on coronary artery aneurysm formation in Kawasaki disease: a meta-analysis of 862 children. *Pediatrics,* Vol.116, No. 4, (December 2005), pp. 989-995, ISSN:00314005.

Yanagawa, B., Kumar, P., Tsuneyoshi, H., Kachel, E., Massad, F., Moussa F., Cohen, G.N. (2010). Coronary artery bypass in the context of polyartiritis nodosa. *Annals of Thoracic Surgery,* Vol. 89, No 2, (February 2010, pp. 623-625, ISSN: 00034975.

Yildiz, M. (2010). Arterial distensibility in chronic inflammatory rheumatic disorders. *Open Cardiovascular Medicine Journal,* Vol.4, No.1, (February 2010), pp. 83-88, ISSN 18741924.

Yiu, K.-H, Wang, S., Mok, M.-Y., Ooi, G.-C., Khong, P.-L., Lau, C.-S., Tse, H.-F. (2011). Relationship between cardiac valvular and arterial calcification in patients with rheumatoid arthritis and systemic lupus erythematosis. Journal of Rheumatology, Vol.38, No. 4, (April 2011), pp.621-627, ISSN: 0315162X.

Yuce, M., Davutoglu, V., Sari, I., Onat, A.M., (2011). Polyarteritis nodosa with multiple coronary aneurysms presenting as acute myocardial infarction. *The American Journal of the Medical Sciences,* Vol.341, No. 5, (May 2011), pp. 409, ISSN: 15382990.

Zaidi, M., Singh, N., Kamran, M., Ansari, N., Nasr, S.H., Acharya, A. (2008). Acute onset of hematuria and proteinuria associated with multiorgan involvement of the heart, liver, pancreas, kidneys, and skin in a patient with Henoch-Schönlein purpura. *Kidney International,* Vol. 73, No.4, (February 2008), pp.503-508, ISSN: 00852538.

Zaidi, M., Singh, N., Kamran, M., Ansari, N., Nasr, S.H., Acharya, A. (2008). Response to multiorgan involvement of vasculitis: Henoch-Schönlein Purpura or polyangiitis overlap syndrome. *Kidney International,* Vol. 74, No.6, (September 2008), pp.828-829, ISSN: 00852538.

14

Occupational Stress and Coronary Artery Disease

Sheng Wang[1] and Dou Chang[2]
[1]*Peking University Health Science Center,*
[2]*China Institute of Industrial Relations,*
China

1. Introduction

Facing fierce competition, complicated interpersonal relationship, and intense social environment in modern society, we are living in a world of tension [1]. Especially for the occupational population, confronting frequent innovation on technology and knowledge and higher requirement on vocational skills, they are under growing occupational stress, which is not only the leading cause of occupational mental diseases (such as anxiety, depression, burnout, post-traumatic stress disorder, and collective mental illness etc.) but also the stimulus or risk factor for raising the chance of getting cardiovascular and cerebrovascular diseases (like coronary artery disease) among workers to damage the health[2].

As one of the risk factors of the potential coronary artery disease, occupational stress has attracted increasing attention from scholars to explore the relation between then and thus lower the change of getting such cardiovascular and cerebrovascular diseases as coronary artery disease by changing people's lifestyle and working habits to improve the quality of our lives.

2. Definition

Stress here refers to the short term physiological, psychological, or behavioral expression caused by emotional strain. There are two kinds of stress, namely "eustress" and "negative stress". Eustress can help our body to adapt to the environmental change by enhancing our consciousness, increasing our vigilance, and producing advanced recognition and behavioral expression. In other words, as a challenge, eustress could promote individual growth and career development. As for negative stress, it could be complicated risk factor to our health. Constantly growing or high level of physiological and psychological stress could be harmful to our body.

Occupational stress is the physical and psychological strain which occurs when there is a discrepancy between the objective or recognitional demands of the environment in certain occupation and the individual's adaptability. It is characterized by the following points:

2.1 Sociality of stressor

Occupational environment is closely related to the social conditions such as community organization, civilization level, and scientific development etc. The composition and influence of stressor always changes with the social development and the corresponding occupation structural reform, which directly causes the change in the spectrum of occupational diseases.

2.2 Persistence of stress load

The stress load caused in occupational environment is always persistent and lasts for a long period, except the acute stress following acute poisoning, accident, or position change and so on. The prolonged high level of stress could result in many kinds of chronic health problems for the cumulative damage effect.

2.3 Collectivity of stress object

For each occupation, there are a considerable number of practitioners, so the stressor in an occupation would influence a group of people. Despite of the individual differences, for which some of them have only slight stress load or no stress, the incidence of disease caused by stress for different occupation remains obviously different.

At present, with the development of science and technology and the change of the mode of production, occupational diseases are gradual shifting from physical ones to psychological. Occupational stress has already been listed as one of the most serious occupational damage in developing countries [3]. Data indicate that the causes of 75% to 90% of the deadly diseases are related to the activation of stress mechanism [4]. Occupational stress could not only damage employee's physiological and psychological health, but also cause organization behavior problem including low satisfaction, high absence, low loyalty, and low efficiency and so on [5-6]. Therefore, it would weaken the productivity. What's worse, it would bring about a large sum of medical cost, compensations for employment injures, and social security cost, and even lawsuit. For instance, the economic damage related to occupational stress in the US is about $15 billion; in the UK, the loss caused by absence from duty related to occupational stress is about £130 million, while the loss caused by illness, reduction of workload, low production efficiency, and medical payment is about £700 million [7]. In 1980s, "karoshi" was first discussed in Japan as a law issue in which the family members of the victims asked for compensation from the enterprise and government because they believe the death was caused by the stress in work and they also found support and evidence from epidemiology. Therefore, the purpose of occupational stress management is not to thoroughly eliminate stressors but to limit it in a certain level to ensure that workers are in the best stress situation.

3. Origin

Occupational stress does not only originate from the characteristics of different occupations and the psychological needs of individuals but also from the social psychological environment of the workplace and even larger areas. The origins of occupational stress at present include: work load (time, complexity, responsibility, shift), interpersonal relationship (between superior and subordinate, among colleagues), career prospect (development opportunity, promotion, lay off, demotion), unfavorable working environment (noise, vibration, chemical poison, pathogenic organisms, bad ergonomics condition), social factors (social relation, social support, social position), individual factors (gender, age, psychological quality, state of health), and so on.

3.1 Originate directly from the stimulus of the occupation

3.1.1 Work load

Overloaded or under loaded, the extent and type of responsibility, and the decision making ability are all important factors to occupational stress.

There are two aspects of work load, quality and quantity. The quality of work load is the level of complexity and difficulty of the work, while the quantity of work load means the intensity and time of the work. Overload of the quality of work can make the workers feel it's hard to finish the complex and difficult work, and thus cause negative physiological and psychological effect, such as high blood cholesterol level and low self esteem. When the quantity of work is overloaded, the workers would feel burdened under the long term highly intensified work. As it is shown in some research, coronary artery disease is related to work overload, as well as smoking, drinking, absence from work, low initiative, and lacking of self esteem. Under loaded work in terms of quality and quantity could also cause stress. Research indicates that lacking of responsibility and engaging in simple and repeated work could cause stress for workers because they cannot realize their ambition and value, and they would be tired of the work and finally lose their creativity.

3.1.2 Work responsibility

High requirement on workers' physical strength, attention, responsibility and personal ability could bring stressor on workers and cause stress, especially when it is related to their life and health. For example, the traffic police working in the area with heavy traffic and lots of accident and the doctor and the nurse working in ICU would face such stressor, and they are facing higher risk for peptic ulcer, miocardial infarction and hypertension than other people.

3.1.3 Duty in an organization

Duty confliction means that it is hard for individuals to satisfy two or more expectation at the same time. For instance, a quality inspector should ensure the quality of the product while try to make both manager and worker content. The major cause for stress is the confusion of duty. Lacking guidance or information for making decision and taking action, it is hard for individuals to have a clear target and evaluate their behaviors. The other kind of stress related to duty happens when there is disparity between individual experience and the expectation of managers and the usable resources, such as lacking time, workers, funds, and the individual can hardly increase the resources and change the target.

3.1.4 Control on work

Lacking control or choice on working method, technique, time and speed could cause stress on workers. For example, when the terminal operators of computer believe the operation is too fast and beyond his control, or when workers on an assembly line should repeat a certain extremely simple job at a fixed speed, they would face stressor both physiologically and psychologically.

3.1.5 Work time

In many departments of public service, like hospital, station, and power department, which adopt shift system, employees have to work at night during night shift. They should sacrifice their time with their family members, friends and others. And this is considered as one of the most important cause of occupational stress.

Shift work is generally acknowledged as a cause of stress in the whole world. It is indicated in some researches that shift work would cause sleep problem, such as lack of sleep, inversion of sleep rhythm, and so on. Shift workers would also face the problem of absent mind and slow reaction, and it would cause higher possibility for making mistakes. Knutsson A and other researchers carried out two cross-sectional studies, and the result shows higher percentage of triglyceride in the blood of shift workers [8]. The case control study by Anders K's team also proves that there is certain relation between shift work and miocardial infarction [9].

3.1.6 Work environment

There might be many potential causes for stress in the physical condition of the work place. Research shows that the unfavorable chemical or physical condition such as noise, poisonous gas, high temperature, and strong or weak light can on the one hand directly influence the physical health of workers; on the other hand, it would disturb their psychological activities. Comfortable and pleasant environment, suitable tools for ergonomics and reasonable methods, and the elimination of risk factors in the environment could be of vital significance in ameliorating and improving the mood, confidence and productivity of workers.

3.1.7 Career prospect

Many turnings and changes in our work, such as transfer, promotion or demotion, employment or lay off, and so on, could be considered as the causing factors of stress. A survey on those unemployed shows that the chance for them to be addicted to alcohol and drugs and have psychological disease is higher than the comparing group, and they have higher rate of peptic ulcer and stress too [10]. Promotion and demotion are also important stressors. Facing new responsibilities, especially those require for new skills, the promoted is unable to do as much as they would like to do. This would trigger anxiety, uncompensated psychological reaction, or bizarre behavior. The investigation on US navy also proves that setbacks and demotion in one's career would cause higher rate of psychological disease [11].

3.2 Personal and social factors

Why would individuals have different reaction under the same stressors?

The susceptibility of individuals to stressors varies for the influence of many personal factors, such as character, family, social status, and social support system etc. In modern society, adults should earn their living by engaging in certain occupation to satisfy their material needs; on the other hand, it is an important part in their social life. Occupation could influence people's daily life from different aspects. For example, the interpersonal relationship in work place would influence people's satisfaction on the job and their level of stress. There are already large amounts of data on this point. In the culture of some society, some occupations are considered inferior and discriminated. Unemployment and retirement would force the employee leave their former post and social environment, and thus cause stress on them. Even the transfer of position could cause stress for the difficulty in adapting to new environment. All these are stressors of occupational stress.

3.3 Organization and interpersonal relationship

The production in industrialized society is carried out in different organizations, and people, as a member of the organization, have the responsibility and obligation to follow the arrangement and regulation of the organization, and then duty relations of different levels are formed. The accompanying conflicts in political interests, difficulty in communication, the assignment of tasks, determination, and regulations, all of them could become the origin of occupational stress.

Any change in the organization, such as the development of new products, the restructuring of group organization, and so on, would change the adaptability of individuals. We can always find anxiety, dropping satisfaction on the work, and low mood in some workers when a new production line was introduced. The change could damage the balance in the inner environment and raise the risk of stress. The relationship with superiors is the most important factor among all the factors influencing people's health. When an employee realizes that he (she) is neglected by his (her) superiors or he (she) can hardly communicate smoothly with his (her) superiors or colleagues, he (she) would feel the stress which is reflected by the dropping satisfaction on his (her) job. On the contrary, if he (she) can receive the support from co-workers, especially the praise from the superior, the stress would be relieved. The result of the research of Kawakami N's group fully proved the relation between psychological health and interpersonal relationship [12]. The conflict between personal opinion and mood and the goal of the organization could also cause stress.

Moreover, workers in some occupations which should be exclusive and apart from the society, such as astronomy, meteorology, hydrology, marine research, atomic research, and ocean navigation, are obviously lacking social activity. They are also vulnerable to stress.

4. Functioning mode

Western researches have already put forward many functioning modes of occupational stress since 1970s. They are mainly as follows:

4.1 Human-environment mode [13-14]

According to this mode, when (1) the ability of human fails to meet the needs ofwork (the angle of need-ability); or when the condition provided by environment (2) cannot satisfy the motivation of human (the angle of motivation-satisfaction), stress is produced. The needs of work include work load and complexity; and motivations include income, participation and self-realization etc.

In this mode, the subjective environment and human are separated from the objective ones. Here subjective refers to the recognition of human. It is assumed that stress is produced when the subjective human cannot adapt to the subjective environment. This explanation is subjective, and stress is considered as a fundamental function of individual perception. It emphasizes the flexibility in job designing and considers the workers as individuals of all kinds of ability, motivation and perception.

It follows the footstep of the cognitive mode of the early stages by emphasizing subjective cognition, and it considers the function of motivation as well. Similar to the cognitive mode, this one denies the function of objective factors except for those in the work place on human cognition. In addition, it believes that once there is inconsistence between need and ability or motivation and satisfaction from both the angle of need-ability and that of motivation-satisfaction, stress could be produced in individuals, yet it didn't tell the relation between the two angles. Therefore, there are apparent limitations in recognizing and forecasting those objective factors causing stress.

4.2 Work requirement: Self control mode [15-16]

Work requirement –self control mode believes that stress comes from work itself but not the subjective cognition, and stress is produced when there is inconsistence between work requirement and the decisional competency (or controlling ability) of the workers in the work place. For the response of individuals, losing control is a kind of stress from the environment. The decisional competency could be divided into two parts which are closely related in work, namely, the control of individuals on making decisions, and the ability in choosing the application of knowledge and technology and operational mode. Investigation on stress syndrome shows that negative stress cannot be produced merely by lacking psychological need and the most important factor is that can he (she) control his (her) behavior when there is a certain requirement.

In a sense, this mode is similar to the definition of stress given by McGrath (the imbalance between requirement and response ability) [17]. Yet the fundamental difference between them is that the environment restricts the individual's response ability when raising the requirement. It is characterized by the relation between requirement and control, namely the high requirement of environment on individuals and their low controlling ability. The investigation on this mode reveals that there is apparent connection among work requirement, decisional competency and stress. Decisional competency adjusts the requirement, and at the same time is a risk factor which can cause stress independently. It is generally accepted that the controlling ability is a decisive factor of occupational stress. This mode provides a dynamic explanation for the cause of stress, yet it neglects the important role of social behaviors of human and animals. Therefore, the function of social supporting factors should be considered in the application of this mode.

4.3 NIOSH mode

By the end of the 1990s, American NIOSH put forward the Occupational stress and health mode based on the previous study. This mode considers occupational stress as an interaction between stressors in the working condition or the comprehensive working environment and the individual characteristics. The long term influence of related restraining factors could cause acute imbalance and disorder of the physiological or psychological stability, which would lead to a series of physical and psychological diseases.

4.4 Ecology mode [18]

Using "theory of human ecology" and considering the macro and micro environment for human development, Salarza's group explored the requirement and adaptation of individuals or groups on work environment in terms of physiology, psychology, humanity and social politics to illustrate the ecology mode of occupational stress.

The cause of occupational stress was dated back to four connected ecological environment system in this mode: (1) Micro environment system. It means the environment directly related to workers, including the specific environment at the work place, structure, content, and conditions of the work, as well as the adaptability of the workers; (2) the related supporting environment system. It refers to the organizational structure, service function and cultural policy orientation of the management system of labor union and teams and groups; (3) the related surrounding organizational environment system. It means the regional economic condition, political atmosphere, and social custom influencing the workers, and the directly related situation in community; (4) the macro social political organizational environment system. It means the culture, social habit, tradition, and political and economical policy which directly or indirectly influence the interest of workers. It also includes the restraining factors of "controlling effects" like individual character, countermeasures on stress, marriage /family status, the interaction between individual factors and the stressors, etc., which could relieve and intensify the unfavorable reaction of body to stressors. In this way, an ecological occupational stress mode of "stressor (by restraint factors)-stress-healthy effect" is constructed, which provide theoretical support for the comprehensive intervening measures in work place to promote health by "stress control".

5. Influence on health

Stress means the integrated physical and psychological reaction of human under the stimulus of stressors. There are generally four aspects: physiological reaction, such as the increase of blood pressure, decline of immunity, cervical spine disease, coronary artery disease, digestive disease, and neurasthenia etc.; psychological reaction, like anxiety, depression, irritability, apathy and so on; behavioral effect, such as irritable, exciting, and accident tendency etc.; organizational effect, like absence from duty, lacking teamwork spirit, low efficiency, high incidence of accident, passive mood, burnout etc.

5.1 Physiological health

According to a survey, there are over 6 million coronary artery disease patient in China, and about 2.6 million people die of cardiovascular and cerebrovascular diseases, which means 1 death for every 12s. After studying the cases of cardiovascular and cerebrovascular diseases, it is revealed that the incidence of these diseases in growing and the patients is becoming younger and younger.

Occupational stress is considered as one of the most important risk factors for these diseases, and there are certain relation between occupational stress and hyper tension and ischemic heart disease [19-20]. Work stress also relate to the increase of carotid artery intima-media thickness in male patients [21].

People with different occupations are exposed to different stressor, for example, the work stress of police is higher than that of teachers and retirees. The related research in China shows that the occurrence of electrocardiogram abnormality in police is significantly higher than that in secondary school teachers and retired personnel, in which there is significant difference ($P < 0.05$) in arrhythmia, ST-T changes, left ventricule high voltage or hypertrophy; the serum cholesterol level in police officers with high occupational stress level is significantly higher than the control ($P < 0.05$)[22]. Two peaks occur in the heart rate and diastolic blood pressure of train crew 0.5 h and 1.5 h after start (the heart rate is 89 beats / min before start, and 92 beats / min at peak), which reflects that the professional stress of crew has significant effect on cardiac function[23].

Research shows that stress is the major risk factor for myocardial infarction. The body is in the state of psychological stress when there is high work stress, the sympathetic nerve becomes excited, and the renin angiotensin system is activated, so the blood pressure increases rapidly. Moller's group found the recent high work stress would increase the risk for myocardial infarction in the following 24 hours by 6 times, and the high stress in the past 12 months would increase the risk by 80% [24]. Shouldering large responsibility, the chance of male to get myocardial infarction would increase by 6 times, while that for female 3 times.

Kuper's team systematically reviewed 13 prospective cohort studies (each of them has more than 500 cases) concerning the relation between work stress and coronary artery disease [25]. Five of them are highly independent associated (the relative risk degree >2.0) regardless of the job category and gender difference ($P > 0.05$). A recent study on the risk factor of the coronary artery disease among young male shows that work stress is related to the existing atherosclerosis [26].

Besides, occupational stress changes the incidence of digestive disease, such as ulcer, intestinal canal function disorder, constipation etc. by influencing the movement of autonomic nervous system.

5.2 Psychological health

Study in Western countries has already proved that such social psychological stress as depression, anxiety, and panic could increase the incidence of cardiovascular event among coronary artery disease patients. The influence of social psychological stress on the physiological function of human body is mainly reflected by the enhanced endocrine response, which is characterized by the increase of HPA axis secrete and the increasing level of blood stress hormone and GCs which is of vital importance in affective behavior, metabolism, cardiovascular efficiency, and inflammation and immune system regulation.

Studies in China have shown that the work stress intensity of white-collars in four cities of Beijing, Shanghai, Guangzhou and Shenzhen is far higher than the average value in national major cities, in which the workload of Beijing is the highest. 15% of the respondents believe that their work stress is very high, they are in the bad state of "burn out"; and 68% of the respondents have physical and mental illnesses related with work stress in a certain extent. Gomez-Caminero, et al reported [27] that the occurrence risk of coronary heart disease in panic disorder patients was almost doubled compared with that in those without panic disorder, and the risk was higher when depression is complicated.

The occurrence of cardiovascular disease is also related with A-type personality. The basic characteristics of A-type personality is impatience, irritability, emotional lability, competitiveness, heart wariness or hostility. The occurrence of coronary heart disease in patients with A-type personality is as more than 2 times as that of those with B-type personality [28]; the incidence of coronary atherosclerosis in patients with A-type personality is 5 times higher than that of those with B-type personality [29].

5.3 Behavior

The temporary behavior changes caused by stress include escaping alcohol reliance, overuse of tobacco and drugs, and so on. Workers always become addicted to alcohol, skip work without valid reason, low initiative, lack confidence, etc. When workers' behavior changes for a long time, he (she) would give up his (her) control over the situation and future, and become passive and evasive---it is called "learned helplessness". The research based on Requirement-control Mode shows that when workers lose their control on work, he (she) would become passive in family and group and reluctant to take part in socialized group activities such as assembly, entertainment, religious activities, etc.

Prolonged stress can cause mental fatigue, lead to reduced nerve excitability, cause reduced attention, memory, manual operation dexterity and psychokinesis stability, decreased responding ability of vision and hearing and other neurobehavioral changes. A survey shows that air traffic control officers (it refers to the personnel who observe and handle the various parameters of aircrafts in the process from takeoff to landing through radar screen, and issue instructions to guide the safe flight of aircrafts) has significantly increased subjective feeling of fatigue after working, reduced flicker fusion frequency and photopie vision durability and prolonged ART; compared with the control, VCRT and ACRT is extended, DM and neurobehavioral function is reduced [30].

Smoking is one of the important risk factors for cardiovascular disease. Smoking can increase hs-CRP level, smoking amount is positively correlated with the increase level of hs-CRP. It is not only an important inflammatory factor in vivo, but also an independent risk factor for lipid disorder and high blood pressure, which can predict the occurrence of cardiovascular events[31]. High concentrations of hs-CRP can promote endothelial cell proliferation, migration and endarterium thickening, and promote the formation and development of atherosclerosis [32].

6. Functioning mechanism

Coronary artery disease is a typical complicated disease which is extremely harmful to people's health. The causes of the disease include two aspects, namely environment factors and hereditary factors, which involve many risk factors. As one of the potential risk factors, occupational stress has attracted more and more attention of the scholars both at home and abroad [33-34]. The functioning mechanism is rather complex, and not entirely clear. One research shows that the effect of occupational stress on coronary artery disease is weakened or lowered when it is mixed with traditional risk factors, so the impact of occupational stress on coronary artery disease could partly be realized through influencing other traditional risk factors [35].

6.1 Direct mechanism

The stimulus of tension can one the one hand make sympathetic nerve excited, increase the secreting of adrenal medulla and the level of CA; on the other hand, it would increase the amount of adrenal cortical hormone and the level of corticosteroid through the HPA system, which would cause hyper tension, hyperlipoidemia, arteriosclerosis and arrhythmia cordis, and thus increase the risk of coronary artery disease.

Some researches show that occupational stress could cause change in human immune index [36-38]. For example, Theorell's team found clear difference of serum IgG level among workers under different stress state; Arnetz and other researchers investigation on laid off women revealed that the reaction of their lymphocyte on phytohemagglutinin was weakened; if the body is under high level of tension during the work, and there are certain factors causing psychological stress (like the high requirement, low control state), Musculoskeletal pain syndrome like lumbago would be caused [39].

6.2 Indirect mechanism

Long term stress could trigger a series of unhealthy lifestyle, like smoking, drinking, high fat diet, and lacking exercise, etc., which would indirectly increase the risk of angiocardiopathy. Research shows that the smoking rate and seriousness of smoking is much higher among workers under occupational stress than others.

Moreover, occupational stress could also lead to functional disorder of blood coagulation system and cause disease. The research of WOLF shows that occupational stress could increase the level of PAI-1 and make the blood in hypercoagulative state. Acute psychological stress could activate the Coagulative and Fibrinolytic System of healthy subjects at the same time, but cause hypercoagulative state among people who suffer from arteriosclerosis and impaired endothelial function. While chronic stress (occupational tension and low social economic position) could increase the number of Fib or VII factor, lower the fibrinolytic activity, and thus cause the hypercoagulative state and CAD.

It is worth noting that some researches abroad believe that occupational stress has little influence on coronary artery disease and it is not a risk factor for the disease. After meta-analysis on the recent prospective cohort study and exploration on the relation between all kinds of social psychological factors including occupational stress and the outbreak and prognosis of coronary artery disease, Kuper and other researchers believe that occupational stress has no apparent influence on the outbreak and prognosis of coronary artery disease [40]. In the research of Framingham Offspring [41], 3039 subjects were observed for ten years, yet they didn't find that occupational stress could increase the risk of coronary artery disease and the death rate. In a research on females, researcher also didn't gain any conclusion to show the close relation between occupational stress and coronary artery disease [42]. After studying the results of previous meta-analysis, experts from Australian Heart Foundation believe that the influence of occupational stress on the outbreak and prognosis of coronary artery disease is still not certain yet, and they are inclined to little or no influence.

7. Evaluation

It is rather hard to evaluate because occupational stress is a relatively subjective feeling. At present, there are mainly three methods to evaluate it: (1) determine the level of stress according to the kind of occupation. It could reflect the stress for a certain group, but not individuals. (2) Field evaluation by expert after checking the work place. The limitation on human resource hinders large scale research, so it is not feasible. (3) Questionnaire, and self evaluation by the workers themselves, and it is widely adopted nowadays. There have been all kinds of theories on occupational stress and their corresponding questionnaires since the 1960s. The most widely used are the questionnaire based on work requirement-level of autonomy-social support mode and that based on ERI mode and ERIQ.

7.1 Work requirement-level of autonomy-social support mode and JCQ

It was firstly put forward by Karasek who believes that the origin of occupational stress lies in the imbalance between work requirement and personal autonomy (control) ability [43]. Here work requirement refers to the stress on workers while realize the work goal, and the level of autonomy means the autonomy of workers in using skills, making decisions, and allocating tasks. This mode can be divided into four types: Active Type (high requirement-high autonomy), Easy Type (low requirement-high autonomy), Stress Type (high requirement-low autonomy), and Passive Type (low requirement-low autonomy). The social support, as the relieve index, shows the active personal relationship between individuals and their superiors and colleagues. When workers face high requirement with low autonomy and not enough social support, the lonely type stress is the worst state to one's health. JCQ based on the work requirement-level of autonomy-social support mode has 27 entries, including work requirement, skill autonomy, decision autonomy, social support, and the stability of work etc. The level of stress is evaluated by the ratio between work requirement and autonomy level. This kind of questionnaire has been successfully used in North Europe and America, especially in the study on the relationship between occupational stress and hyper stress, CAD, and myocardial infarction.

7.2 ERI mode and ERIQ

ERIQ was firstly put forward by Siegrist to emphasis the relationship between effort and return in the work of individuals [44]. The stress state is determined by high efforts and/or low return. ERI mode also include a parameter reflecting the characteristics of individuals—internal investment. The level of stress would be intensified when there is too much effort and return. There are 23 entries in ERIQ. The level of stress is evaluated by the ratio of ERI. The stress level is comparatively high when the ratio is >1 and the converse is lower. It can also be evaluated by the percentiles and median of ERI value. It is also widely used in recent years and shows good value and forecast ability in many researches.

JCQ and ERIQ were widely used in the past 20 years in the evaluation of social psychological factors in work place both in cross sectional study and longitudinal tracing research. Both of them can make excellent prediction and evaluation and was proved effective [45].

8. Measures of prevention

To control the risk factors can effectively prevent the occurrence of coronary artery disease and improve the prognosis. Because it is easy to change the environment factors, recognizing the new risk factors in the environment and then take measures of prevention could lower the incidence and death rate of coronary artery disease.

8.1 Build good work atmosphere and reduce work load

Provide good work condition for workers by ensuring enough personnel, providing study opportunity, and good environment for workers to rest during night shift, show your care about them and encourage them. Moreover, the department in charge should follow the principle of standardized, human based, and reasonable management from recruiting to daily management by establishing long term and fair incentive measures to provide confidence for workers, stabilize the team, and improve the quality of work. A lot of epidemiologic studies abroad have revealed that high requirement on work would increase the incidence and death rate of coronary artery disease [46-47].

8.2 Improve workers character

A type character is one of the most important reasons for coronary artery disease. The susceptibility of people to life varies according to different character. Those who have low sensitivity threshold would fall ill when they face some small incidences; while other who have high sensitivity threshold is not ease to be ill. A type people is characterized by irritable, emulative, ambitious, and highly competitive, but lack of patience and stubborn. They are unwilling to receive others' suggestion, and like to deal with different job at the same time (such as reading files while eating, making phone call etc.); they are eager to finish the work at hand soon so that they can deal with other jobs; they would consider their work even when they are having a rest; they do not have the patience to listen to others and tend to frequently interrupt others; they do not trust others and can hardly enjoy relaxed vocation.

B type person is just contrary to A type. They hold the opinion to enjoy life, experience life and appreciate the nature; they are calm and unflustered; they always follow the rules and do not seek to prevail over others; and they pay little attention to gain and loss. Generally speaking, they make less achievement than A type workers. And many people are in between. Accord to a survey: 85% of the angiocardiopathies related to A type character. The chance for A type character workers to get coronary artery disease is two times higher than that of B type [28]. It is revealed in an autopsy study that the chance for A type character workers to get coronary atherosclerosis is five times higher than that of B type character workers [48].

Therefore, workers should try to change their busy lifestyle and make life easy, listen to others and do not interrupt others, appreciate the nature, and allocate some time for relaxation every day.

8.3 Maintain happy and balanced mood

Maintain stable and happy mood. Firstly, ensure good interpersonal relationship, including the relationship among family members, colleagues, between superior and subordinates, relatives, and neighbors.

Secondly, treat life events properly. Life events generally happen when you are under some mood, large or small. If it is improperly dealt with, it would cause negative mood, like depression, anxiety, upset, anger, fear, sadness, and despair est. Negative mood, especially those accumulated for a long time, could trigger hyper tension and arteriosclerosis. The best way to deal with it is: objectively analyze the reasons and results, and find the correct way to deal with it, or talk with your family, friends, and superiors to gain their help and make a decision rather than stay alone and do nothing but worrying. Bad things can also be changed into good ones.

8.4 Training

Enhance training against occupational stress; actively create opportunities for promotion and further study; strengthen the confidence and self-evaluation of workers; put forward suitable expectation by evaluate oneself; arrange one's work and life properly according to their energy and ability; learn to confide and release your bad feelings and stress; improve the ability to control the mood and sense of achievement while strengthen one's physical and psychological health.

8.5 Exercise

It is well known that exercise can improve your physical health by improving not only your muscle, bone, and ligament, but also the cardiovascular system, respiratory system, gastrointestinal system, urinary system, and nerve system. Frequent exercise of cardiovascular system can directly prevent arteriosclerosis, and the exercise on brain nerve can improve the coordination of human organs and prevent coronary artery disease.

8.6 Others

The first one is quit smoking. There are more than 3000 poisonous materials in the smoke of tobacco. Besides such carcinogens as polycyclic aromatic hydrocarbon and nitrosamine, Nicotine, as an extremely toxic substance, can cause tachycardia, vasoconstriction, elevation of blood pressure, increasing level of cholesterin and low density lipoprotein in blood, and finally arteriosclerosis. It is found in a research that social isolation despondent syndrome could promote the development of atherosclerosis in female patients, whose diameter of coronary artery deceased by 0.18mm, while those of the comparing group decreased only 0.01mm. This has no relation with the vessel diameter, age, smoking history, hyper stress, and high-density lipoprotein [49]. In the research of Lander's team, there is higher rate of smoking and obese among social despondent, both of them can increase the risk of coronary artery disease [50].

Secondly, listen to music can reduce the incidence of coronary artery disease too. Music is extremely infectious to nerve system. Bright and relaxing music, with its pleasant melody, could adjust and improve the nerve organization related to brain and mood to make it more balanced. It could relax the muscle, balance blood pressure, stabilize cardiac rate, control the vessel movement, and thus prevent coronary artery disease.

In conclusion, we should maintain a peaceful mind and avoid tension and stress to prevent the development of coronary artery disease.

9. References

[1] Carl, Z. (1994). Occupational medicine. *Mosby Year Book*, 3rd ed, Inc. St. Louis, pp. 945
[2] Cooper. CL, Marshall, J. (1976). Occupational Sources of Stress. *Occup. Psychol*, Vol. 49, pp. 11-28

[3] Dollard MF, Winefield AH. (1996). Managing occupation stress: A national and international perspective. *Int. J. Stress Manag*, Vol. 3, pp. 69-83

[4] Daley AJ, Parfitt G. (1996). Good health—Is it worth it? *J. Occupat. Organiz. Psychol*, Vol. 69, pp. 121-134

[5] Baba VV, Jamal M, Tourigny L. (1998). Work and mental health: A decade in Canadian Research. *Can. Psychol*, Vol. 39, pp. 94-104

[6] Daniels K. (1996). Why aren't managers concerned about occupational stress? *Work Stress*, Vol. 10, pp. 352-366

[7] Grayham DA. (1997). Work-related stress: implications for the employer. *J. Roy. Soc. Health*, Vol. 117, pp. 81-87

[8] Romon M, Nuttens MC, et al. (1992). Increased triglyceride levels in shift workers. *Am J Med*, Vol. 93, pp. 259—62

[9] Anders K, Johan H., et al. (1999). Shiftwork and myocardial infarction: a case-control study. *Occup Environ Med*, Vol. 56, pp. 46—50

[10] Institute for social research: Termination: The consequences of job loss. *Univ of Michigan Press*,1977

[11] Arthur RJ, Gunderson EK. (1965). Promotion and mental illness in the Navy. *J Occup Med*, Vol. 7, pp. 452

[12] Kawakami N, Haratani T, Araki S. (1992). Effects of perceived job stress on depressive symptoms in blue-collar workers of an electrical factory in Japan. *Scand J Work Environ Health*, Vol. 18, pp.195—200

[13] Caplan RD, et al. (1977). Job demands and worker health. Washington, D.C.:*NIOSH* (publication no. 75—160)

[14] French JR Jr, Caplan RD, Van Harrison R. (1982). The mechanisms of job stress and strain. *Chichester: Wiley*

[15] Karasek R, Theorell T. (1992). Healthy work—stress, productivity, and the reconstruction of working life. *New York: Basic Books*

[16] Karasek RA. (1981). Socialization and job strain: The implications of two related psychosocial mechanisms for job design. *In B Gardell, G Johansson. eds. Working life. London: Wiley*

[17] McGrath JE. (1970). A conceptual formulation for research on stress. In JE McGrath. ed. Social and psychological factors in stress. *New York: Holt, Rinehart, & Winston*, pp. 22—40

[18] Salazar M. K, Beaton R. (2000). Ecological model of occupational stress: application to urban firefighters. *AAOHN Journal*, Vol. 48, No. 10, pp. 470

[19] Pickering TG, Devereux RB, et al. (1996). Environmental influences on blood pressure and the role of job strain. *J Hypertens*, Vol.14 (suppl 5), pp. 179-185

[20] Schwartz JE, Schnall PL, et al. (1996). The effect of job strain on ambulatoty blood pressure in men over 6 years is comparable to other risk factors (abst). *J Hypertens*, Vol. 14 (suppl 1), pp. 54

[21] Hintsanen M, Kivimaki M, Elovaininio M, et al. (2005). Job strain and early atherosclerosis: the cardiovascular risk in young finns study. *Psychosom Med*, Vol. 67, No. 5, pp. 740-747

[22] Songshen C, Peixiang L, etc. (2002). Impact factors of cardiovascular disease and ECG of different occupational groups. *Qingdao Medical Journal*, Vol. 34, No. 5, pp. 373-374

[23] Baoying L, Maoli Z, et al. (1999). Relationship between of Occupational 1 Stress Factors of Train Attendants and Hypertension, Coronary Heart Disease. *Chinese Journal of Hypertension*, Vol. 7, No. 4, pp. 349-351

[24] Moller J, Theorell T, de Faire U, et al. (2005). Work related stressfull life events and the risk of myocardial infarction. Case-control and case-crossover analyses within the stockholm heart epidemiology programme (SHEEP). *J Epidemiol Community Health*, Vol. 59, No. 1, pp. 23-30

[25] Kuper H, Marmot M, Hemingway H. (2002). Systematic review of prospective cohort studies of psychosocial factors in the etiology and prognosis of coronary heart disease. *Semin Vasc Med*, Vol. 2, No. 3, pp. 267-314

[26] Hintsanen M, Kivimaki M, Elovainio M, et al. (2005). Job strain and early atherosclerrosis: the Cardiovascular Risk in Young Finns study. *Psychosom Med*, Vol. 67, No. 5, pp. 740-747

[27] Gomer-Caminero A, Blumentals WA, Russo LJ,et al. (2005). Does panic disorder increase the risk of acute coronary heart disease ? A cohort study of a national managed care database. *Psychosom Med*, Vol. 67, No. 5, pp. 688-691

[28] Lisspers J, Sundin O, Ohnan A, et al. (2005). Long-term effects of style life behavior change in coronary artery disease: effects on recurrent coronary events after percutaneous coronary intervention. *Health Psychol*, Vol. 24, No. 1, pp. 41-48

[29] Lett HS, Blumental JA, Babyak MA, et al. (2005). Social support and acute coronary heart disease, epidemiologic evidence and implications for treatment. *Psychosom Med*, Vol. 112, No. 6, pp. 869-878

[30] Hongbin X, et al. (1995). The research on impact factors of occupational stress of Air traffic control operators. *Industrial Health and Occupational Diseases*, Vol. 21, No. 6, pp. 325

[31] RRidker PM. (2003). Clinical application of C-reactive protein for cardiovascular disease detection and prevention. *Circulation*, Vol. 107, pp. 363-369

[32] Hayaishi-Okano R, Yamasaki Y, Katakami N, et al. (2002). Elevated C-reactive protein associates with early-stage carotid atherosclerosis in young subjects with 1 diabetes. *Diabetes Care*, Vol. 25, pp. 1432-1438

[33] Kuper H, Marmot M. (2003). Job strain, job demands, decision latitude and risk for coronary heart disease within the Whitehall II study. *J Epidemiol Commun Health*, Vol. 57, pp. 147-153

[34] Peter R, Siegrist J, Hallqvist J, et al. (2002). Psychological work environment and myocardial infarction: improving risk estimation by combining two complementary job stress models in SHEEP study. *J Epidemiol Commun Health*, Vol. 56, pp. 294-300

[35] Alterman T, Shekelle RB, Vernon SW, et al. (1994). Psychologic demand, job strain, and coronary heart disease in the Western Electric Study. *Am J Epidemiol*, Vol. 139, pp. 620-627

[36] Henningsen GM, Hurell JJ, et al. (1992). Measurement of salivary immunoglobulin A as an immunologic biomarker of job stress. *Scand J Work Environ Health*, Vol. 18, pp. 133-136

[37] Meijiman TF, van Dormolen M, et al. (1995). Job strain, neuroendocrine activation, and immune status. In : Sauter SL, Murphy LR, eds. Organizational Risk Factors for Job Stress. Washington, DC: American *Psychological Association*, pp. 113-126

[38] Kawakami N, Tanigawa T, et al. (1997). Effects of job strain on helper-inducer (CD4+CD29+) and suppressor-inducer (CD4+CD45RA+) T cells in Japanese blue-collar workers. *Psychother Psydhosom*, Vol. 66, pp.192-198

[39] Bongers P.M. et al. (1993). Psychosocial factors at work and musculoskeletal disease. *Scand. J. Work Environ. Health*, Vol. 19, pp. 297-312

[40] Kuper H, Marmot M, Hemingway H. (2002). Systematic review of prospective cohort studies of psychological factors in aetiology and prognosis of coronary heart disease. *Semin Vasc Med*, Vol. 2, pp. 267-314

[41] Eaker ED, Sullivan LM, Kelly-Hayes M, et al. (2004). Does job strain increase the risk for coronary heart disease or death in men and women? the Framingham Off-spring study. *Am J Epidemio*, Vol 160, No. 10, pp. 1031-1032

[42] Lee S, ColditzG, Berkman L, et al. (2002). A prospective study of job strain and coronary heart disease in US women. *Int J Epidemio*, Vol. 31, No. 6, pp. 1147-1153

[43] Karasek RA. (1979). Job demands, job decision latitude, and mental strain: implications for job redesign. *Admin SciQ*, Vol. 24, pp. 285-308

[44] Siegrist J, Starke D, Chandola T, et al. (2004). The measurement of effort-reward imbalance at work: European comparisons. *Soc SciMed*, Vol. 58, No. 1483-1499

[45] Vegchel NV, Jonge JD, Bosma H, et al. (2005). Reviewing the effort-reward Imbalance model: drawing up the balance of empirical studies. *Soc Sci Med*, Vol. 60, pp. 1117-1131

[46] Kivimaki M, Head J, Ferrie JE, et al. (2006). Why is evidence on job strain and coronary heart disease mixed? An illustration of measurement challenges in the Whitehall II study. *Psychosom Med*, Vol. 68, pp. 398-401

[47] Kivimaki M, Leino-Arjas P, Luukkonen R, et al. (2002). Work stress and risk of cardiovascular mortality: prospective cohort study of industrial employees. *Br Med J*, pp. 325-357

[48] Lett HS, Blumental JA, Babyak MA, et al. (2005). Social support and acute coronary heart disease, epidmiologic evidence and implications for treatment. *Psychosom Med*, Vol. 112, No. 6, pp. 869-87

[49] Wang HX, Mitteleman MA, Leineweber C, et al. (2006). Depression symptoms, social isolation, and progression of coronary artery atherosclerosis: the Stockholm Female Coronary Angiography Study. [J].Psychother *Psychother Psychosom*, Vol. 75, No. 2, pp. 96-102

[50] Lauder W, Mummery K, Jones M, et al. (2006). A comparison of health behaviours in lonely and non-lonely populations. *Psychol Health Med*, Vol. 11, No. 6, pp. 233-245

15

Specific Features of Target Organ Damage in Patients with Arterial Hypertension and Coronary Artery Disease

Corina Şerban, Ruxandra Christodorescu, Alexandru Caraba, Germaine Săvoiu, Carmen Cristescu and Simona Drăgan
University of Medicine and Pharmacy "Victor Babeş" Timişoara, Romania

1. Introduction

Worldwide, nearly 8 million premature deaths, 54% of stroke cases and 47% of ischemic heart disease cases were attributable to high blood pressure (BP >115 mm Hg systolic) (Ruilope, 2011). It is widely known that arterial hypertension has effects on target organs like the brain, the heart and the kidney. Now a large body of evidence on the crucial role of subclinical organ damage in determining cardiovascular risk in individuals with and without high blood pressure is available. New evidence showed that inflammation and activation of immunity are central features in the pathogenesis of atherosclerosis and also in hypertension-induced target organ damage. Recent studies have demonstrated that macrophages and various T-cell subtypes play a pivotal role in the regulation of blood pressure and target organ damage (Muller, 2011). A powerful promoter of inflammation and one of the major mediators of hypertension-induced target organ damage is also Angiotensin (Ang) II (Kvakan, 2009). European guidelines for the management of arterial hypertension from 2007 defined target organ damage by the presence of any of the following:

- electrocardiographic left ventricular hypertrophy (LVH) (Sokolow-Lyon > 38 mm; Cornell >2440 mm x ms)
- echocardiographic LVH (left ventricle mass index in men ≥ 126 g/m^2 and in women ≥ 110 g/m^2)
- carotid wall thickening (IMT > 0.9 mm) or plaque
- ankle/brachial index <0.9
- slight increase in plasma creatinine
- males: 115–133 µmol/l (1.3-1.5 mg/dl)
- females: 107–124 µmol/l (1.2-1.4 mg/dl)
- Low estimated glomerular filtration rate (< 60 ml/min/1.73 m^2) or creatinine clearance < 60 ml/min
- Microalbuminuria 30-300 mg/24 h or albumin–creatinine ratio: ≥22 (males); or ≥31 (females) mg/g creatinine

Since then, other studies proposed *home blood pressure* to be as reliable as ambulatory monitoring in predicting hypertension-induced target-organ damage, because it is superior to carefully taken office measurements (Viazzi, 2002; Stergiou, 2007). Marinakis et al. have demonstrated a relationship between heart rate variability and TOD, thus highlighting its importance in the genesis of subclinical cardiovascular disease (Marinakis, 2003). Recently, inflammation, and in particular tumor necrosis factor-α (TNF-α), has been implied in the cascade leading to TOD in patients with essential hypertension (Navarro-Gonzalez, 2008). Another study proposed the maximum value of home blood pressure to be a novel indicator of target organ damage in hypertension (Matsui, 2011).

Remodeling of small resistance arteries is also considered an early sign of target organ damage in hypertension (Cheng, 2010). The microcirculation is recognized as the site where the earliest manifestations of cardiovascular disease, especially inflammatory responses, that may play a pivotal role in driving the atherosclerotic process in conduit vessels, occur (Lockhart, 2009). Endothelial dysfunction is a predictor of a series of cardiovascular diseases (Heitzer et al, 2001; Halcox et al, 2002), although data on hypertension are still scarce (Taddei et al, 2002). Furthermore, techniques available for investigating endothelial response to various stimuli are invasive, laborious and time consuming. Finally, methods are not yet standardized and no certainty exists, that endothelial function assessed in an organ is representative of other vascular territories. However, current studies on circulating markers of endothelial activity and on endothelial cell progenitors are promising (Werner et al, 2005). This could facilitate evaluation of their prognostic role on a larger scale for more widespread clinical use. Although not traditionally considered a target organ, arterial blood vessels represent the site for the development of the atherosclerotic process that causes cardiovascular events.

Remodeling of large arteries during essential hypertension is also an early sign of organ damage. There are a number of noninvasive screening tests to identify structural and functional abnormalities of large arteries in arterial hypertension. By the time symptoms develop or clinical signs of atherosclerosis can be detected in conduit vessels, the disease process is already at an advanced stage (McVeigh, 2004; Lockhart, 2009). Remodeling of large arteries is characterized by an increase in intima-media thickness (IMT) aimed for maintaining circumferential wall stress, lumen enlargement of proximal elastic arteries, and no change in the lumen diameter of distal muscular arteries. Measurement of IMT by ultrasound examination of carotid arteries, and identification of atherosclerotic plaques, are predictors of both stroke and myocardial infarction (Salonen et al, 1993, Bots et al, 1997; Hodis et al, 1998, O`Leary et al, 1999). There is evidence that in untreated hypertensive patients without target organ damage, these alterations are common and therefore carotid ultrasound examination can detect structural damage at an early stage by routine examination. The relationship between increased carotid IMT and cardiovascular events is known, and value of IMT in the common carotid artery > 0.9 mm is considered the cut-point to emphasize the existence of structural abnormalities also in coronary arteries (Graf, 2009). Increased carotid IMT may be related to intimal or medial hypertrophy or both, and may be an adaptive response to changes in flow, wall tension, or lumen diameter (Vaudo, 2000). It is likely that ultrasound examination limited to the common carotid artery measures vascular hypertrophy only, while the evaluation and examination of bifurcation atherosclerosis and/or internal carotid artery, where plaques are most common, are more reliable for IMT estimation. The presence of atheromatous plaques can be identified by the presence of focal increased thickness of 0.5 mm or 50% of the surrounding IMT (Zanchetti et al, 2002; Zanchetti et al, 2004).

Low ankle-arm index below 0.9 indicates the presence of peripheral arterial disease and, in general, advanced atherosclerosis (Feringa et al, 2006), while the measurement of carotid IMT can detect early changes (Zanchetti et al, 2002). However, a low ankle-arm index correlates with further development of angina, myocardial infarction, heart failure, need for coronary bypass's, stroke, need for carotid surgery and peripheral vascular level (Hiatt et al, 2001, Vogt et al, 1993) and in patients with multivessel coronary involvement it confers additional risk (Burek, 1999).

In the last 10 years, a large amount of data has been accumulated on large artery compliance and pulse wave reflection phenomenon, which have been identified as the most important pathophysiological determinants of isolated systolic hypertension and increased pulse wave velocity (Safar et al, 2003). Measurement of arterial compliance by vascular diameter changes in relation to changes in blood pressure is complex and unsuitable for clinical use. On the other hand, pulse wave velocity measurement between femoral-carotid arteries provides detailed non-invasive assessment of arterial compliance, which is simple and rigorous enough to be considered a procedure (Laurent et al, 2006). This determination is an independent predictor for overall mortality and cardiovascular morbidity, coronary events and strokes in patients with uncomplicated essential hypertension (Laurent et al, 2001, Boutouyrie et al, 2002, Laurent et al, 2003; Willum-Hansen et al, 2006). Although the relationship between aortic stiffness and coronary events is continuous, a threshold value > 12 m/s for pulse wave velocity suggests significant alterations of aortic elastic function in middle-aged hypertensives (Mancia, 2007).

Several methods for detecting vascular lesions cannot be clinically used for a variety of reasons. An elevated media-to-lumen ratio of small resistance arteries dissected from gluteal subcutaneous tissue is an indicator of increased cardiovascular risk (Rizzoni et al, 2003). These measurements can demonstrate early changes in diabetes and hypertension (Korsgaard et al, 1993, Park et al, 2001; Rizzoni et al, 2001, Schofield et al, 2002) and have predictive value for cardiovascular morbidity and mortality (Rizzoni et al, 2003), but the invasive character of the method makes this approach unsuitable for general use. Increased calcium content in coronary arteries, measured by high resolution cardiac CT was also validated by prospective studies as predictor of cardiovascular disease but its availability is limited due to high costs (Greenland et al, 2003).

Other diagnostic procedures such as magnetic resonance, cardiac scintigraphy, coronary angiography and exercise testing are reserved for specific indications. Chest X-ray can be a useful additional diagnostic method, when dyspnea is the main symptom or when looking for information on large intrathoracic arteries of the pulmonary circulation. In recent years, an increased interest was given to assessment of cardiac fibrosis. Basic techniques have used echoreflectivity (Ciulla et al., 1997; Hoyt et al., 1984). Reversed dispersion method (backscattering signal) may reflect to some extent the contractile properties of the myocardium more than collagen content, while echoreflectivity more directly correlates with histologically measured fibrosis. Echoreflectivity showed that left ventricular hypertrophy may vary and that drugs that promote its regression may differ in reducing fibrosis (Ciulla et al, 2004). Now, the most accurate method of assessing cardiac tissue composition is nuclear magnetic resonance, whose cost, however, prevents its widespread use. Also, tissue collagen component markers are currently under investigation (Ciulla et al, 2004), but they have been shown to only partially derive from cardiac tissue.

2. Hypertension-induced retinal damage

Hypertension, if not controlled, causes injuries to blood vessels and thereby causes alterations also in the retinal microcirculation. Advanced retinopathy is nowadays confirmed as hypertension-induced target organ damage (Cohuet, 2006). Signs of hypertensive retinopathy are frequently seen in adults 40 years and older, and are predictive for stroke, congestive heart failure, and cardiovascular mortality—independently from traditional risk factors (Wong, 2007). Mild hypertensive retinopathy signs, such as generalized and focal retinal arteriolar narrowing and arteriovenous kinking, are weakly associated with systemic vascular diseases. Moderate hypertensive retinopathy signs, such as isolated microaneurysms, hemorrhages and cotton-wool spots, are strongly associated with subclinical cerebrovascular disease and predict incident clinical stroke, congestive heart failure and cardiovascular mortality, independent from blood pressure and other traditional risk factors (Wong, 2005). Clinically, signs of hypertensive retinopathy were classified into four grades of increasing severity (Keith, 1974). The correlation between retinal vascular modifications and the severity of hypertension supports the importance of using fundus oculi to improve the diagnosis and to predict future cardiovascular events (Porta, 2005). In fact, assessment of hypertensive retinopathy signs for risk stratification is supported by international hypertension management guidelines, including the US Joint National Committee on Prevention, Detection, Evaluation, and Treatment of High Blood Pressure (JNC) and the British Society of Hypertension (Williams, 2004; Chobanian, 2003).

The pathophysiological mechanism of hypertensive retinopathy is not completely established. It seems that elevated blood pressure and other pathogenic mechanisms may be involved, such as increased oxidative stress or low-grade inflammation. Retinopathy lesions have been associated with hyperglycemia, hypertension, endothelial dysfunction and inflammation in different studies (Wong, 2007). Many studies have linked signs of hypertensive retinopathy with cognitive decline, cerebral white-matter lesions identified by cerebral MRI, lacunar infarctions, cerebral atrophy, and stroke mortality (Wong, 2002; Kwa, 2002; Wong, 2003; Mitchell, 2005; Wong, 2007). Today, retinal examination offers an excellent way to study non-invasively the effects of common vascular risk factors on small vessels and possibly for gaining a better understanding of the pathophysiological processes involved in cerebral small vessel disease (Doubal, 2009).

3. Hypertension-induced cardiac damage

Electrocardiogram is part of all routine assessment of subjects with arterial hypertension. Left ventricular hypertrophy (LVH) is one of the earlier manifestations of TOD and constitutes a powerful predictor of cardiovascular events (Agabiti-Rose, 1998). This simple test provides useful information on conduction disturbances and ischemic heart disease, conditions that might urge the performance of additional investigations and influence the choice of antihypertensive drugs. A main advantage of ECG is to allow the detection of left ventricular hypertrophy (LVH) (Larsen, 2002; Alfakih, 2006; Waeber, 2009). Sensitivity for identifying left ventricular hypertrophy is increased but still Sokolow-Lyon index (SV1 + RV5-6 > 38 mm) or the product of QRS duration times Cornell voltage (with adjustment of 6 mm in women and a partition value of > 2440 mm × ms) are independent predictors of cardiovascular events (Levy et al, 1994). Their use as markers of cardiac damage or regression induced by treatment appears to be valuable, at least in patients over 55 years (Okin et al, 2004, Fagard et al, 2004). ECG can also be used to detect patterns of ventricular overload (indicating a severe risk) (Levy et al, 1994), ischemia, conduction disturbances and arrhythmias, including atrial fibrillation, not rare in elderly hypertensive patients. Holter electrocardiographic monitoring is indicated to detect hypertension when arrhythmias or ischemic episodes exist. It may also provide evidence of reduced heart rate variability, which can occur in severe hypertension (Mancia et al, 1983). However, its negative prognostic significance is not established, although it has been demonstrated for heart failure and post infarction (Kleiger et al, 1987, Bigger et al, 1992, La Rovere et al, 2003).

Echocardiography is more sensitive than electrocardiography in diagnosing left ventricular hypertrophy, in cardiovascular risk prediction and may help stratify global cardiovascular risk more precisely and establish therapy, although it has some technical limitations (differences between operators, poor image quality in obese patients and in patients with obstructive lung disease) (Reichek et al, 1981; Levy et al, 1990). A proper assessment includes measuring the dimensions of interventricular septum, posterior wall thickness and left ventricular end diastolic diameter of left ventricular to left ventricular mass calculation according to Devereux formula (Devereux et al, 1986). Although the relationship between left ventricular mass index and cardiovascular risk is linear, the estimates of left ventricular hypertrophy are widely used: > 134 g/m^2 for men and > 110 g/m^2 for women (Hammond, 1986). Concentric hypertrophy (increased left ventricular mass and relative wall thickness ratio >0.45), eccentric hypertrophy (relative wall thickness ratio < 0.42, with increased left ventricular mass) and concentric remodeling (relative wall thickness ratio ≥ 0.42, with normal left ventricular mass), are predictors for increased incidence of cardiovascular disease, but concentric hypertrophy is shown to provide the most cardiovascular risk increase (Jennings et al, 1997; Muiesan et al, 2004). A major advantage of echocardiography compared with ECG is better sensitivity, enabling the detection of milder degrees of LVH (Waeber, 2009). In addition, echocardiography provides a method to assess left ventricular systolic function. Ejection fraction, fractional shortening as medio-parietal endocardial and were proposed as possible additional predictors of cardiovascular events (De Simone, 1996; Aurigemma, 2001). Left ventricular diastolic filling (a measure of so-called "diastolic function") can be assessed by measuring the ratio wave Doppler E/A of transmitral blood flow, time to relax, protodiastolic pulmonary venous flow and left atrial enlargement (Swedberg, 2005). Useful information can be obtained by tissue Doppler at the mitral ring (Ogunyankin, 2006). All these determinations arouse great interest at present, because a considerable proportion (50%) of heart failures can be explained by "diastolic dysfunction" with an impaired systolic minimum and that the so-called „diastolic heart failure "is a condition with adverse prognosis. Alterations in diastolic function are common in hypertensive and elderly subjects with hypertension, at least one in four patients may be affected (Zanchetti, 2006). These changes may occur in the absence of systolic function alterations and even without left ventricular hypertrophy. There is evidence that diastolic dysfunction increases the risk of atrial fibrillation (Tsang, 2004). Furthermore, two studies have reported that diastolic dysfunction is predictive factor for subsequent heart failure (Aurigemma, 2001) and is associated with an increased incidence of mortality (Redfield, 2003), although in another study it was shown that this combination is not independent (Bella et al, 2002). Echocardiography provides information about the presence and degree of left atrial dilation, which correlates with risk of atrial fibrillation, cardiovascular disease and death (Laukkanen, 2005; Verdecchia, 2003; Kizer, 2006). Also, data can be obtained by kinetic abnormalities of left ventricular segmentation, due to ischemia or previous infarction. A regression of left-ventricular hypertrophy on electrocardiography is indicative of substantial clinical benefit and should be an important objective of treatment (Devereaux, 2004; Okin, 2004).

4. Hypertension-induced renal damage

Diagnosis of hypertension-induced renal damage is based on the discovery of a reduced renal function and/or increased urinary albumin excretion detection (Stevens et al, 2006). Renal failure is now classified according to glomerular filtration rate, calculated by MDRD formula that includes age, gender, and race and serum creatinine of the patient (Hallan, 2004). Glomerular filtration rate values below 60 ml/min/1,73 m^2 indicate chronic kidney disease stage 3, while values below 30 ml min/1,73 m^2 indicate chronic kidney disease stage 4, and values below 15 ml/min/1,73 m^2 indicate chronic kidney disease stage 5 (Moe, 2005). Cockroft-Gault formula estimates creatinine clearance and is based on age, sex, weight and patient's serum creatinine (Cockroft and Gault, 1976). This formula is used for values > 60 ml/min, but it overestimates creatinine clearance in chronic kidney disease stage 3-5 (Moe et al, 2005). Both formulas are helpful in the detection of renal function slightly altered, where serum creatinine is still within normal limits (Moe et al., 2005). Reduced glomerular filtration rate and increased cardiovascular risk are also suggested by elevated levels of cystatin C (Shlipak, 2006). A slight increase in serum creatinine (up to 20%) can sometimes occur when initiating or changing antihypertensive therapy, but it should not be considered as a sign of progressive renal damage. Hyperuricemia is common in untreated hypertensives and has been shown to correlate with decreased renal flow and the presence of nephrosclerosis (Viazzi, 2007). While serum creatinine concentration increased or decreased estimated glomerular filtration rate shows a decrease in glomerular filtration rate, increased urinary excretion of albumin or protein indicates deterioration in the permeability of the glomerular filtration barrier.

Microalbuminuria was associated with a cluster of metabolic and nonmetabolic risk factors, suggesting that it might indicate the presence of generalized microvascular damage in patients with essential hypertension (Pontremoli, 1998). It was shown that microalbuminuria is also a predictor of diabetic nephropathy development in type 1 and 2 diabetes (Parving, 1996), while the presence of proteinuria indicates, in general, the existence of renal parenchymal lesions. In diabetic and non-diabetic hypertensive patients, microalbuminuria is a good predictor of cardiovascular events. It has been reported in some studies a linear relationship between non-cardiovascular mortality and cardiovascular and urinary protein ratio/creatinine > 3.9 mg/g in men and 7.5 mg/g in women. Thus the term microalbuminuria may be misleading (for falsely suggests a minor injury) and should be replaced with "low degree of albuminuria." Microalbuminuria can be measured by urinary albumin concentration reporting urinary creatinine concentration (urine samples per 24 hours or the night should be discouraged because of lack of accuracy), type dipstick tests detect albuminuria above 300 mg/g creatinine and positive dipstick test for microalbuminuria in values above 30 mg/g creatinine. Microalbuminuria assessment is now recommended at the initial evaluation of a patient with hypertension. Two first-morning voided urine samples should be tested for the albumin/creatinine ratio (Redon, 2008). Microalbuminuria assessment is now recommended in a risk stratification strategy for hypertension management, since its presence indicates early organ damage and, rarely, a clustering of cardiovascular risk factors (Mancia, 2007).

5. Hypertension-induced brain damage

Until now, preclinical hypertensive lesions in the brain have not been well characterized. Microcirculation dysfunction may explain the deterioration in cognitive functions in hypertensive subjects (Cohuet, 2006). Cognitive deterioration and its end point overt dementia are, in brief, to be characterized by progressive memory loss, disorientation in time and space, loss of autonomy, and ultimately, depersonalisation/alienation (Birkenhäger, 2006). Consensus criteria recognize various syndromes, including multiple cerebral infarcts (large vessel infarcts), single infarcts, small vessel disease (multiple lacunes dementia), global hypoperfusion, and hemorrhagic dementia in the pathogenesis of vascular dementia (Cohuet, 2006). Silent brain infarction, which is cerebral target organ damage of hypertensive microangiopathies, is frequently seen in hypertensive patients (Kwon, 2007). Indeed, the degree of risk for hypertension-induced cerebrovascular disease increases progressively with the rise in BP levels (Wolf, 1991). An increased risk for cerebrovascular events in uncomplicated patients with hypertension and LVH diagnosed using both electrocardiography and echocardiography was demonstrated in the Progetto Ipertensione Umbria Monitoraggio Ambulatoriale (PIUMA) study (Verdecchia, 2001). A close association has also been shown between silent stroke (evidenced by cerebral white matter lesions) and echocardiographic LVH in 62 asymptomatic middle-aged patients with hypertension (Sierra, 2002). Many epidemiologic studies have indicated a correlation between blood pressure level and cognitive decline or dementia later in life (Starr, 1993; Seux, 1998; Postner, 2002; Hanon, 2003; Piguet, 2003; Whitmer, 2005). The importance of lowering blood pressure in hypertensive subjects is well-known, but the relationship between hypertension and cognitive function is still controversial. It is believed that atherosclerosis resulting from long-standing hypertension, and cerebral hypoperfusion secondary to severe atherosclerosis may be major biological pathways linking both high blood pressure in midlife and low blood pressure in late-life to cognitive decline and dementia (Qiu, 2005).

6. Conclusion

Signs of target organ damage (TOD) should be carefully detected in all hypertensive patients because the likelihood of identifying high-risk individuals increases. Detection of any subclinical target organ damage in the coronary, peripheral, cerebral, and renal arterial beds requires therapeutic objectives and strategies in order to induce regression and improve patient prognosis.

7. References

Agabiti-Rosei E, Muiesan ML. (1998). Cardiac hypertrophy and hypertension. *Current Opinion in Nephrology and Hypertension,* Vol. 7, pp. 211–216.

Aurigemma GP, Gottdiener JS, Shemanski L, Gardin J, Kitzman D. (2001). Predictive value of systolic and diastolic function for incident congestive heart failure in the elderly: The Cardiovascular Health Study. *Journal of the American College of Cardiology,* Vol. 37, No.4, (March, 2001), pp. 1042-1048.

Bella JN, Palmieri V, Roman MJ, Liu JE, Welty TK, Lee ET, Fabsitz RR, Howard BV, Devereux RB. (2002). Mitral ratio of peak early to late diastolic filling velocity as a predictor of mortality in middle-aged and elderly adults, The Strong Heart Study. *Circulation,* Vol. 105, No.16, (April, 2002), pp.1928-1933.

Bigger JT Jr, Fleiss JL, Steinman RC, Rolnitzky LM, Kleiger RE, Rottman JN. (1992). Frequency domain measures of heart period variability and mortality after myocardial infarction. *Circulation,* Vol. 85, No.1, (January, 1992), pp. 164-171.

Bots ML, Hoes AW, Koudstaal PJ, Hofman A, Grobbee DE. (1997). Common carotid intima-media thickness and risk of stroke and myocardial infarction: The Rotterdam Study. *Circulation,* Vol. 96, (September, 1997), pp. 1432-1437.

Boutouyrie P, Tropeano AI, Asmar R, Gautier I, Benetos A, Lacolley P, Laurent S. (2002). Aortic stiffness is an independent predictor of primary coronary events in hypertensive patients: a longitudinal study. *Hypertension,* Vol. 39, No.1, (January, 2002), pp. 10-15.

Burek KA, Sutton-Tyrrell K, Brooks MM, Naydeck B, Keller N, Sellers MA, et al. (1999). Prognostic importance of lower extremity arterial disease in patients undergoing coronary revascularization in the Bypass Angioplasty Revascularization Investigation (BARI). *Journal of the American College of Cardiology,* Vol. 34, No.3, (September, 1999), pp. 716-721.

Cheng, Cynthiaa; Daskalakis, Constantineb; Falkner, Bonitac, Alterations in capillary morphology are found in mild blood pressure elevation, *Journal of Hypertension,*Vol.28, No.11, (November, 2010), pp. 2258–2266.

Ciulla MM, Paliotti R, Esposito A, Diez J, Lopez B, Dahlof B, et al. (2004). Different effects of antihypertensive therapies based on losartan or atenolol on ultrasound and biochemical markers of myocardial fibrosis: results of a randomized trial. *Circulation,* Vol. 110, No.5, (August, 2004), pp. 552-557.

Ciulla MM, Paliotti R, Hess DB, Tjahja E, Campbell SE, Magrini F, Weber KT. (1997) Echocardiographic patterns of myocardial fibrosis in hypertensive patients: endomyocardial biopsy versus ultrasonic tissue characterization. *Journal of the American Society of Echocardiography,* Vol. 10, No.6, (July-August, 1997), pp. 657-664.

Chobanian AV, Bakris GL, Black H.R et al. (2003).The Seventh Report of the Joint National Committee on Prevention, Detection, Evaluation, and Treatment of High Blood Pressure: the JNC7 Report. *Journal of the American Medical Association,* Vol. 289, pp. 2560–2572.

Cockroft DW, Gault MH. (1976). Prediction of creatinine clearance from serum creatinine, *Nephron,* Vol. 16, No.1, pp. 31-41.

Cohuet G, Struijker-Boudier H. (2006). Mechanisms of target organ damage caused by hypertension: therapeutic potential. *Pharmacology and Therapeutics,* Vol. 111, No.1, (July, 2006), pp. 81–98.

De Simone G, Devereux RB, Koren MJ, Mensah GA, Casale PN, Laragh JH. (1996). Midwall left ventricular mechanics, an independent predictor of cardiovascular risk in arterial hypertension. *Circulation,* Vol. 93, No.2, (January, 1996), pp.259-265.

Devereux RB, Alonso DR, Lutas EM, Gottlieb GJ, Campo E, Sachs I, Reichek N.(1986). Echocardiographic assessment of left ventricular hypertrophy: comparison to necropsy findings. *American Journal of Cardiology,* Vol. 57, No.6, (February, 1986), pp. 450-458.

Devereux RB, K Watchell and E Gerdts, et al. (2004). Prognostic significance of left ventricular mass change during treatment of hypertension. *Journal of the American Medical Association,* Vol. 292, No.19, (November, 2004), pp. 2386–2388.

Doubal FN, Hokke PE; Wardlaw, JM. (2009). Retinal microvascular abnormalities and stroke: a systematic review. *Journal of Neurology, Neurosurgery and Psychiatry,* Vol. 80, No.2, (February, 2009), pp. 158–165.

Fagard RH, Staessen JA, Thijs L, Celis H, Birkenhager WH, Bulpitt CJ, et al. (2004). Systolic Hypertension in Europe (Syst-Eur) Trial Investigators. Prognostic significance of electrocardiographic voltages and their serial changes in elderly with systolic hypertension, *Hypertension,* Vol. 44, No.4, (October, 2004), pp. 459-464.

Feringa HH, Bax JJ, van Waning VH, Boersma E, Elhendy A, Schouten O, et al. (2006). The long-term prognostic value of the resting and post exercise ankle-brachial index. *Archive of Internal Medicine,* Vol. 166, No.5, (March, 2006), pp.529-535.

Graf IM, Schreuder, FHBM J.M. Hameleers, JM, Mess WH, Reneman RS Hoeks APG. (2009). Wall irregularity rather than intima-media thickness is associated with nearby atherosclerosis. Ultrasound in *Biology and Medicine,* Vol. 35, No. 6 (2009), (June, 2009), pp. 955–961.

Greenland P, Gaziano JM. (2003). Clinical practice, Selecting asymptomatic patients for coronary computed tomography or electrocardiographic exercise testing, *The New England Journal of Medicine,* Vol. 349, (July, 2003), pp. 465-473.

Halcox JP, Schenke WH, Zalos G, Mincemoyer R, Prasad A, Waclawiw MA, et al. (2002). Prognostic value of coronary vascular endothelial dysfunction, *Circulation,* Vol. 106, No.6, (August, 2002), pp. 653-665.

Hallan S, Asberg A, Lindberg M, Johnsen H. (2004). Validation of the Modification of Diet in Renal Disease formula for estimating GFR with special emphasis on calibration of the serum creatinine assay. *American Journal of kidney disease,* Vol. 44, (July, 2004), pp. 84-93.

Hammond IW, Devereux RB, Alderman MH, Lutas EM, Spitzer MC, Crowley JS, Laragh JH. (1986). The prevalence and correlates of echocardiographic left ventricular hypertrophy among employed patients with uncomplicated hypertension. *Journal of the American College of Cardiology,* Vol. 7, pp. 639–650.

Hanon, O., Seux, M. L., Lenoir, H., Rigaud, A. S., & Forette, F. (2003). Hypertension and dementia. *Current Cardiology Reports,* Vol. 5, pp. 435–440.

Heitzer T, Schlinzig T, Krohn K, Meinertz T, Munzel T. (2001). Endothelial dysfunction, oxidative stress, and risk of cardiovascular events in patients with coronary artery disease. *Circulation,* Vol. 104, pp.2673–2678.

Hiatt WR. (2001). Medical treatment of peripheral arterial disease and claudication. *The New England Journal of Medicine,* Vol. 344, pp. 1608-1621.

Hodis HN, Mack WJ, LaBree L, Selzer RH, Liu CR, Liu CH, Azen SP. (1998). The role of carotid arterial intima-media thickness in predicting clinical coronary events, *Annals of InternalMedicine,* Vol. 128, (February, 1998), pp. 262-269.

Houghton JL, Frank MJ, Carr AA, von Dohlen TW, Prisant LM. (1990). Relations among impaired coronary flow reserve, left ventricular hypertrophy and thallium perfusion defects in hypertensive patients without obstructive coronary artery disease. *Journal of the American College of Cardiology,* Vol. 15, No.1, (January, 1990), pp. 43–51.

Hoyt RM, Skorton DJ, Collins SM, Melton HE. (1984). Ultrasonic backscatter and collagen in normal ventricular myocardium, *Circulation,* Vol. 69, pp.775-782.

Jennings G, Wong J. (1997). Reversibility of left ventricular hypertrophy and malfunction by antihypertensy treatment. In: Hansson L, Birkenhager WH (editors). Handbook of Hypertension. Amsterdam: Elsevier Science; Vol. 18, pp. 184-223.

Keith NM, Wagener HP, Barker NW. (1974). Some different types of essential hypertension: their course and prognosis. *American Journal of Medical Science,* Vol.268, (December, 1974), pp. 336–45.

Kizer JR, Bella JN, Palmieri V, Liu JE, Best LG, Lee ET, et al. (2006). Left atrial diameter as an independent predictor of fi rst clinical cardiovascular events in middle-aged and elderly adults: the Strong Heart Study (SHS). *American Heart Journal,* Vol.151, No.2, (February, 2006), pp. 412-418.

Kleiger RE, Miller JP, Bigger JT Jr, Moss AJ, for the Multicentre Post-Infarction Research Group. (1987). Decreased heart rate variability and its association with increased mortality after acute myocardial infarction, *American Journal of Cardiology,* Vol. 59, No.4, (February, 1987), pp. 256-262.

Korsgaard N, Aalkjaer C, Heagerty AM, Izzard AS, Mulvany MJ. (1993). Histology of subcutaneous small arteries from patients with essential hypertension, *Hypertension* Vol. 22, No.4, (October, 1993), pp. 523-526.

Kvakan H, Luft FC, Muller DN. (2009). Role of the Immune System in Hypertensive Target Organ Damage. *Trends in Cardiovascular Medicine.* Vol. 19, No.7, (October, 2009), pp. 242-246.

Kwa VI, van der Sande JJ, Stam J, Tijmes N, Vrooland JL. (2002). Amsterdam Vascular Medicine G. Retinal arterial changes correlate with cerebral small-vessel disease. *Neurology,* Vol. 59, No.10, (November, 2002), pp. 1536–40.

Kwon H-M, Kim BJ, Oh JY, et al. (2007). Retinopathy as an indicator of silent brain infarction in asymptomatic hypertensive subjects. *Journal of the Neurological Science,* Vol. 252, No.2, (January, 2007), pp. 159–162.

La Rovere MT, Pinna GD, Maestri R, Mortara A, Capomolla S, Febo O, et al. (2003). Short-term heart rate variability strongly predicts sudden cardiac death in chronic heart failure patients. *Circulation,* Vol. 107, No.4, (February, 2003), pp. 565-570.

Lang RM, Bierig M, Devereux RB, Flachskampf FA, Foster E, Pellikka PA, et al. (2006). American Society of Echocardiography's Nomenclature and Standards Committee; Task Force on Chamber Quantification; American College of Cardiology Echocardiography Committee; American Heart Association; European Association of Echocardiography. European Society of Cardiology. Recommendations for chamber quantification. *European Journal of Echocardiography,* Vol. 7, (March, 2006), pp. 79-108.

Larsen CT, Dahlin J, Blackburn H, Scharling H, Appleyard M, Sigurd B, et al. (2002). Prevalence and prognosis of electrocardiographic left ventricular hypertrophy, ST segment depression and negative T-wave; the Copenhagen City Heart Study. *European Heart Journal,* Vol. 23, No.4, (February, 2002), pp.315–324.

Laukkanen JA, Kurl S, Eranen J, Huttunen M, Salonen JT. (2005). Left atrium size and the risk of cardiovascular death in middle-aged men. *Archive of Internal Medicine,* Vol. 165, No.15, (August, 2005), pp. 1788-1793.

Laurent S, Boutouyrie P, Asmar R, Gautier I, Laloux B, Guize L, et al. (2001).Aortic stiffness is an independent predictor of all-cause and cardiovascular mortality in hypertensive patients. *Hypertension,* Vol. 37, (May, 2001), pp. 1236-1241.

Laurent S, Cockcrof J, Van Bortel L, Boutouyrie P, Giannattasio C, Hayoz D, et al. (2006). On behalf of the European Network for non invasive investigation of large arteries. Expert consensus document on arterial stiffness: methodological issues and clinical applications. *European Heart Journal,* Vol. 27, pp.2588-2605.

Levy D, Garrison RJ, Savage DD, Kannel WB, Castelli WP. (1990). Prognostic implications of echocardiographically determined left ventricular mass in the Framingham Heart Study, *The New England Journal of Medicine,* Vol. 322, (May, 1990), pp. 1561-1566.

Levy D, Salomon M, D'Agostino RB, Belanger AJ, Kannel WB. (1994). Prognostic implications of baseline electrocardiographic features and their serial changes in subjects with left ventricular hypertrophy. *Circulation,* Vol.90, (October, 1994), pp. 1786-1793.

Lockhart CJ, Hamilton PK, Quinn CE and McVeigh GE. (2009). End-organ dysfunction and cardiovascular outcomes: the role of the microcirculation. *Clinical Science (London)* Vol. 116, (February, 2009), pp.175–190.

Mancia G, Ferrari A, Gregorini L, Parati G, Pomidossi G, Bertinieri G, et al. (1983). Blood pressure and heart rate variabilities in normotensive and hypertensive human beings. *Circulation Research,* Vol. 53, (July, 1983), pp. 96–104.

Mancia G, De Backer G, Dominiczak A, Cifkova R, Fagard R, Germano G, et al. (2007). Management of Arterial Hypertension of the European Society of Hypertension; European Society of Cardiology. 2007 guidelines for the management of arterial hypertension: The Task Force for the Management of Arterial Hypertension of the European Society of Hypertension (ESH) and of the European Society of Cardiology (ESC). *Journal of Hypertension,* Vol.25, (June, 2007), pp.1105–1187.

Marinakis A.G., G.P. Vyssoulis and E.A. Karpanou, et al. (2003). Heart rate and blood pressure variability are predictors of target organ damage in arterial hypertension. *American Journal of Hypertension,* Vol. 16, p. 246A.

Matsui Y, Ishikawa J, Eguchi K, Shibasaki S, Shimada K, Kario K. (2011). Maximum value of home blood pressure: a novel indicator of target organ damage in hypertension. *Hypertension*. Vol. 57, No.6, (June, 2011), pp.1087-1093.

McVeigh, G. E., Plumb, R. and Hughes, S. (2004). Vascular abnormalities in hypertension: cause, effect, or therapeutic target? *Current Hypertension Reports*, Vol. 6, (June, 2004), pp. 171–176.

Mitchell P, Wang JJ, Wong TY, Smith W, Klein R, Leeder SR. (2005). Retinal microvascular signs and risk of stroke and stroke mortality. *Neurology*, Vol. 65, pp. 1005–09.

Moe S, Drueke T, Cunningham J, Goodman W, Martin K, Olgaard K, et al. (2005). Kidney Disease: Improving Global Outcomes (KDIGO). Definition and classification of chronic kidney disease: a position statement from Kidney Disease: Improving Global Outcomes (KDIGO). *Kidney International*, Vol. 67, (June, 2005), pp. 2089-2100.

Muiesan ML, Salvetti M, Monteduro C, Bonzi B, Paini A, Viola S et al. (2004). Left ventricular concentric geometry during treatment adversely affects cardiovascular prognosis in hypertensive patients. *Hypertension*, Vol. 43, No.4, (April, 2004), pp. 731-738.

Muller DN, Kvakan H, Luft FC. (2011). Immune-related effects in hypertension and target-organ damage. *Current opinion in nephrology and hypertension*. Vol. 20, No.2, (March, 2011), pp.113-117.

Navarro-Gonzalez J.F, C. Mora, M. Muros, A. Jarque, H. Herrera and J. Garcia, (2008). Association of tumor necrosis factor-alpha with early target organ damage in newly diagnosed patients with essential hypertension. *Journal of Hypertension*, Vol. 26, pp. 2168–2175.

O'Leary DH, Polak JF, Kronmal RA, Manolio TA, Burke GL, Wolfson SK Jr. (1999). Carotid-artery intima and media thickness as a risk factor for myocardial infarction and stroke in older adults. Cardiovascular Health Study Collaborative Research Group. *The New England Journal of Medicine*, Vol. 340, pp. 14-22.

Ogunyankin KO, Burggraf GW, Abiose AK, Malik PG. (2006). Validity of revised Doppler echocardiographic algorithms and composite clinical and angiographic data in diagnosis of diastolic dysfunction. *Echocardiography*, Vol. 23, pp. 817-828.

Okin PM, Devereux RB, Jern S, Kjeldsen SE, Julius S, Nieminen MS. (2004). LIFE Study Investigators. Regression of electrocardiographic left ventricular hypertrophy during antihypertensive treatment and the prediction of major cardiovascular events. *Journal of the American Medical Association*, Vol. 292, No.19, (November, 2004), pp. 2343-2349.

Park JB, Schiffrin EL. (2001). Small artery remodeling is the most prevalent form of target organ damage in mild essential hypertension. *Journal of Hypertension*, Vol. 19, (May, 2001), pp. 921-930.

Parving HH. (1996). Initiation and progression of diabetic nephropathy, *The New England Journal of Medicine*, Vol. 335, (November, 1996), pp. 1682-1683.

Piguet O, Grayson DA, Creasey H, et al. (2003). Vascular risk factors, cognition and dementia incidence over 6 years in the Sydney Older Persons Study. *Neuroepidemiology*, Vol. 22, (May-June, 2003), pp. 165–171.

Porta, M., Grosso, A., & Veglio, F. (2005). Hypertensive retinopathy: there's more than meets the eye. *Journal of Hypertension,* Vol. 23, (April, 2005), pp. 683-696.

Pontremoli R, Nicolella C, Viazzi F, Ravera M, Sofia A, Berruti V, et al. (1998). Microalbuminuria is an early marker of target organ damage in essential hypertension. *American Journal of Hypertension,* Vol. 1, (April, 1998), pp. 430-438.

Posner, H. B.; Tang, M. X.; Luchsinger, J., Lantigua, R., Stern, Y., & Mayeux, R. (2002). The relationship of hypertension in the elderly to AD, vascular dementia, and cognitive function. *Neurology,* Vol. 58, No. 8, (April, 2002), pp. 1175- 1181.

Qiu C, Winblad B Fratiglioni, L. (2005). The age-dependent relation of blood pressure to cognitive function and dementia. *Lancet Neurology,* Vol. 4, No.8, (August, 2005), pp. 487–499.

Redfield MM, Jacobsen SJ, Burnett JC Jr, Mahoney DW, Bailey KR, Rodeheffer RJ. (2003). Burden of systolic and diastolic ventricular dysfunction in the community: appreciating the scope of the heart failure epidemic. *Journal of the American Medical Association,* Vol. 289, No.2, (January, 2003), pp. 194-202.

Reichek N, Devereux RB. (1981). Left ventricular hypertrophy: relationship of anatomic, echocardiographic and electrocardiographic findings. *Circulation,* Vol. 63, No.6, (June, 1981), pp. 1391-1398.

Rizzoni D, Porteri E, Boari GE, De Ciuceis C, Sleiman I, Muiesan ML, et al. (2003). Prognostic significance of small-artery structure in hypertension. *Circulation,* Vol. 108, No.18, (November, 2003), pp.2230-2235.

Rizzoni D, Porteri E, Guelfi D, Muiesan ML, Valentini U, Cimino A, et al. (2001). Structural alterations in subcutaneous small arteries of normotensive and hypertensive patients with non-insulin-dependent diabetes mellitus. *Circulation,* Vol. 103, (March, 2001), pp. 1238-1244.

Ruilope LM. (2011). Normotension, blood pressure variability and early target organ damage. *Hypertension research.* Vol. 34, No.10, (July, 2011), pp. 1075.

Safar ME, Levy BI, Struijker-Boudier H. (2003). Current perspectives on arterial stiffness and pulse pressure in hypertension and cardiovascular diseases, *Circulation,* Vol. 107, No.22, (June, 2003), pp. 2864-2869.

Salonen JT, Salonen R. (1993). Ultrasound B-mode imaging in observational studies of atherosclerotic progression, *Circulation,* Vol. 87 (Suppl II), (March, 1993), pp. II56-II65.

Schofield I, Malik R, Izzard A, Austin C, Heagerty A. (2002). Vascular structural and functional changes in type 2 diabetes mellitus: evidence for the roles of abnormal myogenic responsiveness and dyslipidemia. *Circulation,* Vol. 106, No. 24, (December, 2002), pp. 3037-3043.

Seux, M.L.; Thijs, L.; Forette, F.; Staessen, J. A.; Birkenhager, W.H.; Bulpitt, C.J.; et al. (1998). Correlates of cognitive status of old patients with isolated systolic hypertension: The Syst-Eur Vascular Dementia Project. *Journal of Hypertension,* Vol. 16, (July, 1998), pp. 963–969.

Sierra CA. de la Sierra, J.C. Pare, E. Gomez-Angelats and Coca A. (2002). Correlation between silent cerebral white matter lesions and left ventricular mass and geometry in essential hypertension. *American Journal of Hypertension,* Vol. 15, No.6, (June, 2002), pp. 507–512.

Shlipak MG, Katz R, SarnakMJ, Fried LF, Newman AB, Stehman- Breen C, et al. (2006). Cystatin C and prognosis for cardiovascular and kidney outcomes in elderly persons without chronic kidney disease, *Annals of Internal Medicine,* Vol. 145, (August, 2006), pp. 237-246.

Starr, J. M., Whalley, L. J., Inch, S., & Shering, P. A. (1993). Blood pressure and cognitive function in healthy old people. *Journal of the American Geriatrics Society,* Vol. 41, No.7, (July, 1993), 753– 756.

Stergiou GS, Argyraki KK, Moyssakis I, Mastorantonakis SE, Achimastos AD, Karamanos VG, Roussias LG. (2007). Home blood pressure is as reliable as ambulatory blood pressure in predicting target-organ damage in hypertension. *American Journal of Hypertension,* Vol. 20, pp.616–621.

Stevens LA, Coresh J, Greene T, Levey AS. (2006). Assessing kidney function measured and estimated glomerular filtration rate. *The New England Journal of Medicine,* Vol. 354, pp. 2473-2483.

Swedberg K, Cleland J, Dargie H, Drexler H, Follath F, Komajda M et al. (2005). Task Force for the Diagnosis, Treatment of Chronic Heart Failure of the European Society of Cardiology. Guidelines for the diagnosis and treatment of chronic heart failure: executive summary (update 2005). The Task Force for the Diagnosis and Treatment of Chronic Heart Failure of the European Society of Cardiology. *European Heart Journal,* Vol. 26, No.11, (June, 2005), pp.1115-1140.

Taddei S, Salvetti A. (2002). Endothelial dysfunction in essential hypertension: clinical implications. *Journal of Hypertension,* Vol. 20, No.9, (September, 2002), pp. 1671-1674.

Tsang TS, Barnes ME, Gersh BJ, Bailey KR, Seward JB. (2004). Risks for atrial fibrillation and congestive heart failure in patients > 65 years of age with abnormal left ventricular diastolic relaxation, *American Journal of Cardiology,* Vol. 93, No.1, (January, 2004), pp.54-58.

Verdecchia, P. Porcellati, C., Reboldi, G. Gattobigio, R. Borgioni, C. Pearson T.A.Ambrosio, G. (2001). Left ventricular hypertrophy as an independent predictor of acute cerebrovascular events in essential hypertension. *Circulation,* Vol. 104, No.17, (October, 2001), pp. 2039–2044.

Verdecchia P, Reboldi G, Gattobigio R, Bentivoglio M, Borgioni C, Angeli F, et al. (2003). Atrial fibrillation in hypertension: predictors and outcome. *Hypertension,* Vol. 41, No. 2, (February, 2003), pp. 218-223.

Viazzi, F. Leoncini G. Parodi, D. et al. (2002). Pulse pressure and subclinical cardiovascular damage in primary hypertension. *Nephrology Dialysis and Transplant,* Vol. 17, No.10, (October, 2002), pp. 1779–1785.

Viazzi F, Leoncini G, Ratto E, Falqui V, Parodi A, Conti N, et al. (2007). Mild hyperuricaemia and subclinical renal damage in untreated primary hypertension. *American Journal of Hypertension,* Vol. 20, No.12, (December, 2007), pp. 1276–1282.

Vogt MT, Cauley JA, Newman AB, Kuller LH, Hulley SB. (1993). Decreased ankle/arm blood pressure index and mortality in elderly women. *Journal of the American Medical Association,* Vol. 270, No.4, (July, 1993), pp. 465-469.

Vaudo G, Schillaci G, Evangelista F, Pasqualini L, Verdecchia P, Mannarino E. (2000). Arterial wall thickening at different sites and its association with left ventricular hypertrophy in newly diagnosed essential hypertension. *American Journal of Hypertension,* Vol. 13, (April, 2000), pp. 324-331.

Waeber B, de la Sierra A, Ruilope LM. (2009). Target organ damage: how to detect it and how to treat it? *Journal of Hypertension,* Vol. 27 (Suppl 3), (June, 2009), pp.S13 - S18.

Werner N, Kosiol S, Schiegl T, et al. (2005). Circulating endothelial progenitor cells and cardiovascular outcomes. *The New England Journal of Medicine,* Vol. 353, No.10, (September, 2005), pp. 999–1007.

Willum-Hansen T, Staessen JA, Torp-Pedersen C, Rasmussen S, Thijs L, Ibsen H, Jeppesen J. (2006). Prognostic value of aortic pulse wave velocity as index of arterial stiff ness in the general population. *Circulation,* Vol. 113, (February, 2006), pp. 664-670.

Williams B, Poulter NR, Brown MJ, Davis M, McInnes GT, Potter JF, Sever PS, Thom SM. (2004). British Hypertension Society guidelines for hypertension management 2004 (BHS-IV): summary. *British Medical Journal,* Vol. 328, (March, 2004), pp. 634–640.

Whitmer RA, Sidney S, Selby J, Johnston SC, Yaffe K. (2005). Midlife cardiovascular risk factors and risk of dementia in late life. *Neurology,* Vol. 64, No.2, (January, 2005), pp. 277–181.

Wong TY, McIntosh R, Wong TY, McIntosh R. (2005). Hypertensive retinopathy signs as risk indicators of cardiovascular morbidity and mortality. *British Medical Bulletin.* Vol.73–74, (September, 2005), pp. 57 -70.

Wong TY, Klein R, Sharrett AR, et al. (2002). Retinal microvascular abnormalities and cognitive impairment in middle-aged persons: the Atherosclerosis Risk in Communities Study. *Stroke,* Vol. 33, No.6, (June, 2002), pp. 1487–1492.

Wong TY, Klein R, Sharrett AR, et al. (2002). Cerebral white matter lesions, retinopathy, and incident clinical stroke. *Journal of the American Medical Association,* Vol. 288, No.1, (July, 2002), pp. 67–74.

Wong TY, Mosley TH Jr, Klein R, et al. (2003). Retinal microvascular changes and MRI signs of cerebral atrophy in healthy, middle-aged people. *Neurology,* Vol. 61, (September, 2003), pp. 806–811.

Wong TY, Klein R, Nieto FJ, et al. (2003). Retinal microvascular abnormalities and 10-year cardiovascular mortality: a population-based case-control study. *Ophthalmology,* Vol. 110, (May, 2003), pp. 933–940.

Zanchetti A, Agabiti-Rosei E, Ambrosioni E, Chiariello N, Leonetti G, Mancia G, et al. (2006). Left ventricular diastolic dysfunction in a cohort of hypertensive patients attending hospital outpatient clinics in Italy, the APROS-DIADYS project. *Journal of Hypertension,* Vol. 25, No.10, (suppl 6), (October, 2007), pp. 2158-2167.

Zanchetti A, Bond MG, Hennig M, Neiss A, Mancia G, Dal Palu C. (2002). European Lacidipine Study on Atherosclerosis investigators. Calcium antagonist lacidipine slows down progression of asymptomatic carotid atherosclerosis: principal results of the European Lacidipine Study on Atherosclerosis (ELSA), a randomized, double-blind, longterm trial. *Circulation,* Vol. 106, No.19, (November, 2002), pp. 2422-2427.

Zanchetti A, Bond MG, Hennig M, Tang R, Hollweck R, Mancia G. et al. (2004). ELSA Investigators. Absolute and relative changes in carotid intima-media thickness and atherosclerotic plaques during long-term antihypertensive treatment: further results of the European Lacidipine Study on Atherosclerosis (ELSA). *Journal of Hypertension,* Vol. 22, No.6, (June, 2004), pp. 1201-1212.